CRASH COURSE
Pediatrics

S0-BDM-957

Other Titles in the Crash Course Series

There are 23 books in the Crash Course series in two ranges: Basic Science and Clinical. Each book follows the same format, with concise text, clear illustrations and helpful learning features including access to online USMLE test questions.

Basic Science titles
Pathology
Nervous System
Renal and Urinary Systems
Gastrointestinal System
Respiratory System
Endocrine and Reproductive Systems
Metabolism and Nutrition
Pharmacology
Immunology
Musculoskeletal System
Cardiovascular System
Cell Biology and Genetics
Anatomy

Clinical titles
Surgery
Cardiology
History and Examination
Internal Medicine
Neurology
Gastroenterology
OBGYN
Psychiatry
Pediatrics

Forthcoming:
Imaging

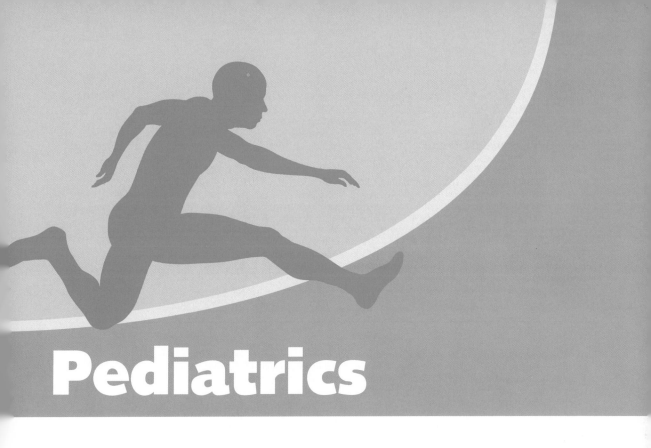

Pediatrics

Jonathan Birnkrant, MD
Pediatrics
Child and Adolescent Psychiatry
Providence, Rhode Island

Anthony J. Alario, MD
Director, Pediatric Ambulatory Medicine
Hasbro Children's Hospital
Professor of Pediatrics
Brown Medical School
Providence, Rhode Island

UK edition authors
David Pang, Tim Newson, Christine Budd, and Mark Gardiner

UK series editor
Daniel Horton-Szar

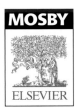

MOSBY
ELSEVIER

1600 John F. Kennedy Blvd.
Suite 1800
Philadelphia, PA 19103-2899

CRASH COURSE: PEDIATRICS
Copyright © 2007 by Mosby, Inc., an affiliate of Elsevier Inc.

ISBN-13: 978-0-323-04795-1
ISBN-10: 0-323-04795-5

All rights reserved. No part of this publication may be reproduced or transmitted in any form or by any means, electronic or mechanical, including photocopying, recording, or any information storage and retrieval system, without permission in writing from the publisher. Permissions may be sought directly from Elsevier's Health Sciences Rights Department in Philadelphia, PA, USA: phone: (+1) 215 239 3804, fax: (+1) 215 239 3805, e-mail: healthpermissions@elsevier.com. You may also complete your request on-line via the Elsevier homepage (http://www.elsevier.com), by selecting 'Customer Support' and then 'Obtaining Permissions'.

Notice

Knowledge and best practice in this field are constantly changing. As new research and experience broaden our knowledge, changes in practice, treatment and drug therapy may become necessary or appropriate. Readers are advised to check the most current information provided (i) on procedures featured or (ii) by the manufacturer of each product to be administered, to verify the recommended dose or formula, the method and duration of administration, and contraindications. It is the responsibility of the practitioner, relying on their own experience and knowledge of the patient, to make diagnoses, to determine dosages and the best treatment for each individual patient, and to take all appropriate safety precautions. To the fullest extent of the law, neither the Publisher nor the Authors assumes any liability for any injury and/or damage to persons or property arising out or related to any use of the material contained in this book.

The Publisher

Adapted from Crash Course: Paediatrics, 2e by David Pang and Tim Newson
ISBN: 0-7234-3374-7 © 2005, Elsevier Science Limited

The rights of David Pang and Tim Newson to be identified as the authors of this book have been asserted in accordance with the Copyright, Designs and Patents Act, 1988.

Library of Congress Cataloging-in-Publication Data
Birnkrant, Jonathan.
   Pediatrics/Jonathan Birnkrant, Anthony J. Alario.—1st American ed.
      p. ; cm.—(Crash course)
   Rev. ed. of: Paediatrics. 2nd ed./David Pang, Tim Newson. ©2005.
   Includes index.
   ISBN 978-0-323-04795-1
   1. Pediatrics.   2. Children—Diseases.   I. Alario, Anthony J.   II. Pang, David. Paediatrics.
III. Title.   IV. Series.
   [DNLM: 1. Pediatrics. WS 100 B6186p 2007]
   RJ48.P36 2007

   616.92–dc22   2006046681

Commissioning Editor: Alex Stibbe
Developmental Editor: Stan Ward
Project Manager: David Saltzberg
Design: Andy Chapman
Cover Design: Antbits Illustration
Illustration Manager: Mick Ruddy

Printed in China

Last digit is the print number:
9 8 7 6 5 4 3 2 1

Working together to grow
libraries in developing countries

www.elsevier.com | www.bookaid.org | www.sabre.org

ELSEVIER   BOOK AID International   Sabre Foundation

Preface

Pediatricians are truly "primary care" physicians: they are faced with the widest range of clinical presentations. Not only charged with understanding all organ systems, pediatricians must also take into account a patient's developmental stage in considering the presentation and management. From neonates and toddlers to latency age, adolescence, and young adulthood, pediatricians treat diseases and disorders at the same time as they keep vigilance on the normal physical, cognitive, and emotional growth of healthy patients through well-child visits. Therefore, the student of pediatrics is faced with the challenge of learning a breadth and depth of information they may not have encountered in other rotations.

Crash Course Pediatrics addresses the primary care challenge through a clear presentation of the fundamentals. The book is divided into three parts. Part I, "The Patient Presents With," is a clinical approach to the symptoms, signs, and problems with which a pediatric patient may present. Part II, "Diseases and Disorders," takes a traditional organ system approach to the clinical features, evaluation, and management of diseases and disorders. Part III, "History, Examination, and Common Investigations," as its name indicates, provides the basic skills with which to approach all pediatric patients. "Hints & Tips" boxes are used to emphasize important points, and tables and algorithms are used to aid the reader in understanding and memorizing the information presented whenever possible. Furthermore, in order to provide a more realistic test-taking experience that closely approximates the conditions for the now computerized USMLE, this U.S. edition of *Crash Course Pediatrics* provides convenient web-based multiple choice questions for self-assessment.

The information brought together in this introduction to pediatrics is intended as a foundation that hopefully will not only help the physician-in-training tackle the discipline's unique challenges, but also inspire them to pursue a future in the tremendously rewarding field of pediatrics.

Dedication

To my parents, mom and Mitch, who are always there for me, thank you. And to my dogs Albert and Jackson (and you too Sax), who are also always there . . . as long as I say "come" or "sit" or "stay."
JB

To my family, my wife Susan and our children and to Judy daSilva, my assistant, who is always there when I need her.
AA

Acknowledgments

In this U.S. edition of *Crash Course Pediatrics*, we would like to acknowledge the English authors for allowing us the opportunity to edit the book for the American market. Furthermore, we would like to acknowledge the many people at Elsevier who have come together to make this U.S. edition a reality—in particular, Alex Stibbe, Stan Ward, and Kate Dimock.

Contents

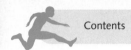

THE PATIENT PRESENTS WITH

1. Fever or Rash

The febrile child

Fever is a common presenting symptom in children and can be a major challenge to pediatricians. Most of the causes are due to benign, self-limiting, viral infections, but skill is needed to distinguish these from serious infection (Fig. 1.1). The latter has the potential to deteriorate rapidly so it is essential that it is identified as early as possible. Clinicians may start antibiotic treatment prior to diagnostic investigations if serious infection is suspected because delay can be associated with significant morbidity and mortality. Clinical assessment is therefore central to the approach of children with fever while awaiting results of diagnostic investigations.

History
How long has the child been febrile?
A duration of more than a week or two suggests viral illness; however, diseases such as tuberculosis (TB), malaria, typhoid, and autoimmune noninfectious disorders must be suspected.

Are there any localizing symptoms?
An infection in certain systems will advertise itself:
- Cough or coryza: suggest respiratory tract infection. ⤷ cold symptoms
- Vomiting and diarrhea: suggest gastrointestinal tract infection, although vomiting alone is nonspecific.
- A painful limb: suggests infection of the bones or joints.
- Lower abdominal pain: suggests urine infection, but lobar pneumonia can also present this way.
- Headache, photophobia, and neck pain: suggest meningism.

Younger children (<2 years of age) may not localize symptoms, and fever may be the only symptom.

Has there been recent foreign travel?
Malaria or typhoid can be overlooked if recent travel abroad is not disclosed in the history.

Examination
Is the child systemically unwell?
The active, playing and communicative child is unlikely to have sepsis. However, any ill child must have an assessment of the airway, breathing, and circulation, and of the vital signs. Clues to serious bacterial sepsis include:
- All children less than 3 months old.
- Poor peripheral perfusion (e.g., capillary refill >3 s).
- Bulging fontanelle.
- White cell count >20 × 10^9/L or <4 × 10^9/L.
- Presence of shock.
- Decreased consciousness or lethargy.
- Persistent tachycardia.
- Apnea.
- Nonblanching rash.

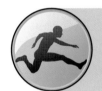

Assume sepsis in all febrile infants aged <3 months until proved otherwise.

Are there local signs of infection?
Tonsillitis, otitis media, pneumonia, meningitis, and septic arthritis can all be revealed on examination (Fig. 1.2); a rash may be diagnostic. Look for a bulging fontanelle in meningitis.

Investigations
In a well child in whom a confident clinical diagnosis has been possible, no investigation is required. However, certain investigations are appropriate in any ill febrile child. These include:
- Markers of inflammation: white cell count (raised or low in overwhelming sepsis), differential (neutrophil predominance in bacterial infection) and C-reactive protein. These are useful if there is uncertainty in diagnosis or for serial measurement of a septic child; however, they cannot rule out serious infection.

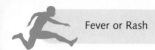
Common causes of a fever	
Minor illnesses	**Major illnesses**
Upper respiratory infection Nonspecific viral infections and rashes Gastroenteritis without dehydration	Meningitis Pneumonia Urinary tract infection Septicemia

Fig. 1.1 Common causes of a fever.

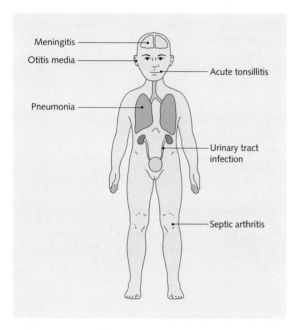

Fig. 1.2 Fever: important sites of local bacterial infection.

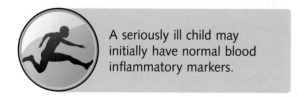

A seriously ill child may initially have normal blood inflammatory markers.

- Samples for microbiologic examination: these can include blood cultures, urine for microscopy and culture, throat swab, and cerebrospinal fluid. Polymerase chain reaction (PCR) is becoming increasingly useful as it provides high sensitivity and specificity.

Causes of fever of unknown origin (FUO)	
Type	**Cause**
Infectious	Tuberculosis Malaria Bone and joint infection Enteric infection (e.g., typhoid) Urine infection
Malignancy	Leukemia
Autoimmune and inflammatory	Systemic lupus erythematosus Kawasaki disease Juvenile idiopathic arthritis Inflammatory bowel disease
Drug-induced	

Fig. 1.3 Causes of fever of unknown origin (FUO).

- Imaging: a chest x-ray (CXR) should be considered if there is any suspicion of lower respiratory tract infection.
- A "septic screen"; infants suspected of severe infection without localizing signs on examination are investigated with a standard battery of investigations before starting antibiotic therapy. These include: blood culture, complete blood count (CBC), lumbar puncture, urine analysis, and CXR.

Management

If a benign viral infection is suspected, then only symptomatic therapy is needed. In the very young, or those who look ill, antibiotics are started before the results of diagnostic testing because quickly ruling out serious infection is often impossible; treatment can be tailored when the results are back. Treating the fever with antipyretics may reduce the risk of febrile convulsions.

Fever of unknown origin (FUO)

The designation FUO should be reserved for a child with a documented protracted fever (more than 7 days) and no diagnosis despite initial investigation (Fig. 1.3). It is frequently misapplied to any child presenting with a fever of which the cause is not immediately obvious. Most are infectious, and 40–60% will resolve without diagnosis.

The child with a rash

Children often present with a rash that may, or may not, be associated with systemic signs. An exact diagnosis is often not possible, but a few rashes are associated with serious systemic disease. Careful clinical history and examination are again essential and investigation is reserved only for certain cases.

History

The history of a rash should ascertain the following:

- Duration, site of onset, evolution, and spread.
- Does it come and go (e.g., urticaria)?
- Does the rash itch (e.g., eczema, scabies)?
- Recent drug ingestion or exposure to provocative agents (e.g., sunlight, food, allergens, detergents).
- Other family members or contacts affected (e.g., viral exanthems, infestations; see Chapter 10).
- Other associated symptoms (e.g., sore throat, upper respiratory tract infection).
- Family history (e.g., atopy, psoriasis).

Examination

Check for nondermatologic features such as:

- Fever.
- Mucous membranes.
- Lymphadenopathy.
- Splenomegaly.
- Arthropathy.

Describe the rash in "dermatologic language," observing the morphology, arrangement, and distribution of the lesions.

Morphology

Describe the shape, size and color of the lesions. There may be:

- Macules, papules, or nodules.
- Vesicles, pustules, or bullae.
- Petechiae, purpura, or ecchymoses.

Arrangement

Are the lesions scattered diffusely, well circumscribed, or confluent?

Distribution

The distribution is important (Fig. 1.4). It can be local or generalized (flexor surfaces: eczema;

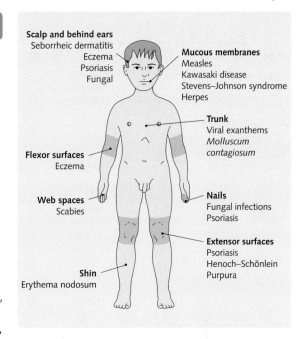

Scalp and behind ears
Seborrheic dermatitis
Eczema
Psoriasis
Fungal

Mucous membranes
Measles
Kawasaki disease
Stevens–Johnson syndrome
Herpes

Flexor surfaces
Eczema

Trunk
Viral exanthems
Molluscum contagiosum

Web spaces
Scabies

Nails
Fungal infections
Psoriasis

Shin
Erythema nodosum

Extensor surfaces
Psoriasis
Henoch–Schönlein
Purpura

Fig. 1.4 Distribution of rashes.

extensor surfaces: Henoch–Schönlein purpura [HSP] or psoriasis) or may involve mucous membranes (measles, Kawasaki disease, Stevens–Johnson syndrome).

It is important to note the distribution as well as the morphology of a rash.

Palpation

Feel the rash for scale, thickness, texture, and temperature; dry skin suggests eczema.

Investigations

Investigations are rarely required but may include skin scrapings for fungi or scabies.

Causes of a rash

The main causative categories are shown in Fig. 1.5.

Causes of a rash	
Type	**Cause**
Infection	Viral Toxin-related Streptococcal Meningococcal
Infestations	Scabies
Dermatitis	Eczema Vasculitis
Allergy	Drug-related Urticaria
Hematologic	Bleeding disorders

Fig. 1.5 Causes of a rash.

Diagnostic features of the more common generalized rashes

The common generalized rashes are: maculopapular rash, vesicular rash, hemorrhagic rash, and urticarial rash.

Maculopapular rash

This is most likely to be caused by a viral exanthem but may be a drug-induced eruption. Common diagnostic features are:

- Measles: prodrome of fever, coryza, and cough. Just before the rash appears, Koplik's spots appear in the mouth. The rash tends to coalesce. *[handwritten: blanching (old ones don't)]*
- Rubella: discrete, pink macular rash starting on the scalp and face. Occipital and cervical lymphadenopathy may precede the rash.
- Roseola infantum: occurs in infants under 3 years. After 3 days of sustained fever, a pink morbilliform (measles-like) eruption appears as the temperature subsides. It is caused by human herpesvirus (HHV)-6 or HHV-7.
- Enteroviral infection: causes a generalized, pleomorphic rash and produces a mild fever.
- Glandular fever: symptoms include malaise, fever, and exudative tonsillitis. Lymphadenopathy and splenomegaly are commonly found.
- Kawasaki disease: causes a protracted fever, generalized rash, red lips, lymphadenopathy, and conjunctival inflammation.

[handwritten margin notes: also known as Roseola; rash shows up after fever; exanthem subitum roseola; central proximal scalp keys; yes conjunctivitis also; adenopathy; high might febrile seizure; 739°; infectious mononucleosis other]

- Scarlet fever: causes fever and sore throat. The rash starts on the face and can include a "strawberry" tongue.

Vesicular rash

Common causes of vesicular rash are:

- Chickenpox: successive crops of papulovesicles on an erythematous base; the vesicles become encrusted. Lesions present at different stages. The mucous membranes are involved.
- Eczema herpeticum: exacerbation of eczema with vesicular spots caused by a herpes infection.

Hemorrhagic rash

Due to extravasated blood these lesions do not blanch on pressure. Lesions are classified by size:

- Petechiae (smallest).
- Purpura.
- Ecchymoses (largest).

Common diagnostic features are:

- Meningococcal septicemia: petechial rash (may be preceded by maculopapular rash).
- Acute leukemia: look for pallor and hepatosplenomegaly.
- Idiopathic thrombocytopenic purpura: the child looks well but may have bruising with, or without, nose bleeds.
- Henoch–Schönlein purpura: distribution is usually on the legs and buttocks. Arthralgia and abdominal pain may be present.

Nonblanching or rapidly spreading rash suggests meningococcal sepsis.

Take care to think of child abuse in traumatic bruising.

Urticarial rash

Urticaria (hives), a transient, itchy rash characterized by raised wheals, appears rapidly and fades; it can recur. Causes include:

- Food allergy (e.g., shellfish, eggs, cow's milk).
- Drug allergy (e.g., penicillin: note that <10% of penicillin allergies are unsubstantiated).
- Infections (e.g., viral: this is the most common and is often self-limiting).

[handwritten bottom note: rash in only 10–15% of patients but if given amoxicillin it is higher is rubella form or any other]

- Contact allergy (e.g., plants, grasses, animal hair).

Two other distinctive rashes that occur in childhood and require special consideration are erythema multiforme and erythema nodosum.

Erythema multiforme
A distinctive, symmetrical rash characterized by annular target (iris) lesions and various other lesions including macules, papules, and bullae.

The severe form with mucous membrane involvement is Stevens–Johnson syndrome. Causes include infections (most commonly herpes simplex, Mycoplasma, or Epstein–Barr virus) and drugs. Mostly it is idiopathic and self-limiting.

Erythema nodosum
Red, tender, nodular lesions usually occur on the shins. Important causes include streptococcal infections and TB.

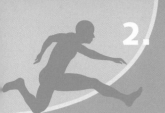

2. Heart, Lung, or ENT Problems

Heart

Congenital heart malformations account for most of the cardiovascular disease seen in pediatric practice. Rare causes include rheumatic fever, viral myocarditis or pericarditis, bacterial endocarditis, and arrhythmias. Kawasaki disease is now the leading cause of acquired heart disease in children in the developed world. Heart disease presents in a limited number of ways:

- An abnormality detected on prenatal ultrasound.
- A murmur noted on routine examination in an asymptomatic infant or child.
- Arrhythmia and/or syncope.
- Cardiac failure with or without low cardiac output.

History
Cardiac symptoms include:

- Poor feeding, cough, and difficulty breathing: cardiac failure in babies.
- Syncope: caused by arrhythmias and on rare occasions by severe aortic stenosis (AS).
- Older children may describe palpitations.
- Rapid weight gain from edema.

 Rapid weight gain is an early sign of cardiac failure in infants.

Examination
The major physical signs are:

- Cyanosis.
- Murmurs.
- Signs of cardiac failure.

Cyanosis
Several varieties of congenital heart disease may present with central cyanosis (a "blue" baby) at, or soon after, birth. Central cyanosis is visible if the concentration of deoxygenated hemoglobin (Hb) in the blood exceeds 5 g/dL. Peripheral cyanosis—blueness of the hands and feet (due to a sluggish peripheral circulation)—is a normal finding in babies who are cold, crying, or unwell from some noncardiac cause.

Central cyanosis due to congenital heart disease is distinguished from that due to respiratory disease by the failure of right radial artery pO_2 to rise above 15 kPa after breathing 100% O_2 for 10 min. Differential cyanosis in the limbs is pathognomic of cardiac disease. It is due to the presence of right to left shunting across the ductus arteriosus.

Causes
In most patients, there is an abnormality that allows a portion of the systemic venous return to bypass the lungs and enter the systemic circulation directly (i.e., a right to left shunt). Right to left shunts result from two general types of cardiac malformation:

1. Lesions with abnormal mixing: desaturated systemic venous blood is mixed with oxygenated pulmonary venous blood so that the blood discharged into the systemic circulation is not fully saturated. Pulmonary vascularity is increased, and increased vascular markings are apparent on chest x-ray (CXR) (e.g., transposition of the great arteries [TGA]) (Fig. 2.1).
2. Lesions with inadequate pulmonary blood flow: these infants often have right outflow tract obstruction and depend on blood flowing to the lungs from left to right across a patent ductus arteriosus (PDA). Severe cyanosis develops when the duct closes, pulmonary vascularity is diminished, and fewer vascular markings are apparent on CXR (e.g., tetralogy of Fallot) (Fig. 2.2).

Murmurs
Cardiac murmurs are common in children of all ages. The majority of these are not associated with pathology (innocent murmurs) and clinical

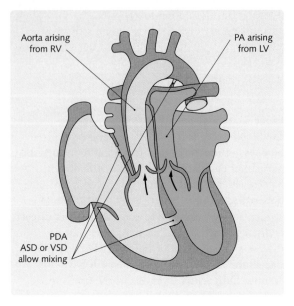

Fig. 2.1 Transposition of the great arteries. There has to be mixing between the two circulations to be compatible with life. As the foramen ovale and the ductus arteriosus begin to close, progressive cyanosis develops.

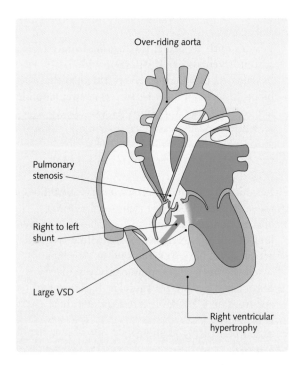
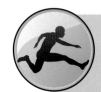

Fig. 2.2 Tetralogy of Fallot: the stenosis of the pulmonary valve causes resistance to flow and shunting of blood through the large ventricular septal defect.

examination will allow most to be distinguished from structural cardiac disease.

Evaluation of a murmur

A murmur is merely one component of the information obtained by examination of the cardiovascular system and cannot be interpreted in isolation. Important features of a murmur include:

- Timing: is it systolic or diastolic? (Most murmurs in children are systolic; diastolic murmurs are rare and always pathological).
- Character: is it pansystolic or ejection systolic?
- Loudness: graded on a scale of 6; grade 4 and above can be palpated.
- Radiation: a murmur that radiates from its site of maximal loudness is more likely to be significant.

Innocent murmurs

The hallmarks of an innocent murmur are:
- An asymptomatic child.
- A normal cardiovascular examination, including normal heart sounds.
- Systolic or continuous (a diastolic murmur by itself is never innocent).
- No radiation.
- Variation with posture.

In most children with a murmur, the heart is normal and the murmur is innocent. Innocent murmurs are generated by turbulent flow in a structurally normal cardiovascular system (CVS). There are two main varieties of innocent murmur, the ejection murmurs and the venous hums.

The ejection murmurs are:
- Generated in the outflow tract of either side of the heart.
- Soft, blowing, systolic.
- Heard in the second or fourth left intercostal space.

The venous hums:
- Are generated in the head and neck veins.
- Are a continuous low-pitched rumble.
- Are heard beneath the clavicle.
- Disappear on lying flat.

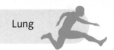

An innocent murmur is more likely to be noted during tachycardia (e.g., with fever, anemia, or exercise).

Significant murmurs

A murmur with any of the following features is significant:
- Symptoms: syncope, episodic cyanosis.
- CVS signs: abnormal pulses, heart sounds, blood pressure (BP), or cardiac impulse.
- Murmur: diastolic, radiating to the back or associated with a thrill.

Significant murmurs, which can be difficult to distinguish from an innocent murmur, include those caused by pulmonary stenosis (PS) and PDA. Refer for echocardiography if in doubt.

Cardiac failure

Cardiac failure is rarely seen in pediatric practice and is usually encountered in babies. The clinical features are different from those in adults. Babies do not climb stairs or need extra pillows at night! Feeding is the only exertion they undertake and, since they are not upright and ambulating at this time of life, their ankles do not swell up.

Clinical features of cardiac failure

The symptoms and signs of cardiac failure are as follows (Fig. 2.3):

- Symptoms: the parents may notice poor feeding and breathlessness, excessive sweating, and recurrent chest infections. There may be failure to thrive.
- Signs: tachycardia, cool periphery, tachypnea, and hepatomegaly. CVS signs can include a third heart sound, murmur, and abnormal pulses.

Causes of cardiac failure

In hemodynamic terms, the cause of cardiac failure is either pressure overload (obstructive lesions) or volume overload (left to right shunts):
- Obstructive lesions usually present in neonates (e.g., severe coarctation of the aorta [COA] or hypoplastic left heart syndrome).
- Volume overload usually presents in infants. The left to right shunt increases (e.g., ventricular septal defects [VSD], PDA) as the pulmonary vascular resistance falls.

Cardiac failure can be confused with the more common respiratory causes of tachypnea, (e.g., bronchiolitis or wheezing associated with a viral infection). A CXR will clarify the situation. Less common causes include supraventricular tachycardia and viral myocarditis.

Investigations for cardiac failure

Useful investigations include:
- CXR.
- Electrocardiogram (ECG).
- Echocardiography.

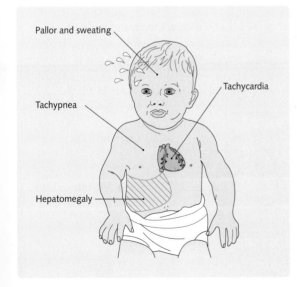

Fig. 2.3 Signs of cardiac failure in an infant.

Lung

Several noises of great diagnostic value emanate from the respiratory tract. A cough is the most obvious. Stridor and wheeze—two other noises associated with breathing and caused by airway narrowing—are also of vital importance.

Pediatric airway anatomy

The pediatric airway differs from the adult and older child:
- The tongue is larger.
- The larynx is higher and more anterior.
- The larynx is funnel-shaped.
- The trachea is short.
- The narrowest portion is at the cricoid (vocal cords in adults).
- The epiglottis is horseshoe-shaped.

Neonates are obligate nose breathers until 5 months of age, although 40% of term babies will convert to oral breathing if nasal obstruction occurs. See Chapter 28 for physiologic respiratory differences.

Cough

A cough is a reflex, involuntary explosive expiration that is a primary defense mechanism of the respiratory tract. In most instances, cough is due to an acute upper respiratory viral infection, but there are important causes of chronic cough. The cough itself is rarely diagnostic except in two instances:
1. The "barking" cough of croup (acute laryngotracheobronchitis).
2. The paroxysmal prolonged bouts of coughing, sometimes ending in a sharp intake of breath (the "whoop"), that occur in pertussis (whooping cough).

History of cough

Find out the following information:
- Duration of the cough: this is usually brief (e.g., less than 1 week). A chronic cough (>3 weeks' duration) raises the possibility of disorders such as chronic infection, suppurative lung disease, postviral cough receptor sensitivity, asthma, whooping cough, inhaled foreign body, or TB. Abrupt onset of symptoms suggests inhaled foreign body.
- Type of cough: whether dry, moist, or productive. The majority are dry (e.g., postviral infection, asthma); a moist or productive cough raises the possibility of suppurative lung disease (e.g., cystic fibrosis). A productive cough is rare in children as any sputum produced is swallowed.
- Association with wheeze: cough without wheeze in children is rarely due to asthma.
- Trigger factors: passive smoking, exposure to daycare, nocturnal cough, or cough on exposure to animals and atopy.

Common causes of a cough are shown in Fig. 2.4. Note that many children with neurologic disorders (e.g., severe cerebral palsy) cannot cough well. This is one of the reasons for their susceptibility to respiratory infections.

Apnea

This is the cessation of breathing for at least 20 seconds. Its presence can signify significant respiratory disease and acute life-threatening events, especially in infants. It is common in preterm infants due to immaturity of the respiratory centers.

Stridor and wheeze
Differences between stridor and wheeze

Stridor is a noise associated with breathing due to narrowing of the extrathoracic airway; wheeze is a noise associated with breathing due to narrowing of the intrathoracic airway. Either noise can occur at any phase of the respiratory cycle. The differences are:
- Stridor is usually worse on inspiration when extrathoracic airways naturally collapse.

Causes of cough		
Type of cough	Cause	Clues to diagosis
Acute	Viral respiratory infection Bronchiolitis Pneumonia Foreign body	Coryzal symptoms Wheeze in <1 year Fever and dyspnea Sudden onset
Chronic	Asthma Tuberculosis Pertussis Suppurative lung disease (e.g., cystic fibrosis) Hyperreactive cough receptors	Associated wheeze Tuberculosis contact Lymphocytosis, apnea Productive cough Usually after upper respiratory tract infection

Fig. 2.4 Causes of cough.

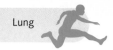

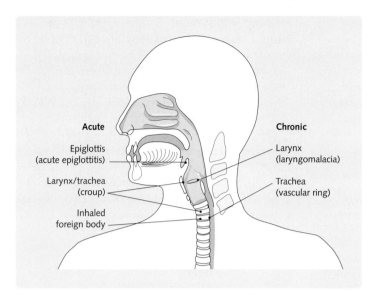

Fig. 2.5 Causes of stridor.

• Wheeze is usually worse on expiration when intrathoracic airways naturally collapse.

It is very important to make a clear distinction between these signs as the likely cause and management of stridor is very different from that of wheeze. Stridor implies an upper airway obstruction, which could be life threatening.

Stridor

There are two types of stridor: the acute and the persistent (Fig. 2.5).

Causes of acute stridor include:
• Acute laryngotracheobronchitis (croup).
• Acute epiglottitis.
• Inhaled foreign body.
• Angioneurotic edema (rare).

Causes of persistent stridor in an infant are:
• Laryngomalacia ("floppy" larynx).
• Anatomic obstructions, such as vascular ring (rare).

The different features of epiglottitis and croup reflect the differences in pathology. In epiglottitis, there is rapid onset of supraglottic swelling (the swollen epiglottis is painful and makes swallowing difficult) and bacteriemia. In croup, involvement of the larynx generates the characteristic hoarse voice and barking cough.

Features of epiglottitis:
• Appearance: toxic.
• Cough: slight/absent.
• Voice: muffled.
• Drooling: yes.
• Able to drink: no.

Features of croup:
• Appearance: well.
• Cough: barking.
• Voice: hoarse.
• Drooling: no.
• Able to drink: yes.

Wheeze

The usual causes are viral lower respiratory tract infections and asthma. In children <1 year old, the tiny airways are easily narrowed by edema and secretions, making wheeze a common feature of infections that involve the bronchi and bronchioles. In children >2 years old, asthma is the most common cause of wheeze. Asthma may have its onset in the first year of life; however, it can be difficult to distinguish from the episodic wheezing induced by recurrent viral infections of the lower respiratory tract. Distinct patterns of wheezing are recognized in childhood asthma: infrequent episodic (75%), frequent episodic (20%), and persistent (5%).

Less common causes of recurrent or acute wheezing in childhood include:

• Cystic fibrosis associated with failure to thrive and frequent chest infections.
• Laryngeal pathology: abnormal voice or cry.
• Gastroesophageal reflux: excessive vomiting.
• Inhaled foreign body: sudden onset is the clue.

Ear, nose, and throat (ENT)

Infections of the ears and the throat are very common in childhood and ENT examination is therefore essential in any febrile child.

 A small child may not localize pain to the ear. The ears must be examined carefully in any febrile child.

Ear
Pain or discharge
Earache is usually caused by infection of the middle ear (acute otitis media). Less common causes include otitis externa, a foreign body, or referred pain from teeth. A discharge may be of wax or purulent material (from otitis externa, otitis media with perforation, or a foreign body).

Hearing impairment
Hearing impairment is classified into two main types: conductive and sensorineural hearing loss (SNHL). The causes of both are illustrated in Fig. 2.6.

• Conductive hearing loss is very common and usually due to otitis media with effusion (OME, also known as "glue ear"). Over half of all preschool children have at least one episode of OME. A much smaller percentage has persistent OME with hearing impairment, which can delay language acquisition. Impedance tests are used to assess middle ear function (Fig. 2.7); they are not a direct measure of hearing.

Causes of impaired hearing	
Type	**Cause**
Conductive	Otitis media with effusion Foreign body Wax
Sensorineural	Congenital infection Prematurity (<32/40) Risk factors: hypoxia 　　　　　　　jaundice 　　　　　　　ototoxic drugs Meningitis Genetic (rare)

Fig. 2.6 Causes of impaired hearing.

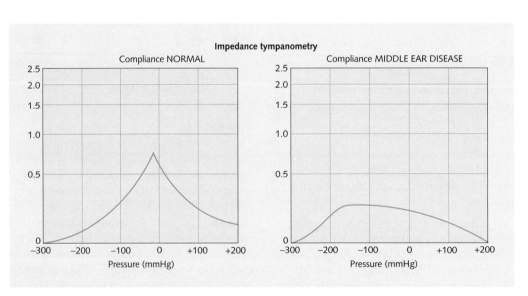

Fig. 2.7 Impedance tympanometry. This tests for middle ear disease. Sound is transmitted across the tympanic membrane if it is compliant (i.e., equal pressure either side). The test measures reflected sound at different pressures. In serous otitis media, compliance is reduced at all pressures because of the fluid present resulting in a flattened curve.

Any child with delayed speech must have a hearing test:
- Speech uses frequencies of 400–4000 Hz.
- Hearing thresholds (in decibels = db):

>70 db = profound hearing loss.
20–70 db = mild/severe hearing loss.
<20 db = normal hearing.

- Sensorineural hearing loss is less common. Routine screening of neonates is now performed in most states (Fig. 2.8). Not all cases will be detected in the neonatal period as, for example, congenital infections and some genetic causes of SNHL are progressive and cannot be detectable at this age.
- Acquired hearing loss occurs after CNS infections (e.g., meningitis), and all affected children should have hearing testing after the acute illness has resolved (Fig. 2.9). Treatment with cochlear implantation may be required.

Tests of auditory function		
Age	**Test**	**Indication**
Newborn	Otoacoustic emission Brainstem-evoked potential audiometry response cradle	Presence of high-risk factors (e.g., prematurity) Newborn screening
7–9 months	Parental questionnaire Distraction test	Used prior to newborn screening
18–24 months	Speech discrimination tests Threshold audiometry (<3 years) Impedance audiometry	Children with suspected hearing loss Children with repeated middle ear disease
School entry	"Sweep test" (modified pure tone audiogram—Fig. 2.9)	Screen all children

Fig. 2.8 Tests of auditory function.

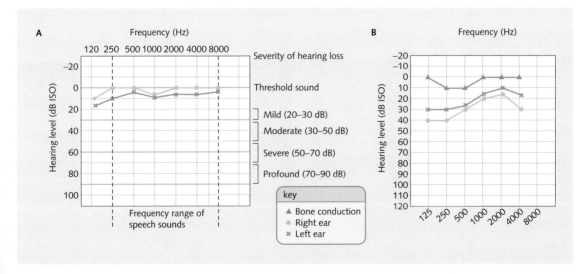

Fig. 2.9 Audiogram demonstrating: (A) normal hearing and (B) bilateral conductive hearing loss. In (B), there is a 20–40 dB hearing loss in both the right and left ears.

- Parental suspicions about possible hearing loss should be taken seriously, with early referral for audiologic testing.
- Children with significantly impaired language development, behavioral problems, or a history of repeated middle ear disease should also be referred.

Nose

Noses can discharge or bleed. The common cold accounts for most acute watery discharges. A chronic discharge may be due to allergic rhinitis or a unilateral foreign body.

Causes of epistaxis (nose bleeds) include:
- Trauma.
- Nose picking.
- Bleeding disorders (especially low platelets).

Throat
Sore throat (pharyngitis)

- Constitutional upset, tonsillar exudates, and lymphadenopathy suggest a bacterial infection: group A β-hemolytic streptococci is a common pathogen ("strep. throat").
- Rarely, a peritonsillar abscess may develop and require incision and drainage.
- Epstein–Barr virus (infectious mononucleosis) is an important cause of exudative tonsillitis.

3. GI Tract or Liver Problems

GI tract

Disorders of the GI tract present with a limited number of symptoms, including abdominal pain, vomiting, diarrhea or constipation, failure to thrive, and bleeding.

Abdominal pain
Acute abdominal pain

The most important issue is whether the pain is being caused by a condition that requires urgent surgical intervention (Figs. 3.1 and 3.2).

History

In babies, abdominal pain is inferred from episodic screaming and drawing up of the legs. In older children, important features in the history are:
- Duration: pain lasting more than 4 hours is likely to be significant.
- Location: the further away from the umbilicus the more likely to be significant (early appendicitis is an exception to this).
- Nature: constant or intermittent/colicky.
- Associated symptoms: vomiting (is there obstruction or gastroenteritis?), stools (pain and bloody stools suggest intussusception in an infant, inflammatory bowel disease in older children), dysuria (urinary tract infection), cough (pneumonia), anorexia (a normal appetite is usually a sign of well-being).

Physical examination

Careful systemic examination is important if the many traps for the unwary are to be avoided. Look for:
- Fever: present in appendicitis, mesenteric adenitis, and urinary tract infections (UTIs).
- Jaundice: infectious hepatitis causes abdominal pain.
- Rash: the abdominal pain of Henoch–Schönlein purpura (HSP) may precede the characteristic purpuric rash.
- Respiratory tract: is there a right lower lobe pneumonia?
- Hernial orifices: is there a strangulated hernia?
- Genitalia: is there a torsion of the testis?

Investigations

Consider the following:
- Complete blood count (CBC): a neutrophil leukocytosis may be present in acute appendicitis or bacterial infection of the urine, lung or throat. A sickle-cell prep should be done in children of African or Afro-Caribbean origin.
- Urinalysis: dipstick for glucose and ketones, urine microscopy and culture.
- Imaging: a plain abdominal film may reveal constipation, renal calculi, or signs of intestinal obstruction. Abdominal ultrasound may reveal obstructive uropathy, an appendix mass intussusception, or ovarian cysts.
- Urea and electrolytes: in a vomiting child, electrolyte disturbances must be identified in advance of anesthesia and surgery.
- Blood glucose.
- C-reactive protein (CRP).

Recurrent abdominal pain

In most children, recurrent abdominal pain does not have an organic cause. In most cases, a positive diagnosis of "functional" abdominal pain can be made without investigations (Fig. 3.3). Further investigation often reinforces anxieties in the parents and child and should be discouraged.

There is a long list of rare causes of recurrent abdominal pain (Fig. 3.4). Careful history and examination will usually provide a clue. Further investigations to exclude a possible organic cause may include:
- Urine microscopy and culture.
- Plain abdominal film.
- Abdominal ultrasound.
- CBC, erythrocyte sedimentation rate (ESR).
- *Helicobacter pylori* serology or hydrogen breath test.

Surgical causes of acute abdominal pain

Cause	Clinical clues
Acute appendicitis	Pattern of migration and right iliac fossa tenderness
Intussusception	Episodic pattern
Torsion of testes	Clinical examination
Strangulated inguinal hernia	Groin mass

Fig. 3.1 Surgical causes of acute abdominal pain.

Medical causes of acute abdominal pain

Abdominal causes	Systemic causes
Colic	Diabetic ketoacidosis
Constipation	Sickle-cell disease
Mesenteric adenitis	Henoch–Schönlein purpura
Hepatitis	Lower lobe pneumonia
Pancreatitis	
Acute pyelonephritis/UTI	

Fig. 3.2 Medical causes of acute abdominal pain.

Features of "functional" recurrent abdominal pain

- Pain is periumbilical, worse on waking, and short-lived
- No associated appetite loss or bowel disturbance
- Family history of migraine, irritable bowel syndrome, or recurrent abdominal pain
- Healthy, thriving child with normal physical examination

Fig. 3.3 Features of "functional" recurrent abdominal pain.

Rare "organic" causes of recurrent abdominal pain

UTI
Urinary calculus
Obstructive uropathy
Inflammatory bowel disease
Duodenal ulcer
Malrotation
Recurrent pancreatitis

Fig. 3.4 Rare "organic" causes of recurrent abdominal pain.

common and benign causes from serious pathology. Vomiting can be caused by a host of illnesses and often indicates disease outside the gastrointestinal tract.

- Acute appendicitis is uncommon under 2 years.
- Consider intussusception in vomiting infants aged 6–12 months.
- Not all abdominal pain originates in the abdomen.
- Diabetic ketoacidosis is often associated with abdominal pain.
- Consider gynecologic causes in a teenage girl.

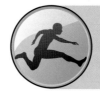

Vomiting is a nonspecific symptom of infection in children.

History

Important points to establish include:
- Does the vomit contain blood or bile? Biliary vomiting must be investigated.

Vomiting

Vomiting is a nonspecific symptom that can be associated with a wide variety of conditions but can also be a normal finding in well babies. A complete clinical assessment often distinguishes the more

Any child with bile-stained vomit requires a surgical consultation.

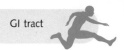

- Duration: is vomiting an acute or a persistent problem?
- Associated symptoms: is vomiting accompanied by fever, abdominal pain, constipation, or diarrhea?

Examination
Examine for the following:
- Signs of dehydration.
- Fever.
- Abdominal distention (visible peristalsis), tenderness or masses.
- Hernial orifices and genitalia.

Common and important causes, considered by age group and divided into medical and surgical conditions, are discussed below.

The neonate
Vomiting can be a sign of systemic infection (e.g., meningitis, UTI) or certain inborn errors of metabolism (e.g., congenital adrenal hyperplasia).

Surgical causes include bowel obstruction, which can be either small or large bowel obstruction. This is often associated with abdominal distention and no bowel movement. Visible peristalsis rarely may be seen.

Causes of small bowel obstruction include:
- Duodenal atresia (associated with Down syndrome).
- Malrotation with volvulus.
- Strangulated inguinal hernia.
- Meconium ileus due to cystic fibrosis.

Causes of large bowel obstruction include Hirschsprung's disease (absence of the myenteric plexus in the rectum and colon). Passage of meconium is often delayed beyond 48 hours.

Infants: 1 month to 1 year
The most common cause of persistent vomiting in babies up to 1 year is gastroesophageal reflux. There is a functional immaturity of the lower esophageal sphincter that resolves spontaneously. Thickening the feeds and positioning head up after feeds are useful maneuvers. Severe reflux is uncommon (it occurs in cerebral palsy and babies with chronic lung disease) and may be complicated by failure to thrive, esophagitis, and recurrent aspiration pneumonia.

Acute medical causes of vomiting include:
- Gastroenteritis.
- Respiratory tract infections such as tonsillitis, otitis media, and whooping cough.
- UTI.
- Meningitis.

Important surgical causes include pyloric stenosis and intussusception:
- Pyloric stenosis causes non-bile-stained projectile vomiting, most commonly in baby boys between the age of a few weeks and 3 months.
- The peak age of intussusception is around 6 months. The vomiting is associated with episodic severe abdominal pain and the eventual passage of bloodstained, "redcurrant jelly" stools.

Older children
Acute vomiting can occur in infections as described or may be one of the symptoms of acute appendicitis. In the older child, recurrent vomiting can occur as part of the symptom complex of abdominal migraine. Rare but important causes include raised intracranial pressure, malrotation of the intestine, inborn errors of metabolism, and eating disorders such as bulimia nervosa.

Hematemesis
The differential diagnosis for vomiting blood varies with the age of the child. In the first few days of life it is usually caused by swallowed maternal blood. Later on, the main causes are esophagitis and gastritis. Esophageal varices are a cause in liver disease, but peptic ulcers in children are uncommon.

Diarrhea
Acute diarrhea
The most common cause is infectious viral gastroenteritis. It commonly occurs in combination with vomiting.

Some infections cause pathology in the lower gastrointestinal (GI) tract. In this case, there may be no vomiting and diarrhea—often with blood and mucus—dominates the clinical presentation (Fig. 3.5). Bloody diarrhea should raise suspicion of specific pathogens and of noninfective conditions such as intussusception and inflammatory bowel disease.

Infectious causes of acute diarrhea
Viral Norwalk agent Adenovirus
Bacterial *Escherichia coli* *Campylobacter* spp. *Salmonella* spp. *Shigella* spp. *Vibrio cholerae*
Protozoa *Giardia lamblia* *Entameba histolytica* *Cryptosporidium parvum*

Fig. 3.5 Infectious causes of acute diarrhea.

Causes of chronic diarrhea	
Infectious causes	Giardiasis Amebiasis
Food intolerance	Disaccharides—lactose intolerance Proteins—cow's milk protein intolerance
Malabsorption	Celiac disease (gluten enteropathy) Cystic fibrosis
Inflammatory bowel disease	Crohn's disease Ulcerative disease

Fig. 3.6 Causes of chronic diarrhea.

Chronic diarrhea in a child who is failing to thrive raises the possibility of several important diagnoses (Fig. 3.6). A description of the stools may suggest steatorrhoea (pale, bulky, and offensive) and the presence of blood or mucus suggests infective causes or inflammatory bowel disease.

Physical examination

Key points include assessment for evidence of malabsorption—anemia, poor weight gain, abdominal distention, and buttock wasting. A thriving child with no associated symptoms is unlikely to have significant disease. Fecal soiling due to constipation with overflow can be mistaken for diarrhea (confirm by rectal examination).

Investigations

These are directed towards the suspected cause and include:
- Stool microscopy and culture.
- Tests for reducing substances.
- Tests for nutrient malabsorption—Hb estimation, serum iron, and red cell folate.
- Jejunal biopsy (celiac disease).
- Sweat test (cystic fibrosis).

Constipation

The term "constipation" refers to infrequent passage of stools, passage of abnormally hard stools, or pain or discomfort on defecation. It may be accompanied by soiling caused by involuntary passage of feces (overflow incontinence) or voluntary passage of feces in an unacceptable place (encopresis).

Bloody diarrhea—consider:
- Infectious causes: *Campylobacter*, *Shigella*, ameba.
- Intussusception: especially 6–9 months.
- Hemolytic–uremic syndrome: check renal function and blood pressure.
- Ulcerative colitis (rare).

On examination, high fever suggests a bacterial gastroenteritis, especially *Shigella* infection. Assessment of dehydration is most important (see Chapter 15).

Chronic diarrhea

The most common cause of persistent loose stools in a well, thriving, preschool child is so-called "toddler diarrhea." A maturational delay in intestinal mobility causes intermittent explosive loose stools with undigested vegetables often present ("peas and carrots" syndrome).
An acute diarrheal episode may become protracted (duration >2 weeks) because of "postgastroenteritis" syndrome due to secondary lactose intolerance. Watery diarrhea returns when a normal diet, including milk, is reintroduced. Stools give a positive Clinitest result for reducing substances. Some infective agents, such as *Giardia*, also cause protracted diarrhea.

Hard stools in a baby may occur with:
• Inadequate milk intake.
• Concentrated formula feeds.
• Changing to cow's milk.
• Formula high in iron content

In infants and children, constipation is often acute and transient and it is important to remember the wide normal variation in stool pattern. Constipation may follow an acute febrile illness and can be prolonged if the hard stools cause a small, superficial anal tear. Though rare, constipation and encopresis can be secondary to child abuse/sexual abuse.

Organic causes of constipation are rare (Fig. 3.7). An organic cause is more likely in infants, with onset at birth or when constipation occurs in the context of additional problems such as failure to thrive.

In childhood, the most common cause of chronic constipation is so-called "simple" constipation (Fig. 3.8) associated with acquired megacolon. Short-segment Hirschprung's disease may present late and should be considered in severe or intractable constipation (Fig. 3.9).

History

Inquire about:
• Frequency and consistency of stools.
• Presence of pain or blood on defecation.
• Presence or absence of soiling (in children).
• Any history of delay in passage of meconium.
• Psychosocial/environmental situation

Organic causes of constipation	
Local causes	Hirschprung's disease Neuormuscular disorders (e.g., cerebral palsy)
Systemic causes	Hypothyroidism Hypercalcemia Renal tubular disorders

Fig. 3.7 Organic causes of constipation.

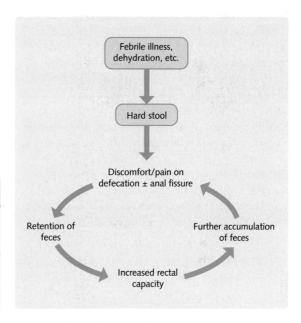

Fig. 3.8 The cycle of simple constipation.

Fig. 3.9 Differences between simple constipation and Hirschprung's disease.

Difference between simple constipation and Hirschprung's disease		
	Simple constipation	Hirschprung's disease
Frequency	Common	Rare—1 : 4500 live births
Onset	Late	85% in first month of life
Passage of meconium	Normal (<24 h)	Delayed
Soiling	Usual	Uncommon
Abdomen	Fecal mass	Distended
Rectum	Loaded and distended	Narrow and empty

Physical examination

Check for the following:

- Systemic signs of failure to thrive or dehydration.
- Abdominal distention, palpable descending colon.
- Presence of anal fissure.
- Rectal examination: anal tone, rectum empty or loaded?

Failure to thrive

The phrase "failure to thrive" is used to describe an inadequate weight gain during the first year of life. Although this may be associated with poor linear growth and short stature, it is better to consider this as a separate problem.

It is the rate of weight gain that is important, and this can only be judged by plotting serial weights on a percentile chart over a period of time; a single observation is difficult to interpret. Much unnecessary anxiety is expended on normal small infants who are proceeding steadily up the third percentile. It is also important to remember that birth weight is determined by the intrauterine environment, and the infant's weight may fall from its birth percentile to a lower, genetically determined percentile (catch down) in the first year. Normal small infants have small appetites, a feature that can cause inappropriate parental anxiety.

Recognition of the constitutionally small child:
- Small parents.
- Low birth weight for gestational age.
- Proportionally small: low percentile for height, weight, and head circumference.
- Normal height and weight velocities.
- Asymptomatic.
- Normal physical examination.

Globally, the most common cause of failure to thrive is inadequate intake of food (i.e., starvation). In the USA, most cases have a nonorganic cause and are associated with psychosocial and environmental deprivation. Organic causes include inadequate food intake, defective absorption of food from the GI tract (malabsorption), protein loss from the gut, and increased energy expenditure (Fig. 3.10).

Extensive investigation is not usually required. The constitutionally small normal child should be recognized and nonorganic failure to thrive can be positively diagnosed. A brief hospital admission to document weight gain on a measured dietary intake may be helpful.

Causes of failure to thrive	
Organic	**Nonorganic**
Inadequate food intake: • Breastfeeding—insufficient milk, poor technique • Bottlefeeding—milk too dilute • Insufficient diet offered • Anorexia: due to chronic illness • Unable to feed: cleft palate, cerebral palsy • Vomiting: gastroesophageal reflux Malabsorption: • Celiac disease • Cystic fibrosis • Short gut (postoperative) Protein-losing enteropathy: • Cow's milk protein intolerance Increased energy requirements: • Chronic illness—cystic fibrosis, congenital heart disease, chronic renal failure	Psychosocial/environmental deprivation Inadequate or inappropriate feeding is usually a component

Fig. 3.10 Causes of failure to thrive.

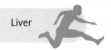

Liver

Liver disease is uncommon in childhood and usually manifests as jaundice or hepatomegaly.

Jaundice

Jaundice is a yellowish discoloration caused by an increase in circulating bilirubin. The bilirubin can be unconjugated or conjugated, depending on the etiology (Fig. 3.11). Mild jaundice is best detected in the sclerae rather than the skin.

Infectious hepatitis is the most common cause of acute jaundice in the older child. However, jaundice is encountered most commonly in the newborn period, at which time its causes range from trivial physiological changes to severe liver disease requiring early recognition and intervention.

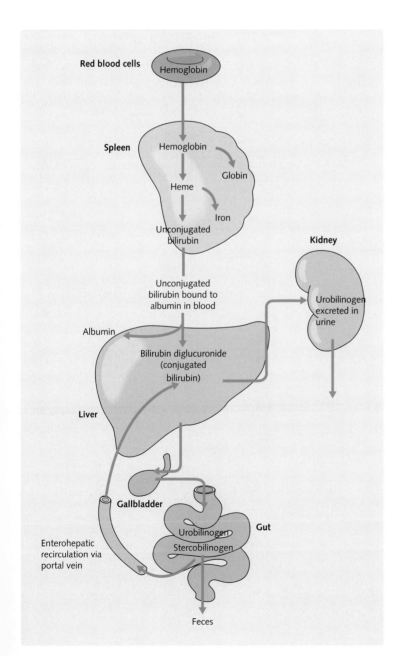

Fig. 3.11 Bilirubin metabolism.

Red blood cells
Hemoglobin

Spleen
Hemoglobin
Globin
Heme
Iron
Unconjugated bilirubin

Kidney

Unconjugated bilirubin bound to albumin in blood

Urobilinogen excreted in urine

Albumin

Bilirubin diglucuronide (conjugated bilirubin)

Liver

Gallbladder

Urobilinogen
Stercobilinogen
Gut

Enterohepatic recirculation via portal vein

Feces

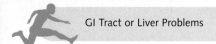

Neonatal jaundice
See Chapter 9.

Jaundice after infancy
Jaundice in childhood usually has an infective cause. Viral hepatitis accounts for most, but other pathogens can involve the liver. Infective hepatitis can be caused by:
- Hepatitis viruses: hepatitis A is the most common cause of jaundice after the neonatal period.
- Epstein–Barr virus (EBV).
- Malaria.
- Leptospirosis (Weil's disease).

Liver injury can be caused by a variety of drugs (e.g., sodium valproate, halothane) and, in overdose, acetaminophen and iron are toxic to the liver. Jaundice with pallor suggests a hemolytic episode (e.g., glucose-6-phosphate dehydrogenase deficiency, spherocytosis, or hemolytic–uremic syndrome). Malaria is an important cause in tropical regions.

Hepatomegaly after infancy
Isolated hepatomegaly is uncommon. In association with jaundice, the causes include biliary atresia and infective hepatitis. In babies, hepatomegaly is an important feature of cardiac failure.

Hepatosplenomegaly can occur in advanced liver disease and in a number of important hematologic diseases (e.g., leukemia, thalassemia) and rare storage disorders (e.g., mucopolysaccharidosis).

In the infant or younger child, urinary tract infection (UTI) is the most common disorder encountered, and it often presents without specific symptoms or signs. Urine abnormalities may also indicate renal pathology, and the diagnostic work-up of some endocrine disorders will require urine collection. Important symptoms are:

- Polyuria (frequency) or enuresis: suggesting UTI or diabetes mellitus.
- Dysuria: suggesting UTI.
- Oliguria: suggesting dehydration or acute renal failure.
- Discolored urine (Fig. 4.1).
- Fever with or without rigors: suggests UTI or pyelonephritis.

- Polyuria and polydipsia suggest diabetes mellitus— test the urine for glucose and ketones.
- Excessive fluid intake is a more common cause of polyuria and polydipsia in a toddler than diabetes insipidus.
- Polyuria may present as secondary enuresis.

Important signs are:
- Hypertension: suggesting glomerulonephritis.
- Edema: suggesting nephrotic syndrome.
- Palpable bladder or kidneys: suggest anatomic abnormalities.

Hematuria

Test strips are very sensitive. Hematuria should be confirmed by urine microscopy and is defined as >10 red blood cells (RBCs) per high power field. The causes are listed in Fig. 4.2.

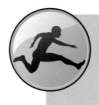

Urine test strips may be positive in hemoglobinuria and myoglobinuria. Dyes and certain foods can discolor the urine. A definite diagnosis of hematuria requires microscopy.

History
Find out the following:
- Duration and recurrence.
- Dysuria and frequency: suggest UTI.
- Associated groin pain: suggests pyelonephritis.
- Recent foreign travel: suggests schistosomyasis.
- Recent sore throat: suggests poststreptococcal glomerulonephritis.
- Family history of stones or deafness: suggests Alport syndrome.

Examination
Examine for:
- Fever: suggests UTI.
- Edema: suggests nephrotic syndrome.
- Hypertension: suggests acute nephritis/chronic renal scarring.
- Rash and joint swelling: suggest Henoch–Schönlein purpura.
- Bruises and purpura: suggest idiopathic thrombocytopenic purpura.
- Abdominal mass: suggests Wilms' tumor.

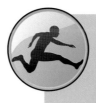

UTI can present with fever and no clues to its origin, especially in infants and young children. Urine microscopy and culture should be undertaken in any infant with unexplained fever.

Investigations

The choice of investigations depends on the renal pathology suspected:

- Microscopy and culture of urine.
- Imaging: nuclear medicine and ultrasound scans.
- Hematology: complete blood count (CBC), coagulation screen, and sickle-cell screen.
- Biochemistry: BUN and electrolytes, creatinine (Cr), Ca^{2+}, PO_4^{3-}, and urate.
- Throat swab.

- Antistreptolysin O titer (ASOT), C3, and hepatitis B antigen.

Transient, benign hematuria can occur but is a diagnosis of exclusion. A renal biopsy may be indicated when there is a need for a diagnosis:

- Persistent proteinuria or hematuria for >6 months.
- Unexplained abnormal renal function.
- Chronic glomerulonephritis.
- Nephrotic syndrome if the child is <1 year or >12 years old at onset.
- Steroid-resistant nephrotic syndrome.

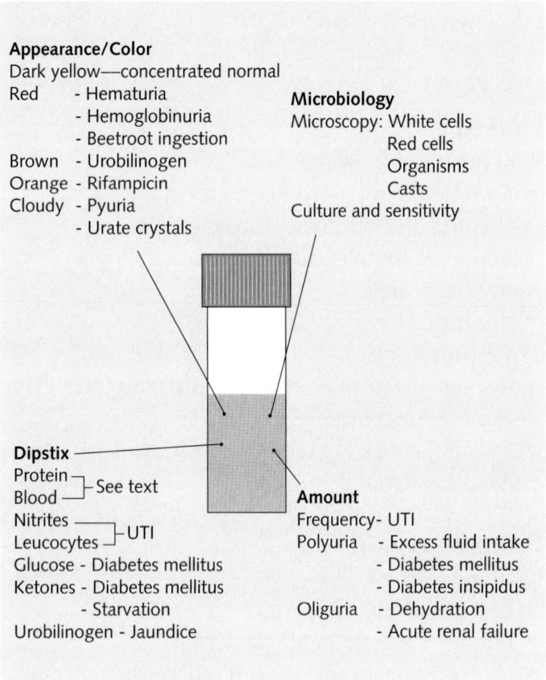

Appearance/Color
Dark yellow—concentrated normal
Red   - Hematuria
     - Hemoglobinuria
     - Beetroot ingestion
Brown - Urobilinogen
Orange - Rifampicin
Cloudy - Pyuria
     - Urate crystals

Microbiology
Microscopy: White cells
     Red cells
     Organisms
     Casts
Culture and sensitivity

Dipstix
Protein ⎤
Blood ⎦ See text
Nitrites ⎤
Leucocytes ⎦ UTI
Glucose - Diabetes mellitus
Ketones - Diabetes mellitus
     - Starvation
Urobilinogen - Jaundice

Amount
Frequency- UTI
Polyuria - Excess fluid intake
      - Diabetes mellitus
      - Diabetes insipidus
Oliguria - Dehydration
      - Acute renal failure

Fig. 4.1 Information available from urine.

Proteinuria

Transient, mild proteinuria is mostly benign. The nephrotic syndrome causes persistent heavy proteinuria. The causes of proteinuria are listed in Fig. 4.3. Normal children produce <60 mg/m^2/24 h of protein in the urine.

Definition

- Early morning urine protein/creatinine ratio >20 mg/mmol (0.2).
- Greater than 5 mg/kg in a 24-hour urine sample.

Examination

Physical examination should include evaluation for the presence or absence of signs of renal disease (especially the nephrotic syndrome), which include:

- Edema: especially periorbital, scrotal, leg, and ankle.
- Ascites.
- Pleural effusions (unusual).
- Blood pressure: low or high.

Causes of hematuria	
Glomerular	**Nonglomerular**
Presence of red cell or white cell casts and proteinuria suggests a glomerular source of the blood—glomerulonephritis: • Acute, poststreptococcal • Henoch–Schönlein purpura • IgA nephropathy (Berger's disease) • Alport syndrome (familial deafness, and nephritis)	Infection • Bacterial UTI • TB • Schistosomyasis Trauma Stones Wilms' tumor Bleeding disorders, especially thrombocytopenia

Fig. 4.2 Causes of hematuria.

Causes of proteinuria	
Transient	**Persistent**
Fever	Nephrotic syndrome
Exercise	(>1 g/m²/24 h)
Orthostatic—proteinuria	UTI
during the day (drops	
when recumbent at night)	

Fig. 4.3 Causes of proteinuria.

Urinary dipstick values	
Stick reading	**Albumin concentration (g/L)**
+	0.3
+ +	1.0
+ + +	3.0
+ + + +	>20

Fig. 4.4 Urinary dipstick values.

Investigations

The investigations include:
- Urine dipstix (Fig. 4.4).
- Early morning protein–creatinine ratio.
- Renal function: BUN, electrolytes, Cr.
- Plasma albumin and lipids.
- Midstream urine for microscopy, culture, and sensitivity.
- Throat swab, ASLO, anti-DNaseB.
- Complement C3, C4.

5. Neurologic Problems

Important symptoms are:
- Paroxysmal episodes (fits, faints, and funny turns).
- Headache.
- Vomiting and ataxia.

Important signs are:
- Focal neurologic signs.
- Altered consciousness or coma.

Global or specific developmental delay can be a manifestation of neurologic disease, as can abnormalities of head size or shape; these are discussed in Chapters 8 and 17.

Fits, faints, and funny turns

Transient episodes of altered consciousness, abnormal movements, or abnormal behavior are a common presenting problem. The first task is to distinguish true epileptic seizures (fits) from faints and funny turns. An accurate account from a witness is essential.

History
Provoking events
Find out exactly when and where the episode occurred.

Description of the episodes
Get an exact description of:
- Any altered consciousness or awareness.
- Abnormal movements (involving limbs or face?).
- Altered tone (rigidity or suddenly flaccid?).
- Altered color (pallor or cyanosis?).
- Eye movements (did they "roll up"?).
- Duration of the episode
- Any trigger (e.g., flashing lights)?

Other important features to establish in the history include:
- Previous history: was the birth normal, was there any developmental delay, has there been any recent head injury?
- Family history: both epilepsy and febrile convulsions run in families.

The paroxysmal episodes (faints and funny turns) that must be distinguished from epileptic seizures are listed in Fig. 5.1 and described below.

- A "seizure" is a transient episode of abnormal and excessive neuronal activity in the brain.
- The term "epilepsy" refers to recurrent seizures.
- Not all convulsions are seizures, and the history from a reliable witness is vital.

Seizures (fits)
Generalized tonic–clonic seizures
These are characterized by:
- Tonic phase of rigidity and loss of posture followed by clonic movements of all four limbs.
- Loss of consciousness.
- Duration: 2–20 minutes.
- Postictal drowsiness.

Febrile seizures are usually of this sort.

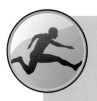
Meningitis or encephalitis must be considered in all children with fever and seizure. Febrile seizures are a diagnosis of exclusion.

Absence seizures
These are characterized by:
- Brief unawareness lasting a few seconds.
- No loss of posture.
- Immediate recovery.
- May be very frequent.
- Associated with automatisms (e.g., blinking and lip-smacking).

Differential diagnosis of seizures by age	
Age	Differential diagnosis
Infants	Jitteriness Benign myoclonus Apnea Gastroesophageal reflux
Toddlers	Breath-holding Reflex anoxic seizures Rigors
Children	Vasovagal syncope (faints) Tics Day-dreaming Migraine Panic attacks, tantrums Night terrors

Fig. 5.1 Differential diagnosis of seizures by age.

Causes of acute seizures	
Common	Uncommon
Febrile seizures Epilepsy Hypoglycemia	Meningitis/encephalitis Head injury Hyponatremia Cerebral tumor or malignant infiltration

Fig. 5.2 Causes of acute seizures.

Fainting (vasovagal syncope)

Features include the following:
- Usually occurs in teenagers.
- Provoked by emotion, hot environment.
- Preceded by nausea and dizziness.
- Sudden loss of consciousness and posture.
- Rapid recovery.

Funny turns
Breath-holding spells

These have the following characteristics:
- They are provoked by temper or frustration.
- The screaming toddler holds his or her breath in expiration, goes blue, then limp, and then makes a rapid spontaneous recovery.

Reflex anoxic seizures

These have the following characteristics:
- They are provoked by pain (usually a mild head injury) or fear.
- The infant or toddler becomes pale and loses consciousness (reflecting syncope, secondary to vagal-induced bradycardia).
- The subsequent hypoxia may induce a tonic–clonic seizure.

Rigors
- Rigors are transient exaggerated shivering in association with high fever.

Examination
The well child

Physical examination is often normal in a well child with idiopathic epilepsy (the majority). However, particular attention should be paid to:
- Skin: neurocutaneous syndromes are associated with epilepsy, especially tuberous sclerosis and neurofibromatosis.
- Optic fundi: fundal changes may be apparent in congenital infections and neurodegenerative diseases.

The seizing child

Physical examination of an infant or child presenting acutely with generalized tonic–clonic seizures has a different emphasis, reflecting the likely causes (Fig. 5.2). Important features on examination include:
- Fever: febrile convulsions or intracranial infection.
- Anterior fontanelle: tense or bulging if the intracranial pressure (ICP) is raised.
- Neck: stiff.
- Optic fundi: swollen discs in raised ICP (changes may occur in congenital infections and neurodegenerative diseases).
- Focal neurologic signs.
- Altered level of consciousness.

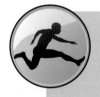

Regarding the seizing child:
- Remember the ABCs: airway, breathing, circulation.
- Always measure blood glucose urgently in a seizing child to identify and treat hypoglycemia.

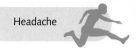

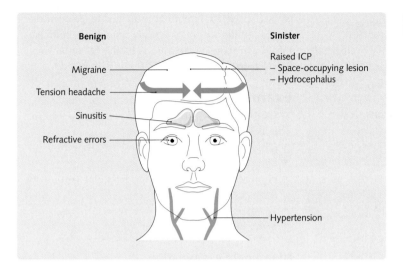

Fig. 5.3 Causes of recurrent headache.

Headache

An acute headache commonly occurs as a nonspecific feature of any febrile illness in a child but is a specific feature of meningitis. Recurrent headaches are very common in children and their causes range from the trivial to the sinister (Fig. 5.3); serious causes are rare.

History
Important features include:
- Site: frontal, temporal, or unilateral?
- Intensity: severe, throbbing?
- Duration and frequency?
- Provoking factors: stress, food?
- Associated symptoms: weakness, paresthesia, nausea or vomiting?

Simple tension headaches
These are characterized by the following:
- Symmetrical and band-like in nature.
- Gradual onset, duration less than 24 hours.
- No associated nausea or vomiting.
- Often recur frequently.
- Affect 10% of school children.

Migraine
- Can be unilateral and throbbing in nature.
- With or without visual aura, area of visual loss, or fortification spectra.
- Associated nausea, vomiting, abdominal pain.
- Duration several hours.

- Trigger factors—stress or relaxation, foods (cheese, chocolate).
- Family history.

Migraine can be classified as:
- Common: no aura.
- Classic: aura preceding headache.
- Complex: associated neurologic deficit (e.g., hemiplegia, ophthalmoplegia).

Headache from raised intracranial pressure
- Worse in recumbent position (i.e., during the night or early morning).
- Associated with nausea and vomiting.
- Pain is usually mild and diffuse.
- Personality changes may develop.

Examination
Attention should be paid to the following signs in a child with recurrent headache:
- Blood pressure: hypertension (e.g., aortic coarctation is a rare cause of headache)
- Pulse: radial-femoral delay (coarctation)
- Visual acuity: refractive errors cause headache
- Papilledema: a late sign of raised ICP
- Focal neurologic deficit: especially cerebellar signs (posterior fossa tumor).

31

Headache is rarely caused by a brain tumor, but 70% of children with a brain tumor present with headache. The headache may wake the child at night, is worst in the morning, and is associated with vomiting. Most are in the posterior fossa and cause raised ICP.

see Chapter 26. It is important not to perform lumbar puncture in an acutely comatose child as raised intracranial pressure is likely. It can always be performed later if a diagnosis is required.

Examination

Systemic examination

This is the priority:

- ABCs: airway, breathing, and circulation.
- Blood glucose.
- Hypertension, bradycardia, irregular respiration (signs of herniation).
- Temperature
- Signs of physical abuse or injury.

Neurologic examination

For a neurologic examination, check the AVPU score; there are four categories:

- **A** = Alert.
- **V** = responds to **V**oice.
- **P** = responds to **P**ain (the Glasgow Coma Scale [GCS] is usually less than 8 at this point).
- **U** = **U**nresponsive.

The unconscious child

The acute development of a diminished level of consciousness is a medical emergency. In the majority of cases a systemic problem rather than a primary brain disorder is responsible (Fig. 5.4). The cause may be evident from the history but, if not, clinical evaluation is the key after emergency management. For investigation and management

When a child is comatose:
- Identify and treat the ABCs and hypoglycemia.
- Establish the degree of unconsciousness (use the GCS or AVPU).
- Look for raised intracranial pressure.
- Establish the possible causes and decide which need immediate treatment.

Causes of coma	
Cause	**Differential diagnosis**
Infection	Meningitis Encephalitis
Trauma	Head injury
Metabolic	Hypoglycemia
Primary CNS disorder	Seizures
Drugs	Opiates Lead

Fig. 5.4 Causes of coma.

Glasgow coma scale			
Score	**Eye opening**	**Best motor response**	**Best verbal response**
1	No response	No response	No response
2	Open to pain	Extension	Nonverbal sounds
3	Open to verbal command	Inappropriate flexion	Inappropriate words
4	Open spontaneously	Flexion with pain	Disoriented and conversing
5		Localizes pain	Oriented and conversing
6		Obeys command	

Fig. 5.5 The Glasgow coma scale: top score = 15.

Check also:
- The Glasgow coma scale (Fig. 5.5).
- The pupils: these may be small (suggests opiate or barbiturate poisoning), large (suggests a postictal state), or unequal (suggests severe head injury or intracranial hemorrhage).

- For meningism.
- The fontanelle.

Further reading

Kirkham FJ. Non-traumatic coma in children. *Archives of Diseases of Childhood* 2001; 85:303–312.

6. Musculoskeletal Problems

Disorders of the musculoskeletal system can present in a variety of ways, including limp, pain in a limb or joint, or variations in posture. Presenting symptoms include:
- Limb or joint pain.
- Fever.

Important signs are:
- Limp.
- Altered posture.
- Point tenderness.
- Reduced range of movement.

Limp

A limp is an abnormality of gait (the term applied to the rhythmic movement of the whole body in walking). It can be painful or painless, and the cause varies with age (Fig. 6.1).

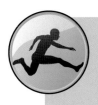

- The most common cause of an acute limp in a well child is toxic synovitis.
- The diagnoses not to miss are septic arthritis or osteomyelitis.

History
The history should establish:
- Duration: chronic pain is unlikely to be caused by infection.
- Any prodromal illness (e.g., sore throat) or trauma.
- Presence and location of any pain.

Examination
Physical examination can begin by observing the child walking, if this can be done without distress. Important physical signs include:

- Fever: suggests bone or joint infection.
- Skin rashes.
- Range of movement.
- Point tenderness or signs of inflammation.
- Unequal leg length.
- Spinal abnormality (e.g., hairy patch).
- Neurologic signs: check tone, strength, and tendon reflexes.

Investigations
Useful investigations may include:
- Imaging: x-rays, ultrasound of hip joint.
- Nuclear medicine: bone scans.
- Complete blood count, acute phase reactants.
- Blood cultures (if febrile).

The painful limb

Pain in a limb can arise from the bone, joint, or soft tissues. In the lower limbs, pain may be associated with a limp (see above). Pain in a joint (arthralgia) is considered separately.

Recurrent limb pain
So-called "growing pains" are common in the lower limbs. Their features are listed in Fig. 6.2.

An important rare cause of limb pain, especially at night, is malignant metastases in the bone (e.g., leukemia).

Limb pain of acute onset
In a young infant this may present as pseudoparalysis. Important causes include:
- Trauma.
- Osteomyelitis.
- Sickle-cell disease ("painful crisis").

Trauma is usually accidental (e.g., sports injury), but nonaccidental injury should also be a consideration. Osteomyelitis usually presents with a painful, immobile limb in a febrile child. The long bones around the knee are the most common site of infection.

35

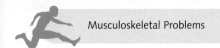

Causes of a limp	
Age group	**Cause**
All ages	Trauma Septic arthritis/osteomyelitis
1–2 years	Congenital dislocation of the hip (developmental dysplasia of the hip) Cerebral palsy
3–10 years	Transient synovitis (irritable hip) Perthes disease Rarities: juvenile idiopathic arthritis, leukemia
11–15 years	Slipped capital femoral epiphysis Osgood–Schlatter disease Rarities: bone tumors, juvenile idiopathic arthritis, hysteria

Fig. 6.1 Causes of a limp.

Features of growing pains
Common between 5 and 11 years of age Occur in evening and night Predominantly lower limbs, calves, shins Normal examination
Never: Functional disability Limp Morning symptoms

Fig. 6.2 Features of growing pains.

The painful joint

Arthralgia usually reflects inflammation, i.e., arthritis. Diagnostic possibilities depend on whether the presentation is acute or insidious, and whether one or several joints are involved. Causes of an acutely painful joint are shown in Fig. 6.3.

Septic arthritis is a medical emergency—joint destruction can occur within 24 h if untreated. X-rays are not helpful in early diagnosis and aspiration of the joint space is indicated if septic arthritis is suspected.

Causes of acute monoarthropathies	
Cause	**Clinical clues**
Septic arthritis	Fever and inability to move
Toxic synovitis	Recent cold
Hemophilia	Easy bruising
Juvenial idiopathic arthritis	Chronic painand swelling
Trauma	Immediate symptoms—no chronicity

Fig. 6.3 Causes of acute monoarthropathies.

Causes of polyarthritis	
Type	**Cause**
Inflammatory	Juvenile idiopathic arthritis Systemic lupus erythematosus Henoch–Schönlein purpura
Infectious/reactive	Viral Mycoplasma Rheumatic fever

Fig. 6.4 Causes of polyarthritis.

Polyarthritis may have an acute onset but is more likely to run a chronic and relapsing course. Causes to consider are shown in Fig. 6.4.

Inequalities of limb length

This is caused by shortening or overgrowth in one or more bones in the leg. Causes include trauma, neuromuscular disorders, and congenital malformations. Treatment is surgical.

Normal postural variants

These are common and most resolve without treatment (Fig. 6.5). They include:
- Bow legs (genu varum): common in infants and toddlers up to 2 years.
- Knock knees (genu valgum): the physiologic knock-knee pattern is seen during the third and fourth years.

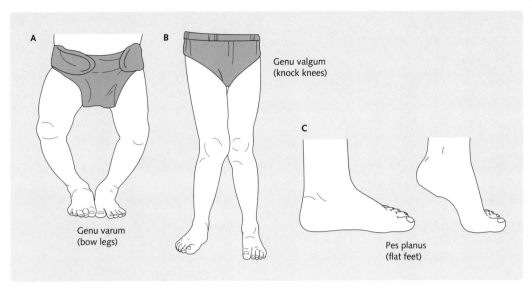

Fig. 6.5 Normal postural variants: (A) genu varum (bow legs), (B) genu valgum (knock knees), (C) pes planus (flat feet). Note the medial longitudinal arch appears when standing on tiptoe.

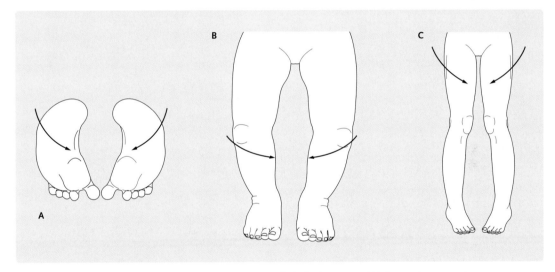

Fig. 6.6 Causes of intoeing: (A) metatarsus varus, (B) medial tibial torsion, (C) femoral anteversion.

- Flat feet (pes planus): often present in toddlers.
- Intoeing: metatarsus varus in infants, medial tibial torsion in toddlers, femoral anteversion in children (Fig. 6.6).

Pathology should be suspected if there is:
- Rapid or severe progression.
- A positive family history.
- Asymmetry.

7. Pallor, Bleeding, Splenomegaly, or Lymphadenopathy

In childhood, disorders of the blood or bone marrow often present with striking physical signs rather than complex symptomatology. The pallor of anemia is the most common sign but abnormal bruising or bleeding, enlargement of the spleen or liver, or a propensity to infection can all reflect an underlying hematologic problem.

Pallor

It is easy to miss mild degrees of anemia, especially in those patients with pigmented skin. Pallor is best diagnosed by observing the conjunctiva and palmar creases. Note that peripheral vasoconstriction also causes pallor (e.g., shock).

Anemia
The history and physical examination will often provide a good idea of the likely cause (Fig. 7.1). Few symptoms will occur unless the hemoglobin decreases below 7–8 g/dL, except in acute blood loss. Infants born preterm have a physiologic anemia at the age of 2 months that can reach as low as 7 g/dL.

History
This should include inquiry about:
- The presence of chronic diseases, especially renal or previous prematurity.
- Gastrointestinal symptoms.
- Dietary history: adequate iron intake? Most anemia in childhood is due to iron deficiency.
- Family history: relatives with inherited disorders such as sickle-cell disease, thalassemia, or hereditary spherocytosis?

Examination
Age and ethnic group
Causes of anemia are very age-dependent, and inherited anemias show a strikingly increased incidence in certain racial groups:
- African-American ancestry: sickle-cell disease.
- Mediterranean and Asian ancestry: thalassemia.

Associated signs
- Jaundice: suggests acute hemolysis.
- Petechiae or bruising: suggest marrow failure.
- Splenomegaly: suggests hemolysis or hemoglobinopathy.

Investigation
The most important initial investigation is examination of the peripheral blood (complete blood count [CBC]) to confirm reduced hemoglobin concentration and document red cell indices (Fig. 7.2). Additional valuable information from the CBC includes:
- Reticulocytes: an increase suggests hemolytic anemia; a decrease suggests marrow aplasia.
- Pancytopenia: a reduction in all cell types suggests marrow failure or hypersplenism.

Depending on the initial results, further investigations to clarify the cause may include:
- Serum iron, ferritin, and total iron-binding capacity.
- Coombs' test: positive in hemolysis caused by immune mechanisms.
- Red cell folate, vitamin B_{12}.
- Hemoglobin electrophoresis.
- Red cell enzyme estimation: glucose-6-phosphate dehydrogenase (G6PD), pyruvate kinase.
- Bone marrow aspiration.

Bleeding disorders

Normal hemostasis requires integrity of the coagulation factors, functional platelets, and their interaction with the vessels. Disorders of the coagulation system are caused by both hereditary and acquired factors. In the past, the coagulation cascade was thought to contain intrinsic and extrinsic pathways; however, it is now thought to comprise a common pathway involving tissue factor activation, with a central role for thrombin and membrane-associated complexes (Fig. 7.3).

Causes of anemia in infants and children	
Cause	Type
Decreased red cell production	
Iron deficiency anemia	Nutritional Occult blood loss (Meckel's diverticulum) Malabsorption (celiac disease)
Hemoglobinopathy	Beta-thalasssemia
Marrow replacement	Malignant disease—acute leukemia Marrow aplasia
Chronic disease	Renal failure, inflammatory disorders
Reduced red cell life span (hemolytic anemia)	
Intrinsic red cell defects	Abnormal membrane—spherocytosis Abnormal hemoglobin—sickle-cell disease, thalassemia Enzyme deficiencies—G6PD (X-linked), pyruvate kinase Immune-mediated
Extrinsic disorders	ABO, rhesus incompatibility Autoimmune response Bacterial infections Malaria Microangiopathy—hemolytic–uremic syndrome Hypersplenism
Excessive blood loss	
Gastrointestinal	Hookworm infestation Meckel's diverticulum
Iatrogenic	Excessive blood draw in babies
Epistaxis	Recurrent, severe
Menstruation	

Fig. 7.1 Causes of anemia in infants and children.

Red cell indices and smear
MCV (mean corpuscular volume) • Microcytic anemia suggests iron deficiency, thalassemia • Macrocytic anemia (normal in neonates) suggests folate, vitamin B_{12} deficiency MCHC (mean corpuscular hemoglobin concentration) • Hypochromic anemia suggests iron deficiency, thalassemia The smear may reveal: • Sickle cells—sickle-cell disease • Microcytic hypochromic cells—iron deficiency • Spherocytes—hereditary spherocytosis

Fig. 7.2 Red cell indices and smear.

Clinical evaluation

The history and examination should answer the following questions:
- Is there a generalized hemostatic problem?
- Is it inherited or acquired?
- What is the likely mechanism: vascular, platelets, coagulation, or a combination?

Investigations will be required to establish the precise nature of the underlying abnormality.

History

- Age of onset: inherited disorders usually present in infancy but, if mild, may not be unmasked until adulthood.

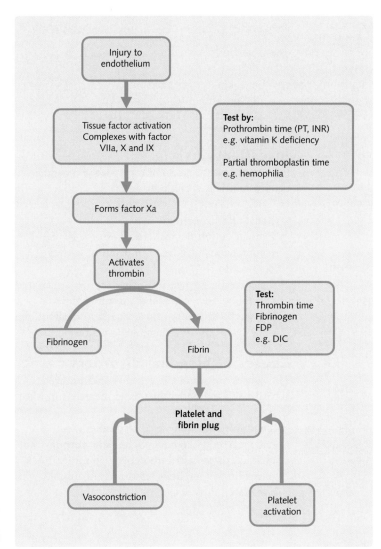

Fig. 7.3 Coagulation cascade: tests and defects.

- If the child has had a hemostatic challenge such as tonsillectomy without excessive bleeding, then a bleeding disorder is unlikely.
- Family history: note that up to one-third of cases of hemophilia are from spontaneous mutation.

- Bleeding into skin and mucous membranes: platelet or vascular disorder.
- Bleeding into muscles or joints: coagulation disorder.

Examination

The most usual clinical manifestation is excessive bleeding into the skin but other sites of spontaneous bleeding include the nasal mucosa (epistaxis), gums, joints (hemarthrosis), and the genitourinary tract (hematuria). Spontaneous bleeding from multiple sites suggests a generalized hemostatic disorder.

Manifestation of skin bleeding

The terms used vary with the size of lesion. Test small lesions using a transparent glass to see if they blanch. Failure to blanch indicates extravasated blood. The terms used when describing manifestations of skin bleeding are:

- Petechiae: small red spots the size of a pinhead.
- Purpura: confluent petechiae.

Bruising—normal and abnormal:
- Mobile toddlers commonly have multiple bruises on shins, but bruises in nonmobile infants need further evaluation.
- Mongolian blue spots in infants can be mistaken for bruising.
- Newborns often have petechiae around the face and forehead.

- Ecchymosis: a large area of extravasated blood (a synonym for a bruise).
- Hematoma: extravasated blood that has infiltrated subcutaneous tissue or muscle to produce a deformity.

An important differential diagnosis of excessive bruising is nonaccidental injury. There are some very important causes of a petechial/purpuric rash (see Chapter 1).

A petechial or purpuric rash in a febrile child must raise the possibility of meningococcal sepsis.

Investigations

Laboratory investigation of a suspected bleeding disorder initially includes:
- CBC, smear.
- Renal and liver function.
- Platelet count: normal is $150–450 \times 10^9/L$ (spontaneous bleeding can occur at counts below $30 \times 10^9/L$).
- Coagulation screen: prothrombin time, activated thromboplastin time, and thrombin time. Further investigation for tissue factors should be done by a tertiary hematologic center.

Causes of bleeding disorders

The causes are set out in Fig. 7.4 and arranged according to the underlying basic mechanism. Most causes are acquired:
- The most common vascular problem encountered is Henoch–Schönlein purpura. The characteristic distribution of purpura (buttocks, lower limbs) and associated features usually allow a clinical diagnosis.

Bleeding disorders in childhood		
Defect	Inherited	Acquired
Vascular defects	Hereditary hemorrhagic telangiectasia (rare) Ehlers–Danlos syndrome (rare)	Henoch–Schönlein purpura Scurvy (vitamin C deficiency) Cushing's disease Meningococcal septicemia
Platelet defects • Thrombocytopenia	Rare	Immune-mediated: idiopathic thrombocytopenic purpura (most common) Peripheral consumption: disseminated intravascular coagulation (DIC), hemolytic–uremic syndrome Marrow failure: aplastic anemia, acute leukemia
• Abnormal function	Rare	Drug-induced (e.g., aspirin, dipyridamole)
Coagulation defects	Hemophilia A (factor VIII) Hemophilia B (factor IX, Christmas disease) von Willebrand disease	Vitamin K deficiency: hemorrhagic disease of newborn, malabsorption, liver disease Drugs—anticoagulant therapy with warfarin, heparin

Fig. 7.4 Bleeding disorders in childhood.

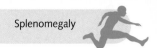

- Excessive bruising with thrombocytopenia in a well child is most commonly due to idiopathic thrombocytopenic purpura (ITP).
- Inherited coagulation disorders are not common but hemophilia must be considered in a male infant or child with a bleeding tendency.
- It is important to rule out bleeding disorders when considering bruising in the context of nonaccidental injury.

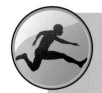

In sickle-cell disease:
- Splenomegaly is present in early life, but splenic infarction subsequently reduces the spleen in size.
- The immunologic function of the spleen is always impaired, regardless of size.

Splenomegaly

In neonates and very thin children, the tip of the spleen is often palpable. The spleen can enlarge during acute infections and splenomegaly is a feature of a number of hematologic diseases. Enlargement of both liver and spleen together suggests a different etiology from that associated with isolated splenomegaly (Figs. 7.5 and 7.6).

Differential diagnosis of a left-sided abdominal mass:
- Splenomegaly.
- Renal masses: Wilms' tumor, hydronephrosis.
- Neoplasia: neuroblastoma (non-renal), lymphoma.

History
- Review of systems: may elicit symptoms related to the many infective causes.
- Family history: inherited anemias, storage disorders (e.g., Gaucher's disease).

Examination
Note coexistent lymphadenopathy, hepatomegaly, pallor (anemia), fever, or rash. In infectious mononucleosis, care must be taken in palpating the spleen because it can rupture.

Investigations
- Abdominal ultrasound scan (USS).
- Infections: monospot, blood cultures, film for malaria parasites.
- Hematologic: CBC, blood smear, reticulocyte count.

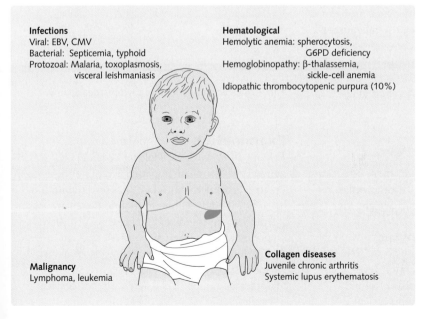

Infections
Viral: EBV, CMV
Bacterial: Septicemia, typhoid
Protozoal: Malaria, toxoplasmosis, visceral leishmaniasis

Hematological
Hemolytic anemia: spherocytosis, G6PD deficiency
Hemoglobinopathy: β-thalassemia, sickle-cell anemia
Idiopathic thrombocytopenic purpura (10%)

Malignancy
Lymphoma, leukemia

Collagen diseases
Juvenile chronic arthritis
Systemic lupus erythematosis

Fig. 7.5 Causes of splenomegaly.

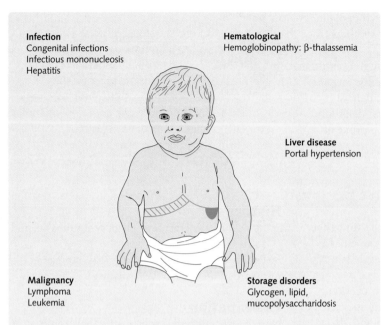

Infection
Congenital infections
Infectious mononucleosis
Hepatitis

Hematological
Hemoglobinopathy: β-thalassemia

Liver disease
Portal hypertension

Malignancy
Lymphoma
Leukemia

Storage disorders
Glycogen, lipid,
mucopolysaccharidosis

Fig. 7.6 Causes of hepatosplenomegaly.

- Malignancy: bone marrow aspiration.
- Liver disease: liver function tests (LFTs), hepatitis serology.

Lymphadenopathy

Lymph node enlargement, particularly in the cervical region, is a common clinical problem in children. Cervical lymph nodes are normally palpable in many children and the first problem is to distinguish this from pathological enlargement.

Local infection is the most common cause of transient regional lymphadenopathy but uncommon sinister causes of persistent or progressive lymphadenopathy do exist (Figs. 7.7, 7.8, and 7.9).

History
The history should establish:
- Duration: less than 4 weeks in most infections; more than 1 year less likely to be neoplastic.
- Constitutional symptoms (e.g., weight loss, fever, night sweats).
- Rash: associated rash suggests viral exanthemata.
- Pets: toxoplasmosis or cat scratch fever.
- Travel contacts and family history of TB.
- Drugs: phenytoin, carbamazepine.

Causes of generalized lymphadenopathy	
Cause	**Example**
Infection	Infectious mononucleosis Rubella Toxoplasmosis Cytomegalovirus HIV infection
Malignancy	Acute leukemia Lymphoma
Immunologic	JCA Sarcoidosis (rare) Kawasaki disease Atopic eczema

Fig. 7.7 Causes of generalized lymphadenopathy.

Examination
Palpate all nodal sites: look for regional or generalized lymphadenopathy. Examine the nodes:
- Size: greater than 1 cm diameter is more likely to be significant. Small, mobile nodes are less likely to be significant than large, firm, fixed nodes.
- Erythema and tenderness: suggest bacterial adenitis.
- Drainage region: ENT and scalp for cervical nodes.

Causes of cervical lymphadenopathy	
Type	**Features**
Acute, short duration	Reactive and secondary to local infection in throat or scalp Cervical adenitis—bacterial infection in gland
Persistent, noninflamed	Reactive and secondary to local infection: Tuberculous adenitis—TB, atypical mycobacteria Neoplasia—lymphoma, neuroblastoma

Fig. 7.8 Causes of cervical lymphadenopathy.

Features of "concerning" lymph nodes
Rapid growth Skin ulceration Fixation to skin or fascia >3 cm with hard consistency >3 cm for more than 6 weeks despite treatment

Fig. 7.9 Features of "concerning" lymph nodes.

- Skin: infective lesions, atopic eczema and exanthemata.
- Abdomen: hepatosplenomegaly.

Also note systemic signs such as weight loss and pallor.

Investigations

The diagnosis is apparent in most children with lymphadenopathy and further investigations to establish the cause are unnecessary. This includes the following common clinical situations:
- Transient node enlargement with local infection.
- Lymphadenopathy in the context of diagnosed systemic illnesses such as rubella, Epstein–Barr virus, atopic eczema, and Kawasaki disease.

By contrast, lymphadenopathy presenting in the following clinical contexts requires investigation to establish an underlying diagnosis.

Persistent significant cervical lymphadenopathy

Initial tests are:
- CBC: to determine infection.
- Chest x-ray: to check for TB, lymphoma.
- Tuberculin skin test: if positive this suggests mycobacteria tuberculosis but weak false positives can be caused by nontuberculous mycobacteria.

If malignancy is suspected, a lymph node biopsy may be indicated.

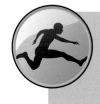

Cervical nodes are quick to enlarge but are slow to resolve with local infection. Consider TB or malignancy in persistent and progressive cervical lymphadenopathy.

Generalized lymphadenopathy

Constitutional symptoms and hepatosplenomegaly may or may not be present.

Initial tests
- CBC plus differential.
- Monospot and Epstein–Barr IgM antibodies.
- Chest x-ray.
- Abdominal US.
- Bone marrow aspiration may be necessary.
- Lymph node biopsy may be necessary.

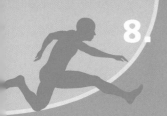

8. Short Stature or Developmental Delay

Growth

Four phases of growth are recognized:
1. Infantile phase (birth to 1 year): dependent on nutrition.
2. Childhood phase (1 year to 5 years): dependent on growth hormone.
3. Mid-childhood phase (5 years to puberty): increased levels of adrenal androgens influence growth.
4. Pubertal phase: growth spurt caused by increased levels of sex steroids.

Growth is assessed by measuring three specific parameters:
- Height (or length in children <18 months).
- Weight.
- Head circumference.

Percentile charts showing the normal range of values for these measurements from before birth to adulthood are available (see Part II). Problems with inadequate weight gain ("failure to thrive") and abnormal head growth (microcephaly and macrocephaly) are considered elsewhere. An approach to the evaluation of "short stature" is presented here. In preterm infants the corrected age (chronological age minus number of weeks preterm) should be used until 2 years of age.

Short stature

A pragmatic definition of short stature requiring further evaluation is:
- A height below the 5th percentile for age.
- A predicted height less than the mid-parental target height.
- An abnormal growth velocity as indicated by the growth curve crossing two percentile lines of the height chart.

Children with short stature can be broadly categorized as having:
- Short but normal growth velocity: treatment is unnecessary but may be investigated for diagnostic purposes.
- Short with abnormal growth velocity: investigation and treatment indicated.

The causes of short stature are shown in Fig. 8.1.

History
This should elicit information about:
- Early childhood illness and systemic disorders.
- Parental height: the genetic height potential is estimated by calculating the mid-parental height (MPH).
- Family history: inherited skeletal dysplasias, parental history of constitutional delay.

To estimate the adult height potential, calculate the mid-parental height (MPH). Then adjust for the sex of the child:

$$\frac{\text{Maternal height} + \text{paternal height (cm)} + 13}{2}$$
$$= \text{boy's eventual height (cm)}$$

$$\frac{\text{Maternal height} + \text{paternal height (cm)} - 13}{2}$$
$$= \text{girl's eventual height (cm)}$$

Target height is MPH + 7.5 cm, ±5 cm for boys and MPH − 7.5 cm, ±5 cm for girls.

Examination
Examine the following:
- Height: measure accurately with a wall-mounted, calibrated stadiometer.
- Growth velocity: a minimum of two measurements, 6 months apart is required. Adjust to inches/year and plot at midpoint in time.
- Dysmorphic features: these may identify a syndrome.
- Weight.
- Visual fields and fundi: may indicate a pituitary tumor.
- Stage of puberty.

An approach to the evaluation of short stature is shown in Fig. 8.2.

Investigations

Investigations that may be of value include the following:

- Bone age: estimated from x-rays of the left wrist (delayed skeletal maturity in constitutional pubertal delay).

- Karyotype: chromosomal analysis to identify Turner syndrome (45, X0) in short girls.
- Skeletal survey: useful if disproportionate; to identify skeletal dysplasias.
- Endocrine investigations: thyroid function tests (T4, TSH) and growth hormone (secretion is pulsatile so a provocation test, e.g., exercise or insulin-induced hypoglycemia, is necessary to identify deficiency).
- Skull x-ray: for suspected craniopharyngioma.

Height should be monitored over 6–12 months in response to parental concern, regardless of current percentile.

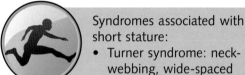

Syndromes associated with short stature:
- Turner syndrome: neck-webbing, wide-spaced nipples, low hairline in a girl.
- Prader–Willi syndrome: obesity, hypotonia, and, in boys, small genitals.
- Skeletal dysplasias: disproportionate limbs and trunk—short limbs (achondroplasia) or short trunk (mucopolysaccharidosis).

Causes of short stature
Familial short stature
Endocrine disorders: • Growth hormone deficiency • Hypopituitarism • Hypothyroidism • Cushing syndrome/steroid excess
Chromosomal disorders/syndromes • Turner syndrome • Silver–Russell syndrome
Skeletal dysplasia: • Achondroplasia
Emotional/psychosocial deprivation
Chronic illness: • Congenital heart disease • Cystic fibrosis • Cerebral palsy • Chronic renal failure

Fig. 8.1 Causes of short stature.

Fig. 8.2 Short stature algorithm.

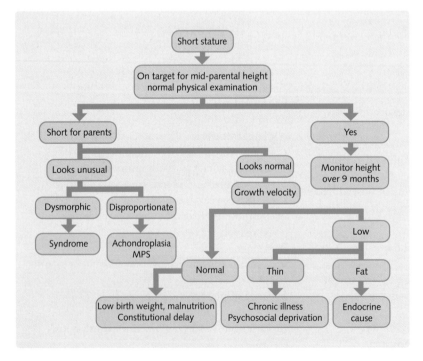

Developmental delay

Normal development depends on genetic potential and on the environment: nature and nurture. There is a wide variation in normal rates of development in all spheres. Delay can be global or specific; normal development is described in Chapter 29.

Delay can present through:
- Parental concern.
- Routine surveillance.
- Concern of teacher, coach, etc.

A list of warning signs shown in developmental delay by age is given in Fig. 8.3.

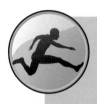

Endocrine causes of short stature are often associated with increased weight; for example:
- Hypothyroidism.
- Growth hormone deficiency.
- Steroid excess.

Warning signs of developmental delay by age	
Age	**Sign**
First 8 weeks	Not smiling in response Poor eye contact Head lag Silent baby—no coos, gurgles
8 months	Poor interaction Not sitting with support Not babbling
18 months	Not recognizing own name Not walking three steps alone Not using first words
24 months	Not giving/receiving affection Unable to build a three-brick tower Not linking two words
Third year	Unable to play Unsteady gait Not using more than 50 words

Fig. 8.3 Warning signs of developmental delay by age.

Development is assessed in four main areas:
- Gross motor.
- Vision and fine motor.
- Hearing and speech.
- Social behavior.

Global delay

A cognitively impaired child is delayed in all aspects of development, but not all children with general delay are cognitively impaired; 40% will have a chromosomal abnormality, 5–10% will have developmental malformations, and 4% will have a metabolic cause.

History

This should encompass:
- Birth history: details of pregnancy and birth including prematurity and hypoxia.
- Family history: of learning disability.
- Developmental milestones.
- Social history: risk factors (e.g., psychosocial deprivation).

Examination

The following should be examined:
- Developmental assessment.
- Appearance: dysmorphic features in syndromes associated with delay, e.g., Down syndrome, Williams syndrome, fragile X syndrome.
- Head circumference: microcephaly.

Investigations

These are directed towards identifying a specific etiology (Fig. 8.4) and will include:
- Karyotype: Down syndrome, fragile X syndrome.
- Thyroid function tests.
- Congenital infection screen.
- Plasma and urine amino and organic acids.
- Brain imaging: MR spectroscopy.

Specific developmental delay

Two common and important examples of delayed development in specific areas are walking and speech.

Causes of global developmental delay	
Type	**Causes**
Perinatal	Hypoxic–ischemic Intracranial hemorrhage Teratogens
Metabolic	Hypothyroidism Inborn errors of metabolism
Infection	Meningitis Encephalitis
Genetic Neurodegenerative disease	Chromosome disorders

Fig. 8.4 Causes of global developmental delay.

Causes of late walking	
Normal variants	Organic causes
Familial	Cerebral palsy
"Bottom shuffler"	Congenital dislocation of the hip
"Commando crawler"	Duchenne muscular dystrophy (boys)

Fig. 8.5 Causes of late walking.

Delayed walking

The percentage of children who are walking unsupported is:
- 50% by 12 months.
- 90% by 15 months.

Further assessment is indicated if a child is not walking unsupported by age 18 months. Many will be normal late walkers, but a small percentage will have an underlying problem (Fig. 8.5).

Examination
- Hips: signs of dislocation (waddling gait, leg length discrepancy, limited abduction).
- Tone, power, and tendon reflexes in all limbs.
- Locomotion: "commando crawler" or "bottom shuffler"?

Investigations
If indicated:
- Imaging of hips or spine.
- Creatine kinase for Duchenne muscular dystrophy.

It is important to distinguish developmental delay from actual regression. Loss of previously acquired skills suggests a serious inherited neurodegenerative disorder or HIV infection.

Speech and language delay

The development of normal speech and language requires:
- Adequate hearing.
- Cognitive development.
- Coordinated sound production.

Speech refers to the meaningful sounds that are made, whereas language encompasses the complex rules governing the use of these sounds for communication. Language can be further divided into language comprehension and language expression, and independent delays can occur in either aspect. As may be expected, the development of language is highly dependent on general intellectual development.

Normal speech and language development:
- 6 months: babbles.
- 12 months: says "mama" or "dada," understands simple commands, and responds to name.
- 18 months: single words with meaning.
- 2 years: speaks in phrases.
- 4 years: conversation.

The causes of delay in speech and language development include:
- Hearing impairment.
- Environmental factors: lack of stimulus.
- Global delay: the most common cause.
- Psychiatric disorders: autism.
- Familial.

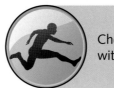

It is worth distinguishing between delay and actual disorders of speech and language such as stammering, dysarthria due to mechanical problems (e.g., cleft palate), or neuromuscular problems (e.g., cerebral palsy).

Check the hearing in any child with delayed speech.

9. Neonatal Problems

Important presenting problems in the term newborn infant include:
- Feeding difficulties.
- Vomiting.
- Jaundice.
- Breathing difficulties.
- Seizures.
- Congenital malformations.
- Ambiguous genitalia.

Feeding difficulties

Difficulties in establishing feeding can occur with both breast- and bottlefed newborn infants.

- Term infants should regain their birthweight by day 7–10.
- Reluctance to feed in an infant who has previously fed normally may indicate serious disease.

Breastfeeding

Breastfeeding should be encouraged by antenatal education and then supported until it is established. Potential problems include:
- Latching on: chin forward and head tilted back (the baby's, not the mother's!). The areola should be in the baby's mouth as this encourages successful feeding and avoids damage to the nipple.
- Cracked nipples: occur commonly and are more likely if the baby does not latch on well.
- Breast engorgement: prevented by demand feeding and alleviated by expression after feeding.
- Rapid intestinal transit: frequent loose stools are common on day four or five when the supply of milk is plentiful. This is normal.

Bottlefeeding

Problems that may occur include:
- Incorrect reconstitution: bowel problems and electrolyte abnormalities.
- Inadequate sterilization: gastroenteritis.

Formulas differ in composition, and age-specific formulas should be used.

Vomiting

Babies often regurgitate small amounts of milk during and between feeds. This is of no pathologic significance and should not be confused with vomiting (the forceful expulsion of gastric contents through the mouth).

Vomiting in the newborn may reflect systemic disease or intestinal obstruction. It is important to establish whether the vomit is:
- Milk.
- Bile-stained.
- Blood-stained.
- Frothy, mucoid.

Important causes are listed in Fig. 9.1. Bile-stained vomit suggests intestinal obstruction. Blood in the vomit may be of maternal or infant origin.

Plain abdominal x-ray is the most useful investigation (supine and lateral decubitus views; Fig. 9.2).

Blood-stained vomit in the newborn may be due to:
- Swallowed maternal blood—predelivery or from a cracked nipple.
- Trauma from a feeding tube.
- Hemorrhagic disease of the newborn—vitamin K deficiency.

Vomiting in the newborn	
Cause	**Features/examples**
Intestinal obstruction	Small bowel: • Duodenal atresia/stenosis (30% have Down syndrome) • Malrotation with volvulus • Meconium ileus (cystic fibrosis)
Tracheoesophageal fistula	Frothy mucoid vomiting occurs if a feed is given
Infections: • Gastroenteritis • Urinary tract infection • Septicemia • Meningitis	Often nonspecific
Necrotizing enterocolitis	Preterm infants
Raised intracranial pressure	Bulging fontanelle
Congenital adrenal hyperplasia	Ambiguous genitalia in a female infant

Fig. 9.1 Vomiting in the newborn.

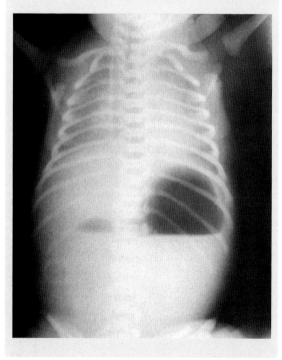

Fig. 9.2 Abdominal x-ray in duodenal atresia showing a "double bubble" from distention of the stomach and duodenum. Air is absent distally.

Jaundice

Neonatal jaundice

Physiologic jaundice occurs in many newborn infants, especially if born preterm. A combination of increased red cell breakdown and immaturity of the hepatic enzymes causes unconjugated hyperbilirubinemia. It is exacerbated by dehydration, which can occur if establishment of feeding is delayed.

Onset of jaundice in the first 24 hours of life is always pathologic; the causes are listed in Fig. 9.3. Recognition and treatment of severe neonatal unconjugated hyperbilirubinemia are important to avoid kernicterus (brain damage due to deposition of bilirubin in the basal ganglia). Evaluation of persistent conjugated hyperbilirubinemia is important to allow early (<6 weeks) diagnosis and treatment of biliary atresia.

- Onset of jaundice in the first 24 hours of life is always pathologic.
- Consider biliary atresia in an infant with persistent neonatal jaundice due to conjugated hyperbilirubinemia and pale stools (rare but treatable).

Causes of neonatal jaundice	
Onset	**Cause**
Less than 24 hours	Excess hemolysis: • Immune-mediated—rhesus or ABO incompatibility • Intrinsic RBC defects—G6PD, pyruvate kinase • Deficiency, or hereditary spherocytosis Congenital infections
Between 24 hours and 2 weeks old	Physiologic jaundice Breast milk jaundice Infection (e.g., UTI) Excess hemolysis, bruising, or polycythemia
Persistent jaundice after 2 weeks old	Unconjugated: • Breast milk jaundice • Infections (e.g., UTI) • Excess hemolysis (e.g., ABO incompatibility, G6PD deficiency) • Hypothyroidism (screened for in newborn) • Galactosemia Conjugated: • Biliary atresia • Neonatal hepatitis

Fig. 9.3 Causes of neonatal jaundice.

Definition of physiologic jaundice:
• Onset after 24 hours of birth.
• Resolves within 2 weeks.
• More than 85% unconjugated.
• Total bilirubin <350 mol/L.

Causes of respiratory distress in term infants	
Pulmonary	**Nonpulmonary**

Transient tachypnea of
  newborn
Pneumonia
Meconium aspiration
Respiratory diaphragmatic
  hernia
Choanal atresia
Pneumothorax
	Septicemia
	Severe anemia
	Congenital heart disease

Fig. 9.4 Causes of respiratory distress in term infants.

Breathing difficulties

In the newborn, breathing difficulties are referred to as respiratory distress. The signs of respiratory distress are:
• Tachypnea: respiratory rate over 60/min.
• Retraction: subcostal or intercostal.
• Nasal flaring.
• Expiratory grunting.
• Cyanosis.

Common breathing difficulties

The most common cause of breathing difficulties in the newborn is the respiratory distress syndrome due to surfactant deficiency, a condition largely confined to preterm infants. The major causes of respiratory distress in term infants are shown in Fig. 9.4.

Respiratory distress syndrome (RDS)

Only 1% of cases of RDS occurs in the term neonate. Such infants are often difficult to ventilate but do respond to surfactant therapy, in a similar manner to the preterm with RDS.

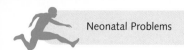

Transient tachypnea of the newborn (TTN)

TTN is believed to be caused by a delay in the normal reabsorption of the lung fluid at birth and is more common after cesarean section. The chest x-ray (CXR) may show a streaky appearance with fluid in the horizontal fissure; it usually resolves within 48 hours.

Meconium aspiration

Approximately 10% of term neonates pass meconium before birth; it is rare in preterm babies. It is associated with birth asphyxia and problems arise from both meconium in the lungs and asphyxia. Meconium should be cleared from the oropharynx and airway at delivery. If the infant inhales meconium into the airways, severe respiratory distress may ensue, caused by bronchial obstruction and collapse, chemical pneumonitis and secondary infection. There is a high incidence of air-leak (pneumothorax, pneumomediastinum) and pulmonary hypertension.

Pneumonia

Risk factors include premature labor and prolonged rupture of the membranes (over 24 hours). Group B streptococcal infection is an important cause of early onset pneumonia.

Pneumothorax

Pneumothorax occurs spontaneously in about 1% of term infants and resolves spontaneously. The cause is mostly iatrogenic in ventilated babies. Diagnosis is by CXR and transillumination in neonates.

Persistent fetal circulation

High pulmonary vascular resistance causes right to left shunting at both atrial and ductal levels with severe cyanosis. It can occur as a primary disorder but is more commonly a complication of birth asphyxia, meconium aspiration, or respiratory distress syndrome. A CXR may show decreased vascular markings. Diagnosis is suggested by differences in PaO_2 on pre- and postductal arterial blood gases (ABGs) and confirmed by echocardiography.

Diaphragmatic hernia

In this uncommon malformation (1 : 4000 births), a hole in the diaphragm (usually on the left) allows the abdominal contents to herniate into the chest. Most diaphragmatic hernias are diagnosed on antenatal ultrasound scan. Initial resuscitation involves early intubation and nasogastric aspiration (to avoid inflation of the bowel). Surgical repair is then undertaken once the neonate is stable. If not diagnosed on antenatal ultrasound, it usually presents with failure to respond to resuscitation at birth. The apex beat and heart sounds are displaced to the right with poor air entry on the left. The relatively high mortality is accounted for by the inevitable pulmonary hypoplasia due to compression of the fetal lung.

Neonatal seizures

Seizures are more common in the neonatal period than any other time of life because the neonatal brain is mostly excitatory. The manifestations of neonatal seizures are rather different from those in older children and it can be difficult to distinguish true seizures from normal baby movements.

Neonatal episodes that are *not* seizures include:
- Jitteriness: the movement is a tremor—rhythmic movements of equal rate and amplitude (in seizures, clonic movements have a fast and slow component). There are no ocular phenomena. It is sensitive to external stimuli and is stopped by holding.
- Benign myoclonus: shock-like jerks when asleep.
- Stretching, sucking movements.

The main types of seizure are:
- Subtle seizures: eye deviation, apneas, autonomic phenomena, and oral movements.
- Clonic seizures: seen as focal rhythmic and slow jerking; generalized clonic seizures are not seen in neonates.
- Myoclonic seizures: rapid isolated jerks.
- Tonic seizures: manifest as flexor or extensor posturing.

Causes of neonatal seizures	
Hypoxia	
Electrolyte and metabolic abnormalities	Hypoglycemia Inborn errors of metabolism
CNS	Hemorrhage Infection Structural abnormality
Drug withdrawal	Opiates Benzodiazepines
Genetic disease	Neurocutaneous diseases
Hyperbilirubinemia	Bilirubin encephalopathy

Fig. 9.5 Causes of neonatal seizures.

The perinatal and birth history together with clinical examination will often indicate the cause.

Initial investigations
- Blood glucose, electrolytes, Ca^{2+}, Mg^{2+}.
- Cerebrospinal fluid (CSF) analysis for infection.
- Cranial ultrasonography for hemorrhages.

As indicated:
- Inborn error of metabolism: blood ammonia, lactate and amino acids, urine amino acids, organic acids, IV pyridoxine test.
- Congenital infection screen.
- Cranial imaging: computed tomography (CT) or magnetic resonance imaging (MRI) (more sensitive).

A detectable cause is present in the majority and varies with the time of onset (Fig. 9.5). The most common causes are neonatal encephalopathy, intracranial hemorrhage, CNS infection, and congenital abnormality.

Congenital malformations

Up to 70% of major congenital malformations can now be detected antenatally using ultrasound. Congenital malformations can affect any of the major organ systems. Some of the most important are described below.

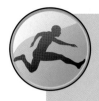

"Congenital" refers to any condition present at birth. The cause may be genetic, environmental, infectious, or idiopathic.

Craniofacial disorders
Cleft lip and palate
This affects about 1 : 1000 babies. It manifests as:
- Cleft lip alone: 35%.
- Cleft lip and palate: 25%.
- Cleft palate alone: 40%.

Inheritance is polygenic, but some cases are associated with maternal anticonvulsant therapy. The cleft lip is usually diagnosed at the 18–20-week scan, but isolated cleft palates can be difficult to diagnose. Some affected infants can be breastfed and special long nipples or other feeding devices may help bottlefed infants. Surgical repair is carried out at 6–12 months of age on the palate, and either early (first week) or late (3 months) on the lip.

Pierre Robin anomaly
This is an association of micrognathia, posterior displacement of the tongue, and midline cleft of the soft palate. Prone positioning maintains airway patency until growth of the mandible is established. The cleft is surgically repaired.

Gastrointestinal disorders
Esophageal atresia
The incidence is 1 : 3500 live births. A tracheoesophageal fistula (TEF) is usually present (Fig. 9.6). As the fetus is unable to swallow during intrauterine life, there is associated polyhydramnios.

Diagnosis should be established before the first feed by attempting to pass a feeding tube into the stomach and checking its location by x-ray. Forty per cent of cases have other associated abnormalities; for example, as part of the VACTERL association:
- **V** = Vertebral
- **A** = Anorectal.
- **C** = Cardiac.
- **TE** = TracheoEsophageal.
- **R** = Renal.
- **L** = Limb (radial).

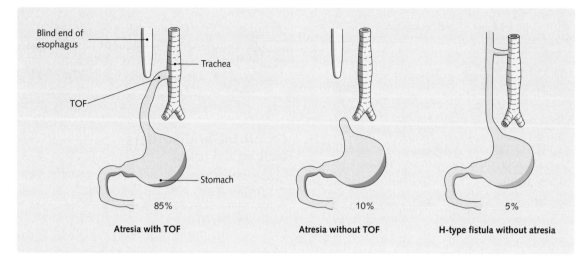

Fig. 9.6 Esophageal atresia and tracheoesophageal fistula (TEF).

Abdominal wall defects

Gastroschisis (1 : 5000)

The bowel protrudes without any covering sac through a defect in the anterior abdominal wall adjacent to the umbilicus. This is usually an isolated anomaly.

Exomphalos (1 : 2500)

The abdominal contents herniate through the umbilical ring and are covered with a sac formed by the peritoneum and amniotic membrane. It is often associated with other major congenital abnormalities.

Neural tube defects

These arise from failure of fusion of the neural plate in the first 28 days after conception. The incidence in the USA has fallen dramatically in the past 25 years. This is probably because of improved maternal nutrition and supplementation to increase folic acid levels (both before conception and in early pregnancy). Antenatal screening and subsequent elective termination have also reduced the incidence of this problem.

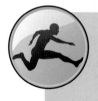

Folic acid supplements should ideally be taken preconception, and all pregnant women are advised to take them during the first trimester.

There are three main types:
- Spina bifida occulta.
- Meningocele.
- Myelomeningocele.

They are usually in the lumbosacral region (Fig. 9.7).

Spina bifida occulta

The vertebral arch fails to fuse. There may be an overlying skin lesion such as a tuft of hair or small dermal sinus. Tethering of the cord (diastomyelia) can cause neurologic deficits with growth.

Meningocele

This is uncommon (5% of cases). The smooth, intact, skin-covered cystic swelling is filled with CSF. There is no neurologic deficit, and excision and closure of the defect are undertaken after 3 months.

Myelomeningocele

This accounts for more than 90% of overt spina bifida. Myelomeningoceles are usually open, with the unfused neural plate, exposed meninges, and leaking CSF. Neurologic deficits are always present and can include:
- Motor and sensory loss in the lower limbs.
- Neuropathic bladder and bowel.

In addition, there is often scoliosis and associated hydrocephalus due to the Arnold–Chiari malformation (herniation of the cerebellar tonsils through the foramen magnum). Surgery is for

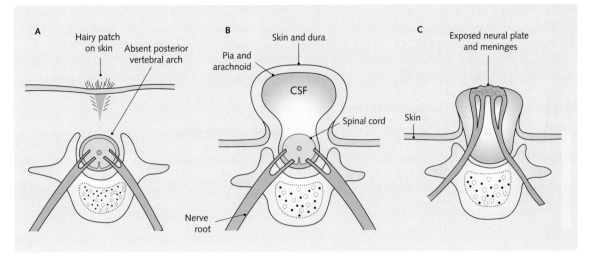

Fig. 9.7 Neural tube defects. Spina bifida occulta (A); meningocele (B); myelomeningocele (C).

preventing infection and not to restore neurologic function.

Congenital talipes equinovarus (club foot)

The entire foot is fixed in an inverted and supinated position (Fig. 9.8). This should be distinguished from "positional talipes," in which the deformity is mild and can be corrected with passive manipulation.

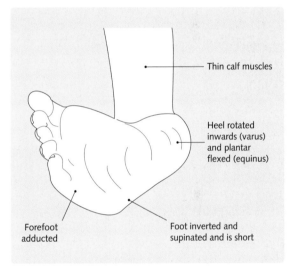

Fig. 9.8 Talipes equinovarus (club foot).

Features of talipes equinovarus:
- 1.5 per 1000 live births.
- Male to female ratio: 2 : 1.
- 50% bilateral.
- Multifactorial inheritance.
- Associated with oligohydramnios, congenital hip dislocation, and neuromuscular disorders (e.g., spina bifida).

Ambiguous genitalia

On occasion, it is not possible to give an immediate answer to the question, "Is it a boy or a girl?" The most common cause of ambiguous external genitalia is congenital adrenal hyperplasia (CAH) leading to a virilized female (see Chapter 21).

- Congenital adrenal hyperplasia (CAH) leading to virilization of a female infant is the most common cause of ambiguous genitalia.
- In two-thirds of children with CAH, a life-threatening, salt-losing adrenal crisis occurs at 1–3 weeks of age, requiring urgent IV treatment with saline and glucose. This may be the first indication in boys.

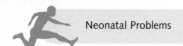
Establishing the definitive cause of ambiguous genitalia takes time, and it is important not to attempt to guess the future sex of rearing. Expert counseling is required. Examination should include measurement of the blood pressure (adrenal problem).

Investigations will include:

- Urgent chromosomal analysis – karyotype.
- Ultrasound imaging of pelvic organs and adrenal glands.
- Electrolyte and endocrine investigations (17-hydroxyprogesterone is increased in CAH).

The chromosomal sex does not necessarily determine the sex of rearing. In many intersex conditions, it is preferable to raise the child as a female because it is easier to fashion female external genitalia than to create a functioning penis.

Further reading

Levene M, Evans D. Neonatal seizures. *Archives of Diseases in Childhood. Fetal Neonatal Edition* 1998; 78: F70–F75.

DISEASES AND DISORDERS

10. Infectious Diseases and Immunodeficiency

Despite the spectacular successes achieved by public health measures and immunization programs in preventing childhood infectious disease, infections remain a major cause of mortality and morbidity in childhood:

- In the developing world, 12 million children under 5 years of age die each year from the combined effects of malnutrition and infections such as gastroenteritis, pneumonia, measles, and malaria.
- In the developed world, major diseases such as diphtheria and polio have been effectively eliminated, and the infection rates of others, such as invasive disease caused by *Haemophilus influenzae* type B, *Streptococcus pneumniae*, measles, mumps, rubella, and pertussis, are greatly reduced.

However, infection remains the most common cause of disease in childhood, and the worldwide resurgence of tuberculosis (TB), together with the growing impact of human immunodeficiency virus (HIV) infection in childhood, leaves no room for complacency

Viral infections

Viral exanthems

The term "exanthem" is applied to diseases in which a rash is a prominent manifestation. Classically, six exanthems with similar rashes were described. They are numbered in the order in which they were described and are listed in Fig. 10.1. The second disease is, of course, bacterial in origin, and the fourth disease is no longer recognized as an entity.

Measles: "first disease"
Incidence and etiology

Measles is caused by infection with a single-stranded RNA virus of the *Morbillivirus* genus. The incidence in the USA declined dramatically after vaccination was introduced, from a pattern of epidemics every 2 years, with up to 450,000 cases, to just 49 cases in 2002.

Clinical features

Fever, cough, coryza, and conjunctivitis are followed (in some cases) by the pathognomonic Koplik's spots on the buccal mucosa and, after 3 or 4 days, by an erythematous maculopapular rash. The rash spreads downward from the hairline to the whole body, becomes blotchy and confluent, and may desquamate in the second week.

Measles is highly infectious. Transmission is by droplet spread and the incubation period is about 10 days. Children should stay out of school for 1 week after appearance of the rash.

Measles is very dangerous in immunocompromised children, such as those in remission from acute leukemia or with HIV. These children are susceptible to giant cell pneumonia and encephalitis. In developing countries, malnutrition and particularly vitamin A deficiency impairs immunity and renders measles a more severe disease. It is estimated that up to 2 million children in developing countries die annually from measles.

Complications

Acute complications include febrile convulsions, otitis media, tracheobronchitis, and pneumonia due either to the primary virus infection or bacterial superinfection (Fig. 10.2). Rarely, severe encephalitis occurs (1 : 5000 cases) about 8 days after onset of the illness. The mortality rate is 15%, and severe neurologic sequelae occur in 40% of survivors. Subacute sclerosing panencephalitis (SSPE) is a very rare immune-mediated neurodegenerative disease that can occur 7–10 years after measles.

Diagnosis

Diagnosis can be confirmed by detection of specific IgM in serum samples ideally taken from 3 days after the appearance of the rash. The disease is reportable.

Management

Treatment is symptomatic.

Viral exanthems		
		Pathogen
First	Measles	Paramyxovirus
Second	Scarlet fever	Group A β-hemolytic streptococci
Third	Rubella	Togavirus
Fourth	"Duke's disease"	—
Fifth	Erythema infectiosum	Parvovirus B19
Sixth	Roseola infantum	Human herpesvirus 6

Fig. 10.1 Viral exanthems.

Complications of measles
Giant cell pneumonia
Conjunctivitis and keratitis
Middle ear infection
Secondary gastrointestinal infections
Encephalitis
Subacute sclerosing panencephalitis

Fig. 10.2 Complications of measles.

Rubella (German measles)

This mild childhood disease is caused by infection with the rubivirus. Its importance lies in the devastating effect maternal infection in early gestation has on the fetus.

Clinical features

Infection is subclinical in up to half of infected individuals. After an incubation period of 14–21 days, a low-grade fever is followed by a pink–red maculopapular rash, which starts on the face and spreads rapidly over the entire body. The rash is fleeting and may have gone entirely by the third day. Generalized lymphadenopathy, particularly affecting the suboccipital and postauricular nodes, is a prominent feature.

Complications

Complications are unusual in childhood but include arthritis (typically affecting the small joints of the hand), encephalitis and thrombocytopenia.

Clinical features of congenital rubella
Growth retardation
Congenital heart disease
• Patent ductus arteriosus
• Pulmonary stenosis
Eye
• Glaucoma
• Cataract
• Retinopathy
Ear
• Sensorineural deafness

Fig. 10.3 Clinical features of congenital rubella.

Diagnosis

Diagnosis is clinical and differentiation from other viral exanthems is often difficult. In circumstances in which it is important, detection of rubella-specific IgM in the saliva or serum is necessary to confirm the diagnosis.

Prevention (immunization)

A live, attenuated vaccine has been available for many years. This has been given as part of the MMR vaccine to all children at 12 months of age. Vaccine failure is rare and, in most people, it provides lifelong protection. The presence of IgG, specific for rubella, indicates immunity as a result of prior infection or immunization.

Congenital rubella
Incidence and diagnosis

The risk and extent of fetal damage are mainly determined by its gestational age at the onset of maternal infection. In the first 8–10 weeks the risk is high; beyond 18 weeks' gestation the risk is minimal.

Maternal infection at up to 10 weeks' gestation confers a 90% risk of some degree of damage that is often severe and includes deafness, congenital heart disease, and cataracts. Between 13 and 16 weeks' gestation, there is a 30% risk of hearing impairment. Although congenital rubella is now rare in the USA, the diagnosis is worth consideration in any growth-retarded newborn or child with unexplained sensorineural deafness.

Clinical features

Clinical features of congenital rubella are shown in Fig. 10.3.

Management

All pregnant women and women contemplating pregnancy should be screened for antirubella IgG. Immigrants to the USA from countries where rubella vaccination is not routine are at particular risk of not being immune. Women found to be seronegative on antenatal screening receive immunization after delivery.

Pregnant women exposed to rubella should be tested for antirubella IgG and IgM regardless of previous history or serological testing. A high likelihood of congenital rubella infection early in pregnancy is an indication for offering termination of the pregnancy.

Erythema infectiosum or slapped-cheek disease: "fifth disease"

This is caused by infection with parvovirus B19, a small DNA virus that is the only parvovirus pathogenic to humans. Transmission can occur via respiratory secretions, from mother to fetus, and by transmission of contaminated blood products.

Clinical features

Asymptomatic infection is common. Erythema infectiosum describes the most common disease pattern of fever followed a week later by a characteristic rash. This starts as a red appearance on the face (hence the name "slapped-cheek disease") and progresses to a symmetrical lacy rash on the extremities and trunk.

The virus suppresses erythropoiesis for up to 7 days. In children with hemolytic anemia, such as sickle-cell disease or hereditary spherocytosis, parvovirus infection can cause an aplastic crisis. Maternal infection during pregnancy can be transmitted to the fetus and causes hydrops fetalis (due to fetal anemia and myocarditis), fetal death, or spontaneous abortion.

Diagnosis and management

Diagnosis is clinical, but if confirmation is important (e.g., in pregnancy), specific IgM can be detected 2 weeks after exposure. Management is symptomatic.

Roseola infantum: "sixth disease"

Roseola infantum is caused by infection with human herpesvirus (HHV)-6 or HHV-7.

Clinical features and diagnosis

Most children acquire the infection between the age of 3 months and 4 years; 65% are seropositive by 1 year of age. There is sudden onset of a high fever (>39°C) with irritability lasting for 3–6 days. The fever then falls abruptly and a widespread maculopapular rash appears on the face, neck and trunk. Other common features include cervical lymphadenopathy, cough, and coryza. Up to one-third of febrile convulsions in children <2 years of age are caused by HHV-6.

Diagnosis is clinical and treatment supportive. Rare complications include aseptic meningitis, encephalitis, hepatitis, and massive lymphadenopathy.

Herpes infections

There are eight human herpesviruses. They cause a number of common and important diseases in children, including chickenpox and glandular fever. A particular hallmark of these viruses is their capacity to become latent with subsequent recurrence, causing, for example, shingles (varicella zoster) and cold sores (HSV1).

The human herpesviruses (HHVs) and their corresponding diseases are shown in Fig. 10.4.

Herpes simplex virus 1 (HHV1, HSV1)
Clinical features

Most primary infections with HSV1 are asymptomatic. The most common clinical manifestation in childhood is gingivostomatitis. The child (usually a toddler) presents with high fever, irritability, and vesicular lesions on the lips, gums, tongue, and hard palate, which may progress to painful, extensive ulceration. The illness can last as long as 2 weeks.

Less commonly, infection can involve the:
- Eye: causing dendritic ulcers on the cornea.
- Skin: causing eczema herpeticum in children with eczema.
- Fingers: causing a herpetic whitlow.
- Brain: causing herpes simplex encephalitis (HSE).

Treatment

Occasionally, IV fluid will be required for gingivostomatitis but in this condition oral acyclovir has only a marginal effect. High-dose IV acyclovir is used in HSE.

The virus becomes latent in the dorsal root ganglion supplying the trigeminal nerve where subsequent reactivation (by UV light, stress or menstruation) can cause labial herpes (cold sores) in later life.

Human herpesviruses (HHV) and their diseases		
	Virus	**Disease**
HHV-1	Herpes simplex virus 1	Oral infection and encephalitis
HHV-2	Herpes simplex virus 2	Neonatal and genital infection
HHV-3	Varicella zoster	Chickenpox and shingles
HHV-4	Epstein–Barr virus	Glandular fever
HHV-5	Cytomegalovirus	Congenital infection and in immunosuppression
HHV-6, -7		Roseola

Fig. 10.4 Human herpesviruses (HHV) and their diseases.

Herpes simplex virus 2 (HHV2, HSV2)

Transmission of HSV2 from the genital tract of a mother can result in neonatal herpes infection. This condition has a very high mortality and morbidity. There may be generalized infection with pneumonia, hepatitis, and encephalitis, with onset usually in the first week of life.

Elective cesarean section is indicated when a mother with active genital herpes goes into labor.

Varicella zoster (HHV3, VZV)

Chickenpox is a common childhood disease caused by primary infection with the varicella zoster virus (VZV). It is highly infectious with transmission occurring by droplet infection (the respiratory route), direct contact, or contact with soiled materials. The average incubation period is 14 days.

Clinical features

A brief coryzal period is followed by the eruption of an itchy, vesicular rash. This starts on the scalp or trunk and spreads centrifugally. Crops appear over 3–5 days and the mucous membranes may be involved.

Complications

Complications are unusual in immunocompetent children but can include secondary bacterial infection of the skin with staphylococci or streptococci and an encephalitis (often affecting the cerebellum), which appears 3–6 days after onset of the rash. Chickenpox can, however, be a very severe disease (mortality 20%) in the immunosuppressed child (children on systemic steroids) and in the newborn infant if the mother develops chickenpox just before delivery.

Diagnosis

Diagnosis is clinical but virus isolated from vesicular fluid can be identified by electron microscopy or culture. The period of infectivity is from 2 days before eruption of the rash until all the lesions are encrusted.

Treatment

Treatment is symptomatic. However, the exposed immunosuppressed child should be given varicella zoster immune globulin (VZIG) if known to be seronegative. VZIG should also be given to newborn babies if the mother develops varicella or herpes zoster in the 7 days before or after birth and to any exposed preterm infant. Acyclovir should be given in severe chickenpox or for clinical infection in an immunocompromised child or newborn infant. Antibiotics are also given concurrently to cover secondary skin infection.

A live, attenuated vaccine is now licensed in the USA, and widespread varicella vaccination has occurred.

Herpes zoster (shingles)

This is due to reactivation of latent varicella zoster and is uncommon in childhood. A vesicular eruption occurs in the distribution of a sensory dermatome. Lesions occur mainly in the cervical and sacral regions, whereas in adults they tend to be thoracic and lumbar. Also, unlike adults, postherpetic neuralgia and malignant association are rare. Treatment with antivirals is not routinely indicated

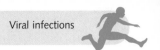

Epstein–Barr virus (HHV4, EBV)

The EBV has a particular tropism for the epithelial cells of the oropharynx and nasopharynx, and for B lymphocytes. It is not only the major cause of the infectious mononucleosis syndrome but is also involved in the pathogenesis of Burkitt's lymphoma and nasopharyngeal carcinoma.

Clinical features

Transmission occurs by droplet transmission or directly via saliva ("the kissing disease"). Most people are infected asymptomatically in childhood. Symptomatic infection (infectious mononucleosis or glandular fever) is most common in adolescents. The incubation period is 30–50 days.

Glandular fever is characterized by fever, malaise, pharyngitis (which may be exudative), and cervical lymphadenopathy. Petechiae may be seen on the palate, and a sparse maculopapular rash may occur. Splenomegaly is present in 50% of cases and hepatomegaly with hepatitis (usually anicteric) in 10%. A florid rash may develop if amoxycillin is given. The infection can persist for up to 3 months.

Diagnosis

Diagnosis is usually clinical. The blood shows atypical lymphocytes (T cells) and a heterophile antibody, which is the basis of slide agglutination tests, including monospot and Paul–Bunnell tests. The latter does not appear until the second week and may not be produced in young children. Specific EBV serology—IgM to viral capsid antigen (VCA)—is available and more reliable. The differential diagnosis is from other causes of infectious mononucleosis (cytomegalovirus, toxoplasmosis) and other causes of pharyngitis.

Management

Management is symptomatic. Rarely, massive pharyngeal swelling can compromise the airway. This is helped by corticosteroid treatment.

Cytomegalovirus (HHV5, CMV)

Cytomegalovirus (CMV) is a common human pathogen. It is transmitted from mother to fetus via the placenta in utero, via the oral or genital routes, and by blood transfusion or organ transplantation.

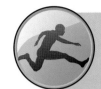

- CMV is a common congenital infection but rarely causes severe disease.
- CMV is an important cause of sensorineural hearing loss.
- CMV-negative blood must be used for transfusion in immunodeficient patients.

Incidence

In the USA, about half of all pregnant women are susceptible to CMV and about 1% of these will have a primary CMV infection during pregnancy. In almost half of these mothers, the infant will be infected, making CMV the most common congenital infection with an incidence of 3 : 1000 live births. However, most infants with congenital CMV are asymptomatic and develop normally.

Clinical features

Infection is mild or asymptomatic in adults or children with normal immunity. It can cause a mononucleosis syndrome with pharyngitis and lymphadenopathy. Severe congenital infection causes:

- Intrauterine growth retardation.
- Hepatosplenomegaly, jaundice and purpura.
- Microcephaly, intracranial calcification and chorioretinitis.
- Long-term sequelae include cerebral palsy, epilepsy, learning disability, and sensorineural hearing loss. Hearing loss may develop later in life without signs of infection in the newborn period.

In the immunocompromised host, CMV can cause severe disease including pneumonitis or encephalitis. It is a particularly important pathogen following organ transplantation.

Diagnosis and treatment

Diagnosis is made by viral isolation, especially from urine or by a strongly positive titer of IgM anti-CMV antibody. To confirm congenital infection, specimens for viral isolation must be taken within 3 weeks of birth.

Treatment with gancyclovir may be effective in immunocompromised patients.

Mumps

Mumps is caused by infection with an RNA virus of the Paramyxovirus family. Routine vaccination at 12–15 months, as a component of the MMR vaccine, has markedly reduced the incidence. Transmission is by droplet spread and the incubation period is 14–21 days.

Clinical features

The clinical manifestations include fever, malaise, and parotitis. Pain and swelling of the parotid gland may initially be unilateral. Parotid gland enlargement is more easily seen than felt. The swelling is between the angle of the mandible and sternomastoid—extending beneath the ear lobe, which is pushed upwards and outwards.

The swelling usually subsides within 7–10 days. Patients are infectious from a few days before salivary gland enlargement to up to 3 days after the enlargement subsides.

The central nervous system is commonly involved. Before vaccination was introduced, mumps was the most common cause of aseptic meningitis. Up to 50% of patients have lymphocytes in their cerebrospinal fluid and 10% have signs of a meningoencephalitis.

Complications

Complications include pancreatitis (abdominal pain and raised serum amylase levels) and epididymo-orchitis. The latter is uncommon in prepubertal males and is usually unilateral. Even when it is bilateral, infertility is very rare. A postinfectious encephalomyelitis occurs in 1 out of 5000 cases.

Diagnosis and treatment

Diagnosis is usually clinical; treatment is symptomatic.

Enteroviruses

The human enteroviruses include:
- Coxsackie virus A and B.
- Echoviruses.
- Poliovirus.

Coxsackie virus A and B

Coxsackie viruses can cause aseptic meningitis, myocarditis, pericarditis, Bornholm disease (pleurodynia), and hand, foot, and mouth disease.

Polio

Poliovirus is an enterovirus with antigenic types 1, 2, and 3. Immunization has rendered poliovirus infection uncommon in developed countries but it remains endemic in parts of the developing world such as Africa and the Indian subcontinent. Transmission is by the fecal–oral route with an incubation period of 7–21 days.

Clinical features

The clinical features vary:
- Over 90% of cases are asymptomatic.
- 5% have a "minor illness"—fever, headache, malaise.
- 2% progress to CNS involvement—aseptic meningitis.
- In under 2%, "paralytic polio" occurs due to the virus attacking the anterior horn cells of the spinal cord.

Diagnosis

Although imported infections and vaccine-associated infections are seen in the USA, they are rare. The differential diagnosis includes other causes of aseptic meningitis and acute paralytic disease such as Guillain–Barré syndrome. Polio is a reportable disease.

Viral hepatitis

This can be caused by:
- Hepatitis virus A, B, C, D, E, or G.
- Arbovirus—yellow fever.
- Cytomegalovirus, Epstein–Barr virus.

Hepatitis A virus (HAV)

This is an RNA virus spread by fecal–oral transmission. The incubation period is 2–6 weeks.

Clinical features

In infants and young children, many infections are asymptomatic or present as a nonspecific febrile illness without jaundice. Older symptomatic children develop fever, malaise, anorexia, abdominal pain (from a tender enlarged liver), and jaundice. Dark urine (due to urobilinogen) may precede the jaundice.

Diagnosis

Diagnosis is often made on the combination of clinical features and history of exposure, but may be confirmed by measurement of IgM anti-HAV antibody. Serum transaminases and bilirubin levels are elevated.

Treatment

There is no specific treatment. The majority of children have a mild, self-limiting illness and recover within 2–4 weeks. The most serious but rare complication is fulminant hepatic failure.

Active immunization is available and may become part of the routine vaccine schedule for infants. Close contacts should be given prophylaxis with intramuscular human immunoglobulin (HIG).

Hepatitis B virus (HBV)

This is a DNA virus of the Hepadnavirus genus. It is a double-shelled particle with an inner core (HBc) and an outer lipoprotein coat comprising the hepatitis B surface antigen (HBsAg).

Transmission is parenteral via blood and other body fluids. In infants, the most important source of infection is vertical perinatal transmission from infected mothers. Most transmission occurs during or just after birth from exposure to maternal blood. The average incubation period is 20 days.

Incidence

HBV is an important cause of liver disease worldwide. The prevalence of infection in the population varies globally. In parts of Africa and Asia, up to 80% of children are infected by adolescence. In the USA, prevalence is under 2% HBsAg positivity in the indigenous population.

Clinical features

In most children, infection is asymptomatic, although features of acute hepatitis may occur; fulminant hepatic failure occurs in 1% of cases. The most important consequence of infection is the risk of becoming a carrier with subsequent development of cirrhosis or hepatocellular carcinoma. The risk of developing carrier status rises with infection at a young age (reaching 90% in those infected perinatally). Between 30% and 50% of carrier children will develop chronic HBV liver disease.

Diagnosis

Diagnosis is dependent on serological testing for antibodies and antigens related to HBV. Acute HBV infection is associated with the presence of HBsAg and IgM antibodies to HBc antigen. Carrier status is defined as HBsAg persisting for more than 6 months. The presence of HBeAg correlates with high infectivity, whereas the presence of antibodies to HBeAg indicates low infectivity (Fig. 10.5).

Management

There is no specific treatment for acute hepatitis B infection at any age. Interferon α treatment is under trial in chronic hepatitis caused by HBV infection.

Prevention

Effective immunization is available and given to infants as part of the routine immunization schedule. It is also recommended:
- After perinatal exposure.
- For individuals at risk (e.g., doctors, dentists, or intravenous drug abusers).
- Postexposure (e.g., needlestick injury).

Perinatal exposure

All pregnant women should have antenatal screening for the HBsAg. All babies born to women known to be HBsAg positive should commence a course of hepatitis B vaccine within 24 hours of birth. Unless the mother is known to be anti-HBe positive, the baby should also receive hepatitis B specific immunoglobulin (HBIG).

Serologic markers of HBV infection				
	HBsAg	Anti-HBs	Anti-HBc IgM	Anti-HBC IgG
Acute HBV infection	+	−	+	+
HBV carrier	+	−	+ or −	+
Immune: previous				
Infection	−	+ or −	−	+
Immune: immunization	−	+	−	−

Fig. 10.5 Serologic markers of hepatitis B (HBV) infection.

Bacterial infections

Staphylococcal infections

The coagulase-positive bacterium *Staphylococcus aureus* is the main pathogen but coagulase-negative bacteria (e.g., *Staphylococcus epidermidis*) are a major problem in intensive care units. Methicillin-resistant *Staphylococcus aureus* (MRSA) causes problems of nosocomial (i.e., hospital-acquired) infection.

Staphylococcus epidermidis is part of the normal skin flora and *Staphylococcus aureus* is found in the nares and skin in up to 50% of children. Infections occur when defenses are compromised. Many infections are therefore caused by the body's own bacteria, but transmission between individuals occurs with close contact.

Staphylococcus aureus most commonly causes superficial infection such as boils and impetigo, but further invasion and spread leads to deep infections (e.g., of the bones, joints, or lungs) (Fig. 10.6). Toxin-producing *Staphylococcus aureus* causes scalded skin syndrome and toxic shock syndrome.

Impetigo

This highly contagious skin infection commonly occurs on the face in infants and young children—especially if there is pre-existing skin disease (e.g., eczema).

Clinical features

Erythematous macules develop into characteristic honey-colored crusted lesions. Some cases are due to streptococcal infection.

Infections caused by *Staphylococcus aureus*

Direct infection	Toxin-mediated
Impetigo	Toxic shock syndrome
Folliculitis/boils	Scalded skin syndrome
Wound infections	Food poisoning
Abscess	
Pneumonia	
Osteomyelitis	
Septic arthritis	

Fig. 10.6 Infections caused by *Staphylococcus aureus*.

Treatment

Topical antibiotics can be used for mild cases (e.g., mupirocin), but more severe infections require systemic antibiotics (e.g., cepholexin or erythromycin). Nasal carriage is an important source of reinfection and can be eradicated by nasal cream containing chlorhexidine and neomycin.

Boils and abscesses

A boil (or furuncle) is an infection of a hair follicle or sweat gland and is usually caused by *Staphylococcus aureus*.

Clinical features

A painful, red, raised, hot lesion develops and usually discharges a purulent exudate heralding spontaneous resolution.

Treatment

Treatment is with systemic antibiotics. Deeper infection can lead to abscess formation in which case incision and drainage are usually required.

Osteomyelitis/septic arthritis

See Chapter 18.

Staphylococcal scalded skin syndrome (SSSS)

This is a potentially life-threatening, toxin-mediated manifestation of localized skin infection.

Clinical features

SSSS results from the effect of epidermolytic toxins produced by certain phage types. They cause blistering by disrupting the epidermal granular cell layer. The lesions look like scalds.

Treatment

Management requires attention to fluid balance and treatment with intravenous oxacillin or nafcillin.

Streptococcal infections

Streptococci are Gram-positive cocci. Important pathogenic types include:
- Group A β-hemolytic streptococci (*Streptococcus pyogenes*).
- Group B streptococci.
- *Streptococcus pneumoniae* (pneumococcus).

These bacteria are responsible for a number of common and important pediatric diseases that can be caused by:
- Direct infection.
- Toxins.

Infections caused by streptococci	
Organism	**Disease caused**
Group A streptococci	Pharyngitis/tonsillitis Cellulitis Osteomyelitis Septicemia Toxin-mediated: • Scarlet fever • Erysipelas • "Toxic shock-like syndrome"
Streptococcus pneumoniae	Otitis media Pneumonia Meningitis Septicemia
Group B streptococci	Neonatal infection (e.g., pneumonia, meningitis, or septicemia)

Fig. 10.7 Infections caused by streptococci.

• Postinfectious immune-mediated mechanisms (acute glomerulonephritis, rheumatic fever).

Infections caused by streptococci are shown in Fig. 10.7. Most of these are described elsewhere: tonsillitis (see Chapter 14), pneumonia (Chapter 14), meningitis (Chapter 17), glomerulonephritis (Chapter 16), and rheumatic fever (Chapter 13).

Scarlet fever

This occurs in children who have streptococcal pharyngitis. The organism produces a toxin, which causes a characteristic rash.

Clinical features

The clinical features include:
• Tonsillitis.
• Strawberry tongue.
• Palatal petechiae.
• Rash: a widespread, erythematous rash starting on the trunk that becomes punctate and desquamates on resolution after 7–10 days (flushing of the face is often associated with circumoral pallor).
• Fever.

Diagnosis

Diagnosis is clinical, but can be confirmed by isolation of the streptococcus from a throat swab, and by elevated antistreptolysin 0 titres.

Treatment

Treatment is with penicillin (or erythromycin if the patient has penicillin allergy).

Erysipelas

This intradermal infection is caused by toxin-producing *Streptococcus pyogenes*.

Clinical features

The face or leg is the usual area affected. The skin is dusky and vesicles or bullae may develop.

Diagnosis and treatment

Skin swabs and blood cultures may be negative; treatment is with parenteral antibiotics.

Preseptal cellulitis

This presents as unilateral periorbital edema in a young child, usually after an upper respiratory tract infection; fever may be present. The common pathogens are *Streptococcus* species and *Haemophilus influenzae* (more common in children under 3 years old).

It is important to distinguish this from the less common, but more serious, orbital cellulitis, in which there is proptosis, limitation of ocular movement, and impaired vision.

Treatment is with IV broad-spectrum antibiotics.

Tuberculosis
Incidence and etiology

Tuberculosis (TB) remains a major global health problem, causing 3–5 million deaths annually. The increasing incidence in patients with HIV, combined with the emergence of multidrug-resistant strains of the causative organism, has generated new concern over this age-old public health problem.

Tuberculosis is a disease of the underprivileged, especially in urban areas, and the immunocompromised. It occurs in all racial groups, but high rates are seen in children whose families have come from endemic areas such as:
• Indian subcontinent (India, Pakistan, and Bangladesh).
• Sub-Saharan Africa.
• Asia.
• Latin America.

Tuberculosis is caused by infection with the acid-fast, slow-growing bacillus *Mycobacterium tuberculosis*. Children are usually infected by

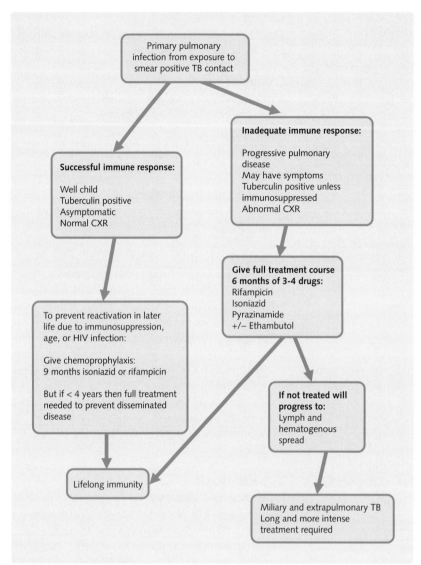

Fig. 10.8 Course of infection in tuberculosis.

inhalation of infected droplet nuclei from an adult who is a regular or household contact. Children with the disease (even with active pulmonary disease) are almost always noninfectious. Therefore once a child is identified as having TB, notification to public health is essential to identify the index case and contact trace.

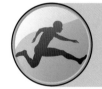

TB contacts <4 years of age are at high risk of disseminated disease and should be evaluated promptly.

Clinical features

The clinical features of TB (Fig. 10.8) reflect the wide variation in outcomes that follow inhalation of the tubercle bacillus or primary infection. Children under 4 years are at particularly high risk of disseminated disease (e.g., TB meningitis).

Tuberculous infection: asymptomatic infection

This is most common. A local inflammatory reaction limits disease progression and the disease becomes latent. Reactivation can occur subsequently.

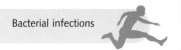

Tuberculous disease: symptomatic infection

Multiplication within macrophages occurs at the peripheral alveolar site (the primary or Ghon focus) and the bacilli spread to the regional lymph nodes causing hilar lymphadenopathy. The peripheral lung lesion and nodes comprise the "primary or Ghon complex." Systemic symptoms can then develop, including fever, anorexia, weight loss, and cough.

The pulmonary pathology can evolve in several different ways. Bronchial obstruction by enlarged lymph nodes may cause segmental collapse and consolidation. Rarer outcomes include development of a pleural effusion or progressive primary pulmonary TB with cavity formation (in adolescents and adults). Spread into the lymphoid system can result in cervical, supraclavicular, or axillary lymphadenopathy.

Hematogenous dissemination

In addition to the above intrathoracic events, hematogenous spread probably occurs in most children, although dormant lesions rather than disease occur in these distant sites. Tubercle bacilli may spread to the bones (especially the vertebral column), joints, kidneys, and meninges. Miliary TB is the most severe result of hematogenous spread. It occurs particularly in small infants or immunosuppressed individuals—lesions are found throughout the lungs, liver, spleen, and bone marrow.

Diagnosis

This can be difficult and requires a high index of clinical suspicion. Because young children <4 years of age are particularly prone to disseminated infection, there is a lower threshold for diagnosis and treatment. A history of close contact to an adult with smear-positive tuberculosis, symptoms (weight loss, night sweats, cough), clinical signs, tuberculin testing, chest x-ray, and examination of appropriate specimens by microscopy and culture (gastric washings) need to be assessed.

Criteria for TB diagnosis include:
- Adult TB contact.
- Signs and symptoms.
- CXR changes.
- Positive Mantoux test.
- Positive cultures (gastric washings or other).

Tuberculin testing

This is done using the Mantoux test, in which an intradermal injection of purified protein derivative (PPD) of tuberculin—for example, 10 units (0.1 mL of 1 : 1000)—is made on the volar aspect of the forearm. The site is read after 48–72 hours by measuring the transverse diameter of induration in millimeters. A 5-mm diameter reaction is considered positive if risk factors are present. When previous BCG immunization has been carried out, a reaction of greater than 10 mm is indicative of infection.

Culture and histology

Isolation of *Mycobacterium tuberculosis* by culture is the gold standard, but positive cultures are obtained in a minority of children. Early-morning gastric washings on 3 successive days are the best specimens. It takes 6–8 weeks for the bacillus to grow. Microscopy is often negative but histological examination of a lymph node biopsy may reveal caseating granulomata and acid-fast bacilli.

Radiology

TB is suggested by hilar or mediastinal lymphadenopathy, especially if it is unilateral, or in combination with a "wedge" of collapse or consolidation. Calcification also suggests TB.

Treatment and prevention

A 6-month triple therapy regimen is most commonly recommended: initially, isoniazid, rifampicin, and pyrazinamide are used. If drug resistance is suspected then ethambutol is added. This is usually changed to isoniazid and rifampicin after 2 months, by which time antibiotic sensitivities may be known from the adult index case. Children with tuberculous infection (asymptomatic with positive Mantoux) but no disease need chemoprophylaxis to prevent future reactivation. In this situation, either a combination of isoniazid and rifampicin for 3 months or isoniazid as a single agent for 9 months is used. The most important preventive measures are prompt treatment of infectious cases and thorough contact tracing.

The BCG (bacilli Calmette–Guerin) vaccine has been used in many countries (but not in the USA) against TB, especially TB meningitis. BCG has been given to:
- Asymptomatic HIV-infected newborns in populations in which the risk of TB is high.

- Mantoux-negative contacts of open TB cases.
- Infants from high-risk households.

Typhoid and paratyphoid fever

Typhoid fever is caused by *Salmonella typhi* and paratyphoid by *Salmonella paratyphi*. Both occur worldwide and the main reservoir is humans; they are invasive, systemic infections. Salmonellosis occurs after infection with *Salmonella enteritidis* or *Salmonella typhimurium*, which usually cause gastroenteritis (food poisoning). Salmonellae are Gram-negative bacilli.

Transmission is by ingestion of food or water contaminated by feces or urine from an infected person. The incubation period is 1–3 weeks.

Clinical features

The clinical presentation is similar in each case but paratyphoid fever is milder. Typhoid (enteric) fever is characterized by slow onset of fever, malaise, headache, and tachypnea. Signs include splenomegaly, and a characteristic rash of "rose spots" on the trunk. Unlike adults, children do not usually develop a relative bradycardia. Paratyphoid is a milder illness but diarrhea is more common.

Diagnosis

Diagnosis is made by culture of organisms from the blood (early in the disease) or from stool and urine (after the first week).

Management

Ceftriaxone for 14 days is effective, as is ciprofloxacin. Family and close contacts should be screened with stool cultures. Three consecutive negative stools signify clearance of infection. Long-term symptomless carriage can occur with a reservoir of infection in the gallbladder and excretion in the feces.

Parasitic infections

Malaria
Incidence and etiology

A child under 5 years of age dies of malaria every 12 seconds, most of them in sub-Saharan Africa. With an estimated 40% of humanity at risk of infection and an annual mortality rate of between 1.5 and 2.7 million, malaria remains a major global health problem.

Malaria is caused by infection with any of the four species of the protozoan parasite *Plasmodium*. Most of the 300 cases of childhood malaria imported to the USA each year are due to *Plasmodium falciparum*, which accounts for 85% of malaria seen in travelers to Africa. Half of these did not take chemoprophylaxis.

Fever in a child who has been to a malarious area is malaria until proven otherwise:
- Most cases are falciparum.
- *Plasmodium falciparum* requires treatment with quinine.

Transmission is vector-borne via the female anopheles mosquito. The onset is usually 7–10 days after inoculation but may be delayed by months or even years. The feeding female mosquito injects sporozoites, which pass to the liver via the bloodstream. After asexual multiplication in hepatocytes, these emerge as merozoites, which invade, multiply in, and destroy the host's red blood cells. Some of the merozoites form gametocytes, which are sucked up by a feeding mosquito; the sexual phase of the life cycle then takes place in the mosquito with the formation of a new generation of sporozoites.

Clinical features

Malaria presents with fever and any child with a fever who has visited a malarious area in the preceding year should be considered to have malaria until proven otherwise. Nonspecific symptoms include headache, rigors, abdominal and muscle pains, cough, diarrhea, and vomiting. Common misdiagnoses include viral influenza, gastroenteritis, or hepatitis.

Apart from the fever, which is rarely periodic, there are no consistent clinical signs. Splenomegaly, anemia, and jaundice can all occur and a number of signs characterize the severe complication of algid malaria (shock), cerebral malaria (coma, seizures), or blackwater fever (hemoglobinuria and renal failure).

Diagnosis

Diagnosis is made by the examination of thick and thin blood films. The former allows rapid scanning of a larger volume of blood per microscopic field. At least three films should be taken as one negative film does not exclude malaria. Both the species and the percentage of parasitemia should be determined; parasitemia >2% indicates moderately severe infection.

Management

Children with confirmed or suspected falciparum malaria require hospitalization and treatment with quinine or mefloquine (for those aged over 2 years). This is given orally in uncomplicated disease or intravenously if the parasite count is high or complications are present. It is advisable to consult experts in tropical hygiene or the Red Book: 2003 Report of the Committee on Infectious Diseases, 26th ed. (American Academy of Pediatrics, Elk Grove Village, Illinois) for up-to-date advice on management. In vivax infection, 2–3 weeks of primaquine is needed to clear dormant hypnozoite hepatic infection; falciparum does not have a dormant life cycle.

Travelers to endemic areas should take chloroquine, mefloquine, or doxycycline from 1 week before to 4 weeks after travel. It is important to warn them that this does not guarantee protection.

Worms (nematodes)

Four important nematodes infect children:
- *Enterobius vermicularis* (pinworm or threadworm).
- *Ascaris lumbricoides* (roundworm).
- *Ancylostoma duodenale* (hookworm).
- *Toxocara canis*.

Threadworm/pinworm

This is very common in preschool children. Transmission is via the fecal–oral route. Adult female worms lay their eggs in the perianal area at night. Scratching results in eggs being carried under the fingernails to the mouth and autoinfection.

Clinical features

Children present with perianal pruritus and vulvovaginitis but tissue invasion does not occur and systemic complications are uncommon. The worms appear like white cotton threads and may be visible at the anus.

Diagnosis

Diagnosis can be made by applying transparent adhesive tape to the perianal region in the morning and examining the tape for eggs with a magnifying glass (Sellotape test).

Management

Treatment is with two doses of piperazine 2 weeks apart or a single dose of mebendazole (for children over 2 years). Reinfection is common and can be reduced by keeping fingernails short and wearing close-fitting pants. Family members should be treated even if asymptomatic.

Toxocariasis

Human toxocariasis is mainly caused by infection with *Toxocara canis*, a common gut parasite of dogs. Toxocara eggs are ingested when a child eats soil, play-pit sand, or unwashed vegetables contaminated with infective dog or cat feces.

Clinical features

There are two distinct forms of disease:
- Visceral larva migrans (VLM): characterized by fever, hepatomegaly, wheezing, and eosinophilia.
- Occular larva migrans: a granulomatous reaction in the retina causing a squint or reduced visual acuity.

Management

Treatment is with thiabendazole for VLM and steroids for the eye disease. Toxocara infection could be prevented by the regular deworming of cats and dogs and by not allowing animals to defecate in public places, including sandpits.

Kawasaki disease

Kawasaki disease (KD), an uncommon systemic vasculitis, is also called mucocutaneous lymph node syndrome. Early diagnosis is important because early treatment may prevent the lethal cardiac complications. It has replaced rheumatic fever as the most common cause of acquired heart disease in children.

Early recognition of Kawasaki disease is vital to reduce the risk of cardiac complications:
- The fever is often unresponsive to antipyretics.
- Characteristically, the child is extremely miserable.
- Think of Kawasaki disease in prolonged fever and rash.

Diagnostic criteria for Kawasaki disease

Fever for 5 days or more
Bilateral (nonpurulent) conjunctival injection
Rash—polymorphous
Lips—red, dry, or cracked and strawberry tongue
Extremities:
- Reddening of palms and soles
- Indurative edema of hands and feet
- Peeling of skin on hands and feet (convalescent phase)
Cervical lymphadenopathy—often unilateral, nonpurulent

Fig. 10.9 Diagnostic criteria for Kawasaki disease.

Incidence

First described in Japan in 1967, KD affects children mainly between the age of 6 months and 4 years (peak at 1 year). It is much more common in children of Asian origin. In the USA 3000–5000 cases occur annually.

Clinical features

The etiology is unknown, but the disease process is a vasculitis affecting the small and medium vessels including, most importantly, the coronary arteries leading to aneurysm formation. Subsequent scar formation causes vessel narrowing, myocardial ischemia, or even infarction, and—occasionally—sudden death. A bacterial toxin acting as a "superantigen" can trigger the vasculitis.

Diagnosis

The diagnosis is based on clinical criteria, which emerge sequentially; five out of six are required to make a diagnosis (Fig. 10.9). Atypical disease is diagnosed if coronary aneurysms are present without all the criteria.

The differential diagnosis includes measles, scarlet fever, rubella, roseola, and fifth disease. The following investigations are undertaken if KD is suspected:
- CBC, ESR.
- Electrolytes, urine analysis, liver function tests.
- Throat swab and ASLO titers.
- Blood cultures and viral titers.
- Echocardiography.
- ECG.

Thrombocytosis, although common, is a late feature and therefore unhelpful in establishing the diagnosis.

Echocardiography is undertaken to detect coronary artery aneurysm formation. These occur in 30% of untreated cases and typically develop within the first 4–6 weeks of the illness. This investigation is repeated at intervals during the first year.

Treatment

The most effective treatment involves a single dose of IV immunoglobulin (2 g/kg). This reduces both the incidence and severity of coronary artery aneurysm formation if given within the first 10 days.

Aspirin is given concurrently to reduce the risk of thrombosis at a high dose initially (100 mg/kg/day in divided doses) until the pyrexia has resolved. A low dose (3–5 mg/kg/day) is continued for 6–8 weeks. Current evidence on steroid treatment is conflicting and their use is now not recommended.

Immunodeficiency

This can be classified into:
- Primary: in which there is an inherited, intrinsic defect in the immune system.
- Secondary: in which a defect in the immune system has been acquired, as occurs in malnutrition, infections (e.g., HIV, measles), immunosuppressive therapy (e.g., steroids, cytotoxic drugs), hyposplenism (e.g., sickle-cell disease, splenectomy).

In acquired immunodeficiency, the cause is usually self-evident. Primary immunodeficiency

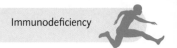

should be suspected in the following clinical circumstances:

- An excess of infections: this is manifest by severe, unusual, or persistent infections, or infections with unusual organisms.
- Unexplained failure to thrive.
- Chronic diarrhea.

See Fig. 10.10 for specific susceptibility conferred by particular defects.

Suspect immunodeficiency in the following circumstances:
- Recurrent bacterial lower respiratory tract infections.
- Neonatal lymphocyte count less than $2.0 \times 10^9/L$.
- Failure to thrive.
- Unusual infection:
  - Recurrent or chronic skin infection.
  - Recurrent or chronic candidal infections.

Primary immunodeficiencies

These can be inherited as X-linked (affecting boys) or autosomal recessive disorders; 40% are diagnosed in first year of life. Examples are given below.

Immune defects and corresponding susceptibility	
Defect	**Susceptibility**
Antibody	Bacteria: *Pneumococcus, Staphylococcus, Streptococcus* spp., *Haemophilus influenzae* Viruses: enteroviruses
Cell-mediated	Viruses: herpesviruses, measles Fungi: *Candida, Aspergillus* spp., *Pneumocystis carinii* Bacteria: *Mycobacteria, Listeria* spp.
Neutrophil function	Bacteria: Gram-positive, Gram-negative Fungi: *Candida, Aspergillus* spp.

Fig. 10.10 Immune defects and corresponding susceptibility.

X-linked agammaglobulinemia (Bruton's disease)

There is a failure of B cell development and immunoglobulin production. It presents with severe bacterial infections in the first 2 years of life.

Severe combined immunodeficiency (SCID)

A heterogeneous group of disorders with profoundly defective cellular and humoral immunity (hence the name "combined"). It presents in the first 6 months of life with failure to thrive, diarrhea, candidal infections, and recurrent, severe, and unusual infections. A blood count often shows lymphopenia. Bone marrow transplantation is curative.

Common variable immunodeficiency (CVID)

This term encompasses a heterogeneous group of patients who have low levels of serum IgG and IgA. Usually present in late childhood with recurrent bacterial infection of sinuses or lungs.

Selective IgA deficiency

This is common (1 : 700 population). Most people with complete absence of IgA are asymptomatic. It is associated with autoimmune diseases in 40% and also with IgG subclass deficiency. Children deficient in IgG_2, the subclass providing immunity against polysaccharide antigens, may be susceptible to infection with encapsulated organisms (e.g., *Streptococcus pneumoniae, Haemophilus influenzae* type B).

Chronic granulomatous disease

An inherited disorder, usually X-linked, in which phagocytic cells fail to produce the superoxide anion. It presents with repeated bacterial and fungal infections involving the skin, lymph nodes, lungs, liver, and bones. Granulomas and abscesses form in these sites. Diagnosis is confirmed by failure to reduce nitroblue tetrazolium (NBT test).

The management of primary immunodeficiency is outlined in Fig. 10.11.

Secondary immunodeficiency
Immunosuppressive therapy

Therapeutic drugs, which cause immunosuppression, include:

- Cytotoxic agents.
- Steroids.

Management of primary immunodeficiency

The following treatment options are available:
• Antibiotic prophylaxis (e.g., cotrimoxazole, to prevent *Pneumocystis carinii* infection)
• Vigorous antibody therapy for infections
• Immunoglobulin replacement therapy—regular IV immunoglobulin can be given for severe defects in antibody production
• Bone marrow transplantation
• Gene therapy—this has been successfully performed for SCID caused by adenosine deaminase deficiency

Fig. 10.11 Management of primary immunodeficiency.

Immunologic test results in AIDS

Reduced DC4 count
Antigen detection (e.g., p24)
Raised IgG antibody
HIV DNA/RNA PCR

Fig. 10.12 Immunologic test results in AIDS.

Cytotoxic chemotherapy for malignant disease (e.g., acute leukemia) causes immunosuppression due to marrow suppression and neutropenia. Febrile children with neutrophil counts less than 0.5×10^9/L are at risk for serious and potentially fatal bacterial and fungal infection.

Children on high-dose corticosteroids (e.g., for nephrotic syndrome) are particularly at risk for disseminated chickenpox infection. Children with organ transplants are prone to infection with cytomegalovirus.

Infection

Worldwide, the two most important infections, which cause immunodeficiency, are:
• Measles.
• HIV infection.

Pediatric HIV infection

Human immunodeficiency virus type 1 (HIV-1), the causative agent of acquired immunodeficiency syndrome (AIDS), is transmitted to infants and children by vertical transmission from HIV-infected women or by HIV-contaminated blood or blood products.

Incidence

WHO estimates that 20 million adults and 1.5 million children have been infected with HIV since the pandemic began; 1500 children in sub-Saharan Africa are infected daily. The incidence of childhood HIV is decreasing in the USA, except for adolescents, among whom the rate is increasing. Mortality has decreased significantly with new antiviral therapies.

Transmission

The main route of transmission to children is vertically from mother to child: intrauterine, intrapartum, or via breastfeeding. Transmission rates vary with geographical area: lower in Europe and North America but higher in Africa. With current management vertical transmission is now <1%.

Diagnosis

All newborns born to HIV-infected women will have circulating maternal HIV antibodies but only a proportion of these are infected with the virus. Passively acquired antibody disappears at 15–18 months of age so this is not a reliable test for infection under 18 months.

Two approaches exist for diagnosis in children younger than 18 months:
• HIV viral culture: the gold standard but not widely available.
• Detection of viral genome by polymerase chain reaction.

Clinical manifestations: progression to AIDS

The incubation period from infection to disease varies but appears to be shorter in perinatally infected children than in adults. Mortality and hospital admissions have decreased since the introduction of combination antiviral therapy.

Changes in immune function are shown in Figs. 10.12 and 10.14, and the clinical manifestations are shown in Figs. 10.13 and 10.15.

Management

Cotrimoxazole prophylaxis against *Pneumocystis carinii* pneumonia is given for children with HIV infection. The primary immunization course should be given. BCG is not recommended, but MMR should be deferred only if severely immunosuppressed.

Clinical manifestations of HIV infection in children

Category	Severity	Manifestation
Category N	Asymptomatic	
Category A	Mild	Lymphadenopathy Hepatosplenomegaly Parotitis
Category B	Moderate	Severe bacterial infection Chronic diarrhea Candidiasis Lymphocytic interstitial pneumonitis (LIP)
Category C	Severe (AIDS)	Wasting (severe failure to thrive) Opportunistic infections (e.g., *Pneumocystis carinii* pneumonia [PCP]) Encephalopathy Severe bacterial infections Malignancy (rare)

Fig. 10.13 Clinical manifestations of HIV infection in children.

CD4 percentage

>25%	No evidence of suppression
15–25%	Moderate immunosuppression
<15%	Severe immunosuppression
Viral load	Unlike adults, does not correlate well with disease course

Fig. 10.14 Immunologic categories.

Noninfectious complications of AIDS

Neurologic	Encephalopathy Motor defects Seizures
Gastrointestinal	Anorexia Nausea Diarrhea Weight loss
Lymphoid hyperplasia syndrome	Lymphoid interstitial pneumonitis Polygrandular enlargement
Cutaneous	Kaposi's sarcoma

Fig. 10.15 Noninfectious complications of AIDS.

Antiretroviral treatment is recommended when the child becomes symptomatic or there is a low or rapid fall in the CD4 count (<15%). This treatment comprises a combination of reverse transcriptase inhibitors with protease inhibitors.

Coordinated psychological and social support for the whole family is a vital aspect of managing an HIV-infected child. Issues include:
- Telling children the diagnosis.
- Retaining confidentiality.
- Two (mother and child) members of the family may be sick or dying at the same time.
- Social or cultural isolation.
- Stigma of diagnosis.
- Major problem with increasing costs of antiviral drugs in developing countries.

Prevention

Zidovudine, given to the mother in pregnancy and during delivery and to the neonate for the first 6 weeks of life reduces the risk of vertical transmission of HIV-1. Cesarean section is recommended but if the maternal viral load is low than vaginal delivery appears to be safe. Antenatal HIV testing therefore confers potential benefits. Education campaigns can reduce but not eliminate the spread of HIV.

- What is the clinical course of TB?
- Who are at highest risk of disseminated disease?
- How is Kawasaki disease diagnosed?
- What are the complications of Kawasaki disease?
- How is antenatal HIV managed?
- How is HIV diagnosed in children?
- How do noninfectious complications of AIDS manifest?
- What features would suggest immunodeficiency?
- How is the diagnosis of malaria made?
- When should malaria be suspected?
- What are the complications of chickenpox?
- What are the complications of herpes simplex virus?

11. Allergy and Anaphylaxis

Allergy can be defined as a hypersensitive reaction initiated by immune mechanisms. This is mediated primarily by antibodies from the IgE isotype but in some reactions non-IgE mechanisms are responsible. The typical IgE-mediated response is biphasic. This is characterized by an early response (within 20 minutes) and a late response at 3–6 hours. Typical allergic reactions include:

- Asthma.
- Food allergy.
- Allergic rhinoconjunctivitis.
- Atopic eczema.
- Anaphylaxis

This chapter will cover mainly food allergy and anaphylaxis, as the others are discussed elsewhere.

Epidemiology

The increasing prevalence of allergy in children over the past 20–30 years has led to an increased need for specialized services dealing in childhood allergy. Although part of the increase in cases of allergy stems from greater awareness and reporting, population-based studies have shown a significant rise in allergic diseases. Approximately 6–8% of all children experience food allergy and 6% of all asthmatics have food-induced wheeze. In atopic eczema, approximately 60% will have a reaction to certain foods.

 Many allergies improve as the child grows older.

The natural history of allergy changes with increasing age. In early childhood, food reactions predominate, with manifestations in the skin and respiratory and gastrointestinal tracts. With increasing age, inhaled allergens become more important; initially this tends to involve indoor allergens (house-dust mite and pets) and then outdoor allergens (moulds and pollens) later. Note that 85% of children outgrow cow's milk allergy at the age of 3 years, but peanut allergy is lifelong.

Cross-reaction to allergens

It is important to note that children sensitized to one allergen can develop reactions to another even though previous exposure has not occurred. This is because certain allergens share the same binding site (epitope) to IgE and one mimics the other. Examples are:

- Grass and peanut.
- Peanuts, soy beans, and lentils.
- Latex and banana.

It is rare to have IgE-mediated reactions to more than three foods and allergy testing results that show cross-reaction should be confirmed by food challenge.

Clinical aspects of allergy

Diagnosis

The aim of the history is to ascertain what allergens the child reacts to and to discover if non-allergy mechanisms may be the cause of symptoms. An example is that 90% of cases of penicillin reaction obtained from the history are not caused by allergic mechanisms. The history should include:

- Age of onset.
- Diurnal and seasonal variations.
- Family history.
- Dietary history.
- Time between exposure and reaction.
- Reproducibility of reaction.
- Housing conditions and school.

Examination of the child must include the skin; ears, nose, and throat (ENT); respiratory and

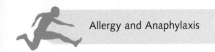

Examining a child for allergy	
Respiratory	Asthma/wheeze Stridor and angioedema Hoarseness Rhinoconjunctivitis
Gastrointestinal	Nausea, vomiting, and diarrhea Abdominal distention Failure to thrive
Cardiovascular	Hypotension and shock Dizziness
Skin	Pruritus Urticaria Atopic dermatitis Angioedema

Fig. 11.1 Examining a child for allergy.

gastrointestinal tracts; and some cardiovascular tests (Fig. 11.1). The nutritional status must be noted.

Symptoms that are severe, persistent or recurrent are an indication for allergy testing. This is commonly in the form of skin-prick testing or specific serum IgE levels. Food challenge is the gold standard and is used when doubts remain about the role of particular allergens. There is no lower age limit on testing and it must be noted that the severity of reaction from skin-prick tests or levels of specific IgE have a poor correlation with severity of clinical symptoms. Neither of these tests diagnoses non-IgE-mediated reactions and only a food challenge is diagnostic.

- Skin-prick testing is useful in all ages but not over areas of eczema.
- Food challenge is indicated in cases of doubt.

Skin-prick testing

This is the most common test because it is cheap and quick and has a good safety profile. For most allergens (except soy) a negative test means that it is unlikely that the patient will react to the allergen tested. Unfortunately, a positive test means only a 50–60% chance that the child will react and therefore the test result must be interpreted with a good clinical history. If there is a strong history of

food reaction and a positive skin-prick test then a food challenge is not needed to confirm the allergen is responsible for symptoms.

Serum-specific IgE

This is commonly referred to as RAST testing because it describes the type of assay that is performed on the serum. It measures levels of IgE that are food specific. This type of test is useful if skin-prick testing cannot be used (e.g., active eczema, patients on steroids or antihistamines and the drug cannot be stopped). Like skin-prick tests, a negative result is good for ruling out allergens but a positive result is useful only in the context of a positive history.

Food challenge

This is the gold standard and is used when uncertainties about the role of particular allergens or when non-IgE mechanisms are implicated. This is the only investigation that can accurately predict what clinical reactions will occur with food exposure. All food challenges should be performed in hospital because there is a risk of severe reactions.

Management of allergy

Children with suspected food allergy should be assessed by a pediatrician experienced in allergy: a specialist nurse and a dietician should be available. Liaison between hospital and community staff, and the education of both family and school play an important part.

A major consideration in management is the anxiety that affects both child and carers. Avoidance of the allergen may be difficult and it is often hard for parents to identify suitable foods; the help of an experienced dietician is essential in these matters. Inhaled allergen avoidance is difficult and various methods are available. Their effectiveness remains controversial, however.

Pharmacologic treatment remains standard for asthma and eczema. Antihistamines can be useful and immunotherapy may play a greater role in the future.

Anaphylaxis

Anaphylaxis is a severe allergic reaction that manifests with respiratory difficulty (wheeze or

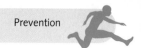

upper airway obstruction) and/or cardiovascular symptoms (shock, hypotension, or dizziness).

It is caused by prior exposure to antigen-sensitizing mast cells and basophils, leading to systemic release of inflammatory mediators resulting in capillary leak, mucosal edema, and smooth muscle contraction.

Anaphylaxis can be mediated by IgE, when the term "allergic anaphylaxis" should be used; when IgE is not implicated or is unclear, the term "nonallergic anaphylaxis" should be used. The term "anaphylactoid" is no longer used.

Anaphylaxis has an increasing incidence and, in children, foods are the most common cause, followed by drugs and hymenoptera (bee/wasp) venom. In adults the common causes are drugs, insect venom, foods, and latex.

Foods

Foods are the most common cause of anaphylaxis in children. Peanuts are the most common food to cause a reaction.

Insect venom

Anaphylaxis to venom is rare in children but it is associated with the greatest anxiety. The reaction to insect stings decreases with age.

Latex

Anaphylaxis to latex is rare in children and is usually found in those who have had numerous surgical procedures. Note its cross-reaction with banana.

Drugs

Vaccines and penicillins account for the majority of reactions but are rare. Note that MMR immunizations can be given to children with egg allergy, although if there has been previous anaphylaxis to egg, or severe coexisting asthma, the vaccine can be given in hospital. Influenza vaccine should not be given to children with egg allergy.

Recognition

Respiratory difficulty is more common than cardiovascular collapse. Foods tend to cause respiratory and airway symptoms whereas injections and stings cause cardiovascular symptoms. Initial symptoms can be subtle and progression rapid.

Respiratory symptoms and signs
- Cough.
- Stridor, hoarseness, and drooling.
- Facial swelling.
- Wheeze.

Cardiovascular symptoms and signs
- Feeling faint/dizziness.
- Syncope.
- Pallor.
- Tachycardia.

Note that the cutaneous signs, such as rash, are not life-threatening and may be absent.

Treatment

Treatment is intramuscular adrenaline (epinephrine). This acts on the α-adrenoreceptors to cause peripheral vasoconstriction and on β-receptors to cause bronchodilation and inotropic effects; it also reduces airway swelling. It should be given to all children with respiratory or cardiovascular symptoms. The intramuscular route is preferred because intravenous administration is thought to have contributed in some deaths. IV hydrocortisone and antihistamines should also be administered.

Prevention

Allergen avoidance is the only preventive measure and all children with suspected anaphylaxis should be referred for allergy testing. The use of an Epipen, which allows subcutaneous administration of adrenaline, can be life saving but it is essential that carers are trained in its use. Only 32% of parents were able to correctly demonstrate correct use in one study. The Epipen is only one part of managing severe allergic reactions. Management should also include:
- Identifying causes.
- Education on allergen avoidance.
- Treatment plan.
- Training of carers and school.
- Annual reinforcement.

Epipens in anaphylaxis are useful if carers are trained in their use.

- What is the natural history of most allergies?
- Describe the respiratory symptoms of allergy.
- What are the important points in the history?
- What is cross-reactivity?
- How does skin-prick testing compare with blood testing?
- What is the long-term management of children with anaphylaxis?

Further reading

Clark AT, Ewen PW. The prevention and management of anaphylaxis in children. *Current Paediatrics* 2002; 12:370–375.

Host A, Halken S. Practical aspects of allergy testing. *Paediatric Respiratory Reviews* 2003; 4:312–318.

Ives A, Hourihane J. Evidence-based diagnosis of food allergy. *Current Paediatrics* 2002; 12:357–364.

Johansson SGO et al. A revised nomenclature for allergy. An EAACI position statement from the EAACI nomenclature task force. *Allergy* 2001; 56:813–824.

Rosenthal M. How a non-allergist survives an allergy clinic. *Archives of Diseases in Childhood* 2004; 89:238–243.

12. Skin Disorders

Eczema (dermatitis)

The term "dermatitis" refers to an inflammation of the skin and is synonymous with eczema (the word eczema literally means to "to boil over"). Three main varieties occur in infants and children:
- Infantile seborrheic eczema.
- Atopic eczema.
- Diaper dermatitis.

Infantile seborrheic eczema
This mild condition presents in the first 2 months of life with a scaly, nonitchy rash initially on the scalp ("cradle cap"); this may spread to involve the face, flexures, and diaper area (Fig. 12.1). Treatment is with emollients and mild topical steroids.

Atopic eczema
Atopic eczema is very common and affects 10–20% of children, usually beginning in the first 6 months of life. There is often a family history of atopic disorders (eczema, asthma, and hay fever), reflecting a genetic predisposition that confers an abnormal immune response to environmental allergens. Early diagnosis and treatment of atopic children with antihistamines can reduce the risk of developing asthma in later life.

Clinical features
A dry, red, itchy rash occurs that usually starts on, and has a predilection for, the extensor surfaces and face in infants and young children, and the flexures (the antecubital and popliteal fossa) in older children (Fig. 12.2). However, the skin appearance can vary from an acute, weeping papulovesicular eruption to the chronic, dry, scaly, thickened (lichenified) skin that develops in older children. Itching is the most important and troublesome symptom.

Affected children may have an eosinophilia and raised plasma IgE concentration. Histopathologic changes include epidermal edema and vesicle formation, vascular dilatation, and cellular infiltration.

Diagnosis
The diagnosis is clinical (see Fig. 12.3 for a comparison of atopic and infantile seborrheic eczema). RAST and food challenges are useful in children with associated difficult to manage asthma.

Management
It is important that the skin is kept hydrated and inflammation is reduced. The treatment options are:
- Important general measures.
- Topical preparations.
- Specific treatment for complications such as secondary infection.

General measures
Advice should be given on avoiding aggravating factors such as:
- Synthetic or woolen fabrics (cotton clothes are preferable).
- Biologic detergents or fabric conditioners.
- Cigarette smoke.
- Dander from furry pets.
- House dust.
- Grass pollen.

Nails should be kept short and excessive heat avoided.

Topical preparations
The mainstays of management are:
- Emollients.
- Topical steroids.

Emollients moisturize and soften the skin. They are safe and should be used frequently. A daily bath using bath oil and aqueous cream as a soap substitute is advisable, with regular application of an emollient two or three times daily.

Mild topical steroids, such as 1% hydrocortisone (ointment rather than cream when the skin is dry), applied to the affected areas twice daily are highly effective. More potent preparations can be used short term for exacerbations but only weak steroids should be applied to the face. Severe eczema can be treated with wet wraps in hospital to maximize hydration.

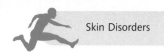

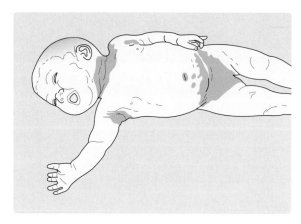

Fig. 12.1 Distribution of infantile seborrheic eczema.

A new class of drug—topical immunomodulators (e.g., tacrolimus cream)—is available and has the advantage of few side effects and low systemic absorption.

In atopic eczema:
- Treat dry skin with emollients.
- Inflamed skin with topical steroids.
- Consider infection if not responding to treatment.

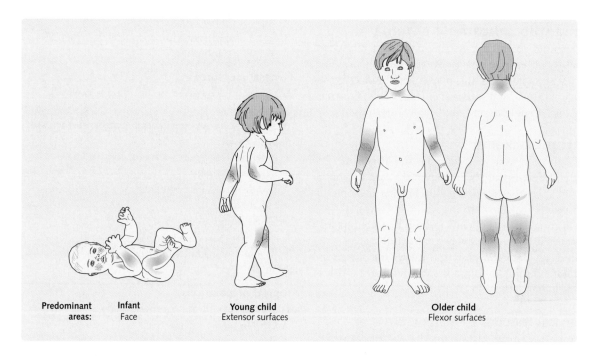

| Predominant areas: | Infant Face | Young child Extensor surfaces | Older child Flexor surfaces |

Fig. 12.2 Distribution of atopic eczema.

Fig. 12.3 Differences between infantile seborrheic eczema and atopic eczema.

Differences between infantile seborrheic eczema and atopic eczema		
	Infantile seborrheic eczema	Atopic eczema
Age	<3 months (usually)	>3 months (usually)
Sleeping	Undisturbed	Affected
Pruritus	Nil	Significant
Family history of atopy	Usually negative	Often positive
Course	Self-limiting	Chronic, relapsing

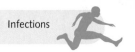

Complications

The most important is secondary infection with either viruses or bacteria. Infection with herpes simplex (eczema herpeticum) is potentially serious and should be treated with acyclovir. Bacterial superinfection is usually caused by staphylococci or streptococci and requires systemic antibiotic treatment.

Atopic dermatitis persists into adulthood in up to 60% of all children and particularly in those with early onset, severe disease and associated asthma and hay fever.

Diaper dermatitis

Rashes in the diaper area are common and can be due to:
- An irritant contact dermatitis (diaper rash).
- Candidiasis.
- Seborrheic dermatitis.

Clinical features

Diaper rash

Ordinary diaper rash is due to the prolonged contact of urine and feces with skin. Particular causes include skin wetness and ammonia from the breakdown of urine by fecal enzymes. The skin is red and moist and may ulcerate. The inguinal folds are spared.

Diaper rash can be prevented by frequent diaper changes (easier with disposable diapers) and barrier creams such as zinc. Exposure to air can speed recovery but can be impractical to implement at home.

Causes of an "itchy" rash:
- Atopic eczema.
- Scabies.
- Papular urticaria.
- Urticaria (hives).
- Chickenpox.

Candidiasis

Candidiasis is also common and is distinguished by bright red skin with satellite lesions and involvement of the skin folds. Candidal infection can be treated with an antifungal, such as miconazole and fluconazole.

Infections

Bacterial

Bacterial infections of the skin in children include common and important entities such as:
- Impetigo.
- Boils and furuncles.
- Staphylococcal scalded skin syndrome.
- Erysipelas.

These are considered in Chapter 10.

Viral

Viral warts

Hands and feet

The human papilloma virus (HPV) causes viral warts. Two types are seen:
- Skin warts are common on the fingers and soles in school-age children.
- Plantar warts (verrucae) are flat, hyperkeratotic lesions on the soles of the feet.

Most viral warts resolve within a year when immunity develops. Treatment options include:
- Salicylic and lactic acid topical solutions.
- Cryotherapy with liquid nitrogen.

Repeat treatments over many weeks are required.

Other sites

Viral warts also occur in other locations:
- Laryngeal papillomas are found on the vocal cords.
- Genital warts (condylomata acuminata) are papular or frond-like growths in the perineal area.

These can be a sign of sexual abuse in young children.

Molluscum contagiosum

This common eruption in children is caused by the mollusci poxvirus.

Clinical features

Smooth, pearly papules with an obvious central dimple arise in crops (often on the trunk). They are not irritating and are of low infectivity.

Management

The papules resolve spontaneously without scarring usually within 6 months to 2 years and treatment is not required, although cryotherapy can be used if rapid removal is required.

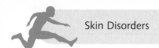

Fungal

These include dermatophytosis (ringworm) and candidiasis (thrush).

Dermatophytoses (tinea capitis, corporis, pedis, and unguium)

Dermatophytes are filamentous fungi that infect the outer layer of the skin and also the hair and nails. They also affect some animal species (e.g., cattle and cats).

Clinical features

Clinical features vary with the site of infection:

- Tinea capitis (scalp ringworm): on the scalp, tinea causes patchy alopecia and occasionally a boggy inflammatory mass called a kerion.
- Tinea corporis (body ringworm): on the trunk, tinea appears as annular lesions with central clearing and a palpable, erythematous border.
- Tinea pedis (athlete's foot): presents as itchy, scaling, and cracking of the skin of the feet, especially between the toes.

Diagnosis

Examination under ultraviolet light (Wood's lamp) shows a green-yellow fluorescence of infected hairs with certain fungal species. Diagnosis can be made by microscopic examination of skin scrapings for fungal hyphae. Culture of the organism is definitive.

Treatment

This varies with the severity of infection:

- Mild infections are treated with topical antifungal preparations such as clotrimazole or miconazole.
- Severe infections require systemic treatment with griseofulvin for several weeks.

Candidiasis (thrush, moniliasis)

Candida albicans, a yeast (budding, unicellular organism), is the most common pathogen. The organism colonizes the skin and mucous membranes. Transmission is via person-to-person contact, contaminated feeding bottles, etc.

Clinical features

In infants, candidal infections frequently involve the oral cavity (thrush) or the diaper area. It is acquired from the mother's vaginal flora. It can also affect the nipples of breastfeeding mothers.

Diagnosis

Diagnosis is clinical:

- Oral thrush presents as white plaques on the tongue and buccal mucosa.
- Monilial dermatitis: localized shiny redness typically affecting moist areas and *not* sparing flexural skin creases (this may occur in the absence of oral thrush).

Management

Topical nystatin is first-line therapy. Oral treatment should be given as well as direct treatment to lesions in perineal disease.

Prevention requires good hygiene and rigorous disinfection of feeding bottles.

Chronic or recurrent mucocutaneous candidiasis should raise the suspicion of immunodeficiency.

Infestations

Papular urticaria

This term describes crops of itchy, erythematous papules or small blisters. They are caused by insect bites, most commonly by fleas or mites; bedbugs can also be the culprits. Secondary infection may occur.

Scabies

Scabies is caused by the mite *Sarcoptes scabiei*. It is transmitted by skin-to-skin contact. In the first infestation, the incubation period can be up to 8 weeks. The fertilized adult female mite burrows deep in the stratum corneum laying two or three eggs a day until she dies after about 5 weeks. The eggs hatch after a few days and larvae move on to the skin surface, maturing into adults in 10–14 days.

Clinical features

The first symptom is pruritus, which is worse at night and is related to hypersensitivity to the mite or its feces. The presence of burrows is pathognomonic. Common sites for burrows are the interdigital webs and the anterior aspects of the wrists. In infants, the soles of the feet, head, and neck are commonly affected.

The rash consists of vesicles, weals, and papules, which may become excoriated and secondarily infected.

Diagnosis

Diagnosis is clinical and may (if necessary) be confirmed by identification of mites or ova in scrapings from burrows or vesicles.

Suspect scabies when:
- There is itching in the family.
- Itchy papules or blisters are present on the soles of the feet.

Treatment

Treatment is permethrin cream 5%. This is for two consecutive days and all close contacts should be treated with lotion—covering the body from the neck down. In infants, the scalp and face should be included. Laundering of clothes and bedding is important. It can take several weeks for the pruritus to subside after successful treatment as hypersensitivity persists. This can be managed with oral antihistamines and topical steroids.

Head lice (Pediculosis capitis)

Pediculosis capitis is a blood-sucking arthropod that infests the scalps of up to 10% of school children in some urban areas. Transmission is by head-to-head contact. The head louse prefers clean hair and does not discriminate between socioeconomic status.

Clinical features and diagnosis

The louse egg is attached to the base of the scalp hair and is visible as a small, white, grain-like particle. Eggs hatch after a week and the louse lives for 2–3 months. Many infestations are asymptomatic but the most common manifestation is severe itching of the scalp often accompanied by enlarged cervical lymph nodes. Nits are the egg cases and only finding a louse is diagnostic.

Treatment

Treatment is with 0.5% malathion lotion, which should be left on for 12 hours. The hair is then washed with ordinary shampoo and the dead nits removed with a fine-toothed metal comb. All the family should be treated. Clothing and bedding is disinfected by machine washing (cycles over 50°C inactivate lice and nits).

Other childhood skin diseases

Pityriasis rosea

This common, acute, benign, and self-limiting condition is thought to be of viral origin. It begins with a "herald patch," an oval or round, scaly, erythematous macule on the trunk, neck or proximal part of limbs. This is followed within 1–3 days by a shower of smaller dull pink macules on the trunk in a so-called "Christmas tree" pattern following the lines of the ribs. Spontaneous resolution occurs within 6–8 weeks.

No treatment is required.

Acne vulgaris

This is a chronic inflammatory disorder of the sebaceous glands and probably reflects an abnormal response to circulating androgens. It is an almost universal problem of adolescence, peaking in severity at age 16–18 years.

Clinical features

A variety of lesions occur on the face and upper trunk. Characteristically, comedones occur: plugs of keratin and sebum within the dilated orifice of a hair follicle. These can be open (blackheads) or closed (whiteheads). They progress to papules and pustules (bacterial superinfection) and in severe cases to cystic and nodular lesions, which can cause scarring.

Treatment

Treatment options include:
- Topical treatment with keratolytic agents (e.g., benzoyl peroxide).
- Ultraviolet light therapy: exposure to natural sunlight should be encouraged.
- Oral antibiotics: low-dose therapy with minocycline, tetracycline (>12 years age) or erythromycin is useful for moderate to severe pustular acne. Antibiotics are given for at least 3 months.
- The vitamin A analog, 13-*cis*-retinoic acid: for severe acne that has not responded to conventional treatment. This should be prescribed only by a dermatologist. Retinoic acid is a teratogen, and extreme precaution needs to be taken.

Urticaria (hives)

Urticaria is a transient, itchy, erythematous rash characterized by the presence of raised weals

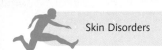

(hives). It is induced by mast cell degranulation, in which histamine and other vasoactive mediators are released causing vasodilatation and an increase in capillary permeability. Most cases are caused by viral infections but an allergy history is needed to exclude allergic causes.

Clinical features

Urticaria can be accompanied by edema of the lips and eyes (angioedema). Involvement of the lips and tongue is an emergency because there is a risk of respiratory obstruction. Chronic urticaria can occur and usually clears spontaneously in about 6 months.

Management

Acute urticaria usually resolves spontaneously within a few hours. If itchy, it can be treated with an antihistamine (e.g., diphenhydramine). Precipitating factors should be avoided.

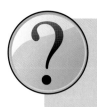

- How is atopic eczema distinguished from seborrheic eczema?
- What general measures can be used in atopic eczema?
- What are the drug therapies available for atopic eczema?
- How is scabies diagnosed?
- What is the treatment of acne?

13. Cardiovascular Disorders

In developed countries, congenital heart disease (CHD) accounts for the majority of cardiovascular problems in infants and children. With improved cardiac surgery, 80–85% of children with congenital cardiac disease survive into adulthood. Ischemic heart disease is rare in children, in contrast to its incidence in adults, although it can occur in Kawasaki disease. Arrhythmias are very rare, with the exception of supraventricular tachycardias (SVTs). Important infections that affect the cardiovascular system (CVS) are infective endocarditis and viral myocarditis.

Congenital heart disease (CHD)

CHD comprises the most common group of structural malformations, affecting 6–8 out of 1000 live-born infants. A number of important causative factors are recognized (Fig. 13.1) but, in the majority of cases, the cause is unknown. CHD presents or may be diagnosed in a limited number of ways. These include:
- Antenatal diagnosis by ultrasound.
- Heart murmur.
- Cyanosis.
- Shock: low cardiac output.
- Cardiac failure (see Chapter 2).

Although there are over 100 different cardiac malformations, a small number account for the majority of cases (Fig. 13.2). These are conveniently classified into:
- Acyanotic forms.
- Cyanotic forms.

Initial evaluation should include a chest x-ray (CXR) and electrocardiogram (ECG), although these investigations do not usually provide a lesion diagnosis. Diagnosis is usually achieved by a combination of echocardiography and Doppler ultrasound. Common investigations are shown in Fig. 13.3.

Acyanotic congenital heart disease

These conditions are caused by lesions that allow blood to shunt from the left to the right side of the circulation or that obstruct the flow of blood by narrowing a valve or vessel:

Left-to-right shunts
Atrial septal defect (ASD)
There are two types of ASD:
- The most common ASD (6 in 10,000 live births) is a foramen secundum defect, high in the atrial septum. It is more common in girls (F : M ratio = 2 : 1) and accounts for 6% of all cases of CHD.
- Much less common is the ostium primum type, which occurs lower in the atrial septum (often associated with mitral regurgitation) and is a common defect in Down syndrome.

Secundum defects are usually asymptomatic in childhood. The left-to-right shunt develops very slowly and pulmonary hypertension is extremely uncommon. It is important to distinguish ASDs from patent foramen ovale (PFO), which is present in one-third of all children. The patent foramen opens only in conditions of raised atrial pressure or volumes, whereas ASDs are large and always open.

Clinical features. The clinical features include:
- Abnormal right ventricular impulse.
- Widely split and fixed second sound (S2).
- Tricuspid flow murmur: rumbling mid-diastolic murmur at the left sternal edge.
- Pulmonary flow murmur: soft, ejection systolic murmur in the pulmonary area.

No murmur is generated by the low velocity flow across the ASD. A significant left-to-right shunt generates flow murmurs at the tricuspid and pulmonary valves.

Diagnosis. The CXR shows increased pulmonary vascular markings, and the ECG shows right ventricular hypertrophy with incomplete right bundle branch block. Echocardiography is diagnostic without cardiac catheterization.

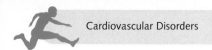

Management.   Treatment is surgical and aims to prevent right cardiac failure and arrythmias in later life. This is best done at 3–5 years of age and 30% can be done in the cardiac catheter laboratory. Endocarditis prophylaxis is not required for children with isolated secundum ASD.

Causes of congenital heart disease
Genetic chromosomal disorders
Down syndrome (e.g., atrioventricular septal defect)
Turner syndrome (e.g., aortic stenosis, coarctation of the aorta)
Chromosome 22 deletions
Williams syndrome (e.g., supraventricular aortic stenosis)
Teratogens
Congenital rubella (e.g., PDA, pulmonary stenosis)
Alcohol (e.g., ASD, VSD)

Fig. 13.1 Common causes of congenital heart disease.

Ventricular septal defect (VSD)

Most are single, although multiple defects do occur and other heart defects coexist in about one-third of children. The natural history and prognosis depends on the following:

- Size and position of the defect.
- Development of changes due to blood shunting from left to right through the defect. This includes narrowing of the right ventricular outflow tract and progressive pulmonary hypertension, both of which reduce the size of the shunt.

 A ventricular septal defect is the most common variety of congenital heart disease. It accounts for one-third of all cases.

Common forms of congenital heart disease			
Type	**Name**	**Abbreviation**	**% of CHD**
Acyanotic	Ventricular septal defect	VSD	32
	Patent ductus arteriosus	PDA	12
	Pulmonary stenosis	PS	8
	Atrial septal defect	ASD	6
	Coarctation of the aorta	COA	6
	Aortic stenosis	AS	6
Cyanotic	Tetralogy of Fallot	—	6
	Transposition of the great arteries	TGA	5

Fig. 13.2 Common forms of congenital heart disease.

Investigations in congenital heart disease	
Investigation	**Demonstrates**
CXR	Cardiac shadow—may be enlarged or abnormal Lung fields—pulmonary vascular markings may be • Increased (plethora): significant left-to-right shunt (e.g., VSD) or • Decreased (oligemia): reduced pulmonary blood flow
ECG	Rate and rhythm of heart Mean QRS axis Hypertrophy of either ventricle
Echocardiogram	Precise anatomic abnormality
Cardiac catheter	Physiologic/hemodynamic status rather than anatomy

Fig. 13.3 Investigations in congenital heart disease.

The clinical features, treatment, and outcome are best considered separately for the different sizes of defect.

Small VSD (maladie de Roger). The child is asymptomatic and the murmur is often first noted on routine examination. The only abnormality is a pansystolic murmur (sometimes with a palpable thrill) at the lower left sternal border. Antibiotic prophylaxis against bacterial endocarditis is necessary for dental extractions, but no other treatment is required. Spontaneous closure may occur.

Medium VSD. These usually present with symptoms during infancy including slow weight gain, difficulty with feeding and recurrent chest infections. In time, symptoms may actually disappear due to relative or actual closure of the defect. On examination, there may be:

- An increased cardiac impulse.
- Palpable thrill.
- Harsh pansystolic murmur, loudest in the third and fourth left intercostal spaces.

If the pulmonary blood flow is high, a mid-diastolic murmur occurs due to blood flow across the normal mitral valve.

A CXR will show moderate cardiac enlargement, a prominent pulmonary artery, and increased vascularity of the lungs.

Echocardiography will show the position of the defect. The shunt is measured by Doppler studies.

Heart failure, if present, should be treated with diuretics and angiotensin-converting enzyme (ACE) inhibitors. Spontaneous improvement occurs in many childhood cases and surgical correction can be avoided. However, if there is still evidence of a significant shunt at 4 years, closure should be considered before the child starts school.

Large VSD. Heart failure develops early on, especially if a chest infection occurs. The cardiac signs are similar to those of a medium VSD but it is worth noting that the systolic murmur may be soft in a very large defect. The defect tends to be larger than the cross-sectional area of the aortic valve.

Initial medical treatment of the heart failure is required and surgical closure under cardiopulmonary bypass is usually necessary. In young infants with multiple defects, banding of the pulmonary artery allows a temporary respite until the child is big enough for definitive correction. An example of a VSD is shown in Fig. 13.4.

Patent ductus arteriosus (PDA)

The ductus arteriosus connects the aorta to the left pulmonary artery and usually closes by the fourth day of life. A PDA is diagnosed if the duct does

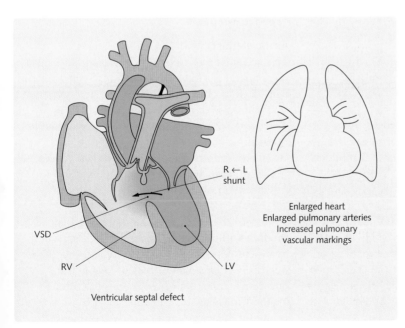

Fig. 13.4 Ventricular septal defect and chest x-ray changes.

R ← L shunt

Enlarged heart
Enlarged pulmonary arteries
Increased pulmonary vascular markings

VSD

RV

LV

Ventricular septal defect

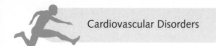

not close after 1 month of life. Risk factors include preterm infants, Down syndrome and high altitudes. PDA seen in preterm infants is a distinct clinical entity from congenital PDA in term infants.

 The risk of developing pulmonary vascular disease or infective endocarditis is higher in PDA than VSD and surgical closure is recommended for all PDAs. This can be achieved by division, ligation, or transvenous umbrella occlusion.

Clinical features. A shunt develops between the aorta and pulmonary artery. The clinical features include:
- "Bounding" pulses: wide pulse pressure.
- Murmur: initially systolic. As pulmonary vascular resistance falls, a continuous run-off from the aorta to the pulmonary artery occurs with a continuous "machinery" murmur.

The PDA is commonly asymptomatic. If the duct is large, a significant left-to-right shunt develops as pulmonary vascular resistance falls and cardiac failure occurs.

Diagnosis. CXR and ECG changes with a large symptomatic PDA are similar to those seen in a patient with a large VSD. The CXR is usually normal but in large PDAs increased pulmonary markings are seen. A PDA can be directly visualized by two-dimensional echocardiography and the ductal shunt can be confirmed by Doppler ultrasound.

Management. The duct can be closed in the cardiac catheter laboratory at 1 year of age but, if large, it may need surgical closure at 1–3 months.

Obstructive lesions
Coarctation of the aorta (COA)
COA accounts for about 6% of CHDs and has a male preponderance (M : F ratio = 2 : 1). There is a narrowing of the aorta, which can be preductal or postductal. The site and severity of the coarctation determine the clinical features, which range from a severely ill newborn to an asymptomatic child, or adult, with hypertension.

 The key to clinical diagnosis of coarctation of the aorta is weak or absent femoral pulses.

Preductal coarctation in symptomatic infants. The abnormal circulation is often diagnosed antenatally but after birth it presents as a sick neonate with absent femoral pulses. While the ductus arteriosus is open the right ventricle can maintain adequate cardiac output to the systemic circulation. There is usually no murmur and cardiac failure occurs when the duct closes. On diagnosis, prostaglandin infusion to maintain ductal patency and transfer to a cardiac center for surgery is indicated.

Postductal coarctation in asymptomatic children. Although usually asymptomatic, there may be leg pains or headache. On examination, there is hypertension in the arm and weak or absent femoral pulses. There may be an ejection click (due to an associated bicuspid aortic valve) and a systolic ejection murmur audible in the left interscapular area.

Surgical correction is required. Options include:
- Balloon dilatation.
- Resection of the coarcted segment with end-to-end anastomosis.

Aortic stenosis (AS)
This accounts for 5% of all CHDs and has a male preponderance (M : F ratio = 4 : 1). Symptoms and signs depend on the severity of the stenosis:
- Children with mild or moderate stenoses present with an asymptomatic murmur and a thrill.
- Severe stenosis can present with heart failure in the infant or with chest pain on exertion and syncope in older children.

Sustained, strenuous exercise should be avoided in children with moderate to severe AS. Surgical treatment depends on the severity and site of the stenosis. Options include balloon or surgical valvotomy. Aortic valve replacement is often required for neonates and children with a significant stenosis requiring early treatment.

Pulmonary stenosis (PS)

This accounts for about 8% of CHDs and may be valvular (90%), subvalvular (infundibular), or supravalvular. Infundibular PS occurs in association with a large VSD as part of the tetralogy of Fallot.

Most cases are mild and asymptomatic. The clinical features include:

- Widely split S2, with soft pulmonary component (P2).
- Systolic ejection click (valvular PS).
- A systolic ejection murmur maximal at the upper left sternal border, radiating to the back.

Treatment options include transvenous balloon dilatation or pulmonary valvotomy.

Cyanotic congenital heart disease

There are two principal pathophysiologic mechanisms for cyanosis in congenital heart disease:

- Decreased pulmonary blood flow with shunting of deoxygenated blood from the right side of the circulation to the left (systemic circulation) (e.g., tetralogy of Fallot).
- Increased pulmonary blood flow with abnormal mixing of systemic and pulmonary venous return (e.g., transposition of great arteries [TGA]).

Tetralogy of Fallot

This represents 6–10% of all CHDs and is the most common cause of cyanotic CHDs presenting beyond infancy. The four cardinal anatomical features are shown in Fig. 13.5.

Clinical features

Most patients present with cyanosis in the first 1–2 months of life. Hypoxic (hypercyanotic) spells are

---

The four cardinal anatomic features of tetralogy of Fallot
A large VSD
Right ventricular outflow tract (RVOT) obstruction
• Infundibular stenosis (50%)
• Pulmonary valve stenosis (10%)
• Combination of above (30%)
Aorta overriding the ventricular septum
Right ventricular hypertrophy

Fig. 13.5 The four cardinal anatomic features of tetralogy of Fallot.

a characteristic feature, as is squatting on exercise which develops in late infancy.

Clinical signs include:

- Cyanosis with or without clubbing.
- Loud and single S2.
- Loud ejection systolic murmur maximal at the third, left intercostal space.

Diagnosis

The ECG shows right axis deviation and right ventricular hypertrophy but normal at birth. The CXR shows a characteristic "boot-shaped" heart caused by right ventricular hypertrophy and a concavity on the left heart border where the main pulmonary artery and RV outflow tract normally create a convexity (Fig. 13.6). Pulmonary vascular markings are diminished. Congestive cardiac failure does not occur in tetralogy of Fallot.

Management

Prolonged hypercyanotic spells require treatment with:

- Morphine—relieves pain and abolishes hyperpnea.
- Sodium bicarbonate (IV) to correct acidosis.
- Propranolol to cause peripheral vasoconstriction and relieve infundibular spasm. Oral propranolol can prevent hypoxic spells.

Definitive treatment is surgical. Palliative procedures may be required in infants with severe cyanosis or uncontrollable hypoxic spells. Pulmonary blood flow is increased by creating a shunt between the subclavian and the pulmonary arteries. Corrective total repair can now be carried out from 4–6 months of age. This involves patch closure of the VSD and widening of the right ventricular outflow tract.

Transposition of the great arteries

This accounts for about 5% of CHDs and is more common in males (M : F ratio = 3 : 1). In complete or D-transposition:

- The aorta arises anteriorly from the right ventricle.
- The pulmonary artery arises posteriorly from the left ventricle (Fig. 13.7).

Clearly, if completely separate, two such parallel circulations would be incompatible with life, but defects allowing mixing of the two circulations coexist. These include ASD, VSD, or PDA.

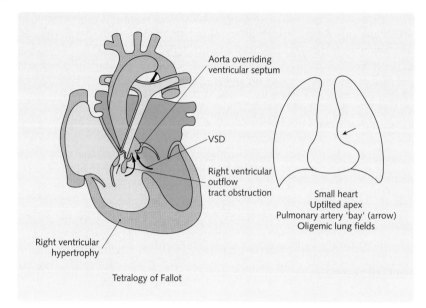

Fig. 13.6 Tetralogy of Fallot and CXR changes.

Aorta overriding ventricular septum

VSD

Right ventricular outflow tract obstruction

Right ventricular hypertrophy

Small heart
Uptilted apex
Pulmonary artery 'bay' (arrow)
Oligemic lung fields

Tetralogy of Fallot

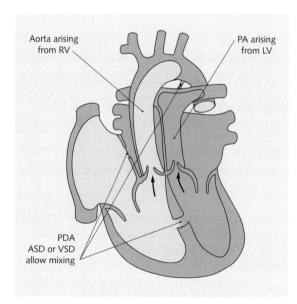

Fig. 13.7 Transposition of the great arteries.

Aorta arising from RV

PA arising from LV

PDA
ASD or VSD allow mixing

The second sound is single and loud. If the ventricular septum is intact, no heart murmur is audible. The systolic murmur of a VSD or PDA may be present.

Management

The immediate aim is to improve mixing of saturated and unsaturated blood. In the sick, cyanosed newborn, an infusion of prostaglandin (PG) E_1 is started to reopen the ductus arteriosus. Emergency cardiac catheterization and therapeutic balloon atrial septostomy (Rashkind procedure) is a life-saving palliative procedure. Definitive repair is usually achieved with an arterial switch procedure, which can be performed at a few weeks of age. The pulmonary artery and aorta are transected and switched over.

Clinical features

Most cases present with severe cyanosis, often within the first day or two of life. Spontaneous closure of the ductus arteriosus reduces mixing of the systemic and pulmonary circulations. Arterial hypoxemia is often profound (PaO_2 = 1–3 kPa, PaO_2 <60 mmHg) and unresponsive to O_2 inhalation.

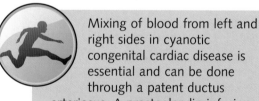

Mixing of blood from left and right sides in cyanotic congenital cardiac disease is essential and can be done through a patent ductus arteriosus. A prostaglandin infusion can open the ductus, allowing mixing.

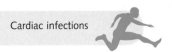

Rheumatic fever

Acute rheumatic fever is a sequela of group A β-hemolytic streptococcal infection, usually a tonsillopharyngitis. It is caused by an abnormal immune response that occurs in less than 1% of patients with streptococcal infection. Although the disease has largely been eradicated in developed countries with improved sanitation and the use of antibiotics for tonsillitis, it remains the most common cause of cardiac valvular disease worldwide. It mainly affects children aged between 5 and 15 years.

Clinical features

Polyarthritis, fever and malaise develop 2–6 weeks after the pharyngeal infection. The arthritis is "flitting," lasting less than a week in individual joints and commonly affects the large joints such as the knees and ankles.

There is a pancarditis in 50% of patients:
- Pericarditis can cause a friction rub and pericardial effusion.
- Myocarditis can cause heart failure.
- Endocarditis commonly affects the left-sided valves leading to murmurs, e.g., of mitral incompetence.

Erythema marginatum—pink macules on the trunk and limbs—is an uncommon painless, early manifestation. Hard subcutaneous nodules occur on the extensor surfaces in a minority of cases.

Sydenham's chorea is a late manifestation occurring 2–6 months after streptococcal infection in 10% of patients. There is emotional lability followed by involuntary, random, jerky movements lasting 2–3 months. Recovery is usually complete.

Diagnosis

The diagnosis is clinical and is based on a modified version of the Duckett Jones criteria (Fig. 13.8).

Diagnosis requires evidence of a preceding streptococcal infection together with two major criteria or one major and two minor criteria. The former is usually done serologically by finding an increase in antibodies to various streptococcal antigens, e.g. antistreptolysin 0 titre. Throat swab is often negative at the time of presentation.

Laboratory investigations in a suspected case include:
- ESR, C-reactive protein (CRP): elevated.
- Antistreptolysin 0 titer: may be elevated.

Modified Duckett Jones criteria (2 major or 1 major and 2 minor)	
Major	**Minor**
Carditis	Fever
Polyarthritis	Arthralgia
Chorea	Previous rheumatic fever
Erythema marginatum	Positive acute-phase reactant
Subcutaneous nodules	(ESR, CRP)
	Leukocytosis
	Prolonged P-R interval on ECG

Fig. 13.8 Modified Duckett Jones criteria for diagnosis of rheumatic fever.

- Throat swab: usually negative at time of presentation.
- ECG: prolonged P-R interval.
- Echocardiography: may show evidence of carditis.

Management

The acute episode is treated by:
- Bed rest.
- High-dose aspirin to suppress fever and arthritis.
- Steroids for severe carditis.
- Diuretics and ACE inhibitors for heart failure.
- Antibiotics if there is evidence of persisting streptococcal infection.

Recurrent attacks should be prevented by prophylactic penicillin (given either orally or as monthly intramuscular injections of benzathine penicillin). Lifelong prophylaxis has been advocated.

Complications

Rheumatic valvular disease is the most common form of long-term damage, its severity increasing with the number of acute episodes. There is scarring and fibrosis of valve tissue, most commonly affecting the mitral valve.

Cardiac infections

These are uncommon and include:
- Infective endocarditis.
- Myocarditis.

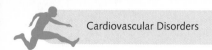

Infective endocarditis

This may be defined as infection of the endocardium or endothelium of the great vessels. It is a cause of great morbidity and prevention in high-risk groups by using prophylactic antibiotics is essential.

Antibiotic prophylaxis against infective endocarditis is essential for dental or surgical treatment in all children with congenital heart disease except osteum secundum defects.

All children with congenital heart disease are at risk of bacterial endocarditis.

Clinical features

Endocarditis should be suspected in any child with fever and a significant cardiac murmur. The clinical features are caused by:

- Bacteremia: fever, malaise.
- Valvulitis: cardiac failure and murmurs.
- Immunologic causes: glomerulonephritis.
- Embolic causes: CNS abscess, splinter hemorrhages.

Noncardiac manifestations are less common in children than in adults.

Diagnosis

It is important to stress that endocarditis is a clinical and laboratory diagnosis.

- Blood cultures: at least three should be obtained in the first 24 hours of hospitalization. The causative organism—most commonly *Streptococcus viridans* (α-hemolytic streptococcus)—is identified in 90% of cases.
- Cross-sectional echocardiography: although this may confirm the diagnosis by the identification of vegetations, it cannot exclude it. Vegetations may persist after successful antibiotic treatment has been completed.
- Acute-phase reactants: elevated.

Management

Treatment comprises 4–6 weeks of intravenous antibiotic (e.g., high-dose ampicillin with an aminoglycoside). Surgical removal of infected prosthetic material may be required.

Myocarditis

This uncommon disease primarily affects infants and neonates. Coxsackie and echoviruses, as well as rubella, have been associated with myocarditis. It can present acutely with cardiovascular collapse or slowly with a gradual onset of congestive cardiac failure.

Treatment is supportive. Most children recover but some develop a chronic dilated cardiomyopathy.

Cardiac arrhythmias

Sinus arrhythmia is more pronounced in children and shows as an increase in heart rate during inspiration and slowing during expiration. Normal sinus rhythm can be up to 210 beats/minute and premature atrial and ventricular contractions are common and benign.

Supraventricular tachycardia

The child has a heart rate >220/minute and often is asymptomatic, although infants can develop cardiac failure. An accessory connection can be present in up to 95% of all young children and infants.

Clinical features

Most children are asymptomatic but infants may present with signs of cardiac failure, such as poor feeding, sweating, and irritability. Older children may describe palpitations.

Diagnosis

The ECG usually shows a narrow complex tachycardia with P waves discernible after the QRS complex. In sinus rhythm, the Wolff–Parkinson–White syndrome may be evident if there is an accessory bundle allowing premature activation of the ventricles. The P-R interval is short and there is a wide QRS with slurred upstroke (delta wave).

Management

An acute episode can be terminated and sinus rhythm restored by:
• Vagal stimulation: applying ice-cold compress to the face or carotid sinus massage.
• Intravenous adenosine; safe and effective.
• Synchronized DC cardioversion: if the above fail.

The prognosis is good in the majority of cases. Ninety percent of children will have no further episodes after infancy (over 1 year old). Radiofrequency ablation of the bypass tract has been used for those with persistent, frequently recurring paroxysms.

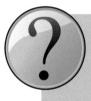

• What are the types of cyanotic congenital heart disease?
• How is a ventricular septal defect managed?
• What are the clinical manifestations of a patent ductus arteriosus?
• How is rheumatic fever diagnosed?
• Who is at risk of endocarditis?
• What are the diagnostic features of endocarditis?
• What is the treatment of supraventricular tachycardia?

Further reading

Ferrieri P et al. Unique features of endocarditis in childhood. *Pediatrics* 2002; 109(5):931–944.

Johnson Jr WH, Moller JH. *Pediatric Cardiology.* Philadelphia: Lippincott Williams & Wilkins, 2001.

14. Disorders of the Respiratory System

Respiratory tract infections are the most common infections of childhood and range from trivial to life-threatening illnesses; 90% of these infections are caused by viruses. They are classified into upper respiratory tract infections (URTIs) and lower respiratory tract infections (LRTIs). The other common and important diseases of this system are asthma and cystic fibrosis.

Children are mores susceptible to respiratory tract infections than adults for many reasons:

- Chest wall is more compliant than that of an adult.
- Fatiguability of respiratory muscles.
- Increased mucous gland concentration.
- Poor collateral ventilation.
- Low chest wall elastic recoil.

Parental smoking should be discouraged because passive smoking worsens symptoms of all respiratory disease.

Upper respiratory tract infections

The upper respiratory tract comprises the ears, nose, throat, tonsils, pharynx, and sinuses, together with the extrathoracic airways.

The common cold (acute nasopharyngitis)

This is a viral infection causing a clear or mucopurulent nasal discharge (coryza), cough, fever, and malaise. Although over 200 viral types are known, 25–40% of colds are caused by rhinoviruses. Symptomatic treatment (e.g., acetaminophen) is all that is required for this self-limiting illness as no known treatment affects clinical outcome. Young infants, who are obligate nose-breathers, may experience feeding difficulties.

Sore throat (pharyngitis and tonsillitis)

These are commonly viral, especially in the under-3-year-olds, but may also be caused by group A β-hemolytic streptococci. Children present with a sore throat, fever, and constitutional upset. It is very difficult to distinguish viral and bacterial infection clinically. However, a purulent exudate, lymphadenopathy, and severe pain suggest a bacterial cause.

Treatment

Most treatment is symptomatic as there is no evidence that antibiotics prevent complications.

Complications

These include:

- Retropharyngeal abscess.
- Peritonsillar abscess.
- Poststreptococcal glomerulonephritis or rheumatic fever.

Tonsillectomy is now less commonly performed than it used to be. Indications include recurrent tonsillitis, or obstructive sleep apnea.

Acute otitis media

The cause of this can be viral—e.g., respiratory syncytial virus (RSV) influenza—or bacterial (*Pneumococcus* species, *Haemophilus influenzae*, group B streptococci, *Moraxella catarrhalis*). It is very common in preschool children, who present with fever, vomiting, and distress. It is important to examine the eardrums in any ill and febrile toddler, as only older children will localize the pain to the ear.

Clinical features

Examination reveals a red eardrum with loss of the light reflex and poor mobility. The eardrum may bulge, and perforation may occur, with a purulent discharge.

Management

Symptomatic treatment is usually all that is needed; amoxicillin can reduce symptoms but not complications.

Recurrent infections are associated with otitis media with effusion. Mastoiditis and meningitis are now uncommon complications of acute otitis media.

Otitis media with effusion (OME, secretory otitis media, glue ear)

In young children who are prone to recurrent upper respiratory tract infections, it is common for the middle ear fluid to persist (an effusion), causing a conductive hearing loss and an increased susceptibility to reinfection. An effusion can also occur without a history of acute infections and is probably due to poor eustachian tube ventilation due to enlarged adenoids or allergy. The effusion and resulting hearing impairment are often transient, but persistence can be an indication for surgical drainage of the middle ear with grommet insertion. A grommet is a hollow plastic tube that ventilates the middle ear and remains effective only while patent. Ultimately it is extruded from the tympanic membrane. Decongestants and antibiotics are widely used but have unproven value. A low-power hearing aid may be required.

Obstructive sleep apnea (OSA)

This is increasingly recognized in children. There is usually a history of snoring and associated apnea. It can be associated with failure to thrive, daytime somnolence, behavioral problems, and poor school performance. Long-term complications include cor pulmonale. Gold standard diagnosis is by polysomnography. Children at high risk of OSA include those with craniofacial abnormalities. Treatment is by adenotonsillectomy with nocturnal continuous positive airway pressure (CPAP) if there is no improvement with surgery.

Croup

Croup, or viral laryngotracheobronchitis, is most commonly caused by the parainfluenza virus. It has a peak incidence in winter in the second year of life.

Clinical features

Symptoms of upper respiratory tract infection (coryza, fever) are usually present for a day or two before the onset of a characteristic barking ("sea lion") cough and stridor (which is caused by subglottic inflammation and edema). Symptoms typically start, and are worse, at night.

Management

Most children are mildly affected and improve spontaneously within 24 hours. Management at home is symptomatic and duration of symptoms 3 days. About 1 in 10 children require hospitalization because of:

- More severe illness.
- Young age (under 12 months).
- Signs of dehydration and fatigue or respiratory failure.

There is evidence that a single dose of dexamethasone, 0.15 mg/kg, or nebulized budesonide, 2 mg, has a beneficial effect in croup. This should be used if stridor is present. Humidifiers and steam therapy are ineffective.

Nebulized adrenaline provides transient improvement by constricting local blood vessels and reducing swelling and edema. It should be given only under close supervision in hospital, where it can provide rapid, if transient, relief of airway obstruction, allowing time for transfer to the intensive care unit (ICU) and intubation in a child with severe airways obstruction.

Diphtheria

This potentially fatal and highly infectious disease is caused by a toxin produced by *Corynebacterium diphtheriae*. In the USA, this infection has been eliminated by an effective immunization program, but it remains endemic in some countries and imported cases occur.

Acute epiglottitis

Acute bacterial epiglottitis is an uncommon life-threatening emergency caused by infection with *Haemophilus influenzae* type B. It has become rare since the introduction of Hib immunization. It is most common in children aged 1–6 years.

Clinical features

The onset is rapid over a few hours with the development of an intensely painful throat. The characteristic picture is of an ill, toxic, febrile child who is unable to speak or swallow, with a muffled voice and soft inspiratory stridor. The child tends to sit upright with an open mouth to maximize the airway, and may drool saliva.

Management

It is vital to distinguish this illness from viral croup because the management is different:

- Minutes count if death is to be avoided.
- Urgent hospital admission should be arranged.
- No attempt should be made to lie the child down, to examine the throat with a tongue depressor, or to take blood, as these maneuvers can precipitate total airway obstruction and death.

Examination under anesthetic should be arranged without delay (preferably in the presence of a senior anesthetist, pediatrician, and ENT surgeon) to allow confirmation of the diagnosis, followed by intubation. Once the airway is secured, blood should be taken for culture and intravenous antibiotics started, using a third-generation cephalosporin (e.g., cefuroxime). Intubation is not usually required for longer than 48 hours.

 Do not examine the throat if epiglottitis is suspected: complete airway obstruction may be provoked.

Lower respiratory tract infections

A minority of infections involve the lower respiratory tract, but these are more likely to be serious than infections of the upper respiratory tract and are more common in infants. Causative agents include viruses and bacteria. They vary with the child's age and the site of infection. Infection can occur by direct spread from airway epithelium or via the bloodstream.

A number of well-defined clinical syndromes (determined by the predominant anatomical site of inflammation) are recognized (e.g., bronchiolitis and pneumonia) and often provide a clue to the likely pathogen. The term "chest infection" should be avoided. The hallmarks of a lower respiratory tract infection are apparent on inspection (Fig. 14.1).

Pneumonia

Pneumonia is characterized by inflammation of the lung parenchyma with consolidation of alveoli. It can be caused by a wide range of pathogens and different organisms affect different age groups (Fig. 14.2).

Clinical features

Usually, following an URTI the patient develops pallor, worsening fever, cough, and breathlessness.

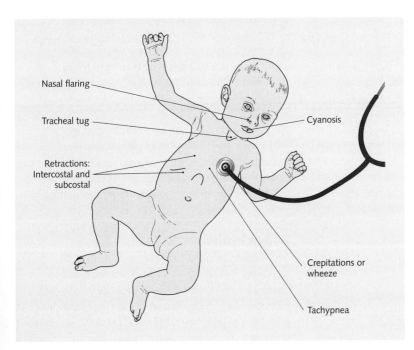

Fig. 14.1 Signs of lower respiratory tract infection in the infant.

Nasal flaring

Tracheal tug

Retractions: Intercostal and subcostal

Cyanosis

Crepitations or wheeze

Tachypnea

Pathogens causing pneumonia in infants and children	
Age	**Pathogens**
Neonates (<1 month)	Group B streptococci E. coli Chlamydia trachomatis
Infants	Respiratory viruses (e.g., RSV, adenovirus) Streptococcus pneumoniae Haemophilus influenzae Bordetella pertusis
Children	Streptococcus pneumoniae Haemophilus influenzae Group A streptococci Mycoplasma pneumonia

Fig. 14.2 Pathogens causing pneumonia in infants and children.

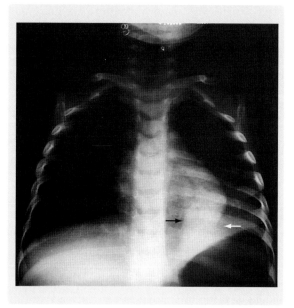

Fig. 14.3 CXR of lobar pneumonia. Consolidation is seen in the lower left lobe obscuring the left hemidiaphragm.

Tachypnea is a key sign. The classic signs of consolidation (dullness to percussion, decreased breath sounds, and bronchial breathing) may be present but they are difficult to detect in infants; crackles may also be present. In bacterial pneumonia, pleural inflammation causing chest (or abdominal) pain and an effusion more commonly develops.

Diagnosis

A chest x-ray (CXR) can help confirm the diagnosis. A complete blood count (CBC), blood culture, and nasopharyngeal aspirate for viral isolation should be carried out in hospitalized children as blood cultures are negative in over 90% of cases.

It is often difficult to distinguish between viral and bacterial infections clinically. Young children and babies are not good providers of sputum and definitive diagnosis of bacterial infection remains difficult. However, the following all suggest bacterial pneumonia:

- Polymorphonuclear leukocytosis.
- Lobar consolidation (Fig. 14.3).
- Pleural effusion.

Mycoplasma infection can be diagnosed reliably by acute and convalescent serology or by demonstration of cold agglutinins.

Management

Antibiotics are usually given if a diagnosis of bacterial pneumonia is made; the choice is dictated by the child's age and the severity of illness (e.g., toxic or requires O_2):

- Amoxicillin is first line in most children.
- Cefuroxime is indicated in severe illness.
- If mycoplasma is suspected, azithromycin should be given.

Rarely, pneumonia can be complicated by empyema, which needs drainage or surgery. Recurrent or persistent pneumonia should raise the possibility of an inhaled foreign object (Fig. 14.4), congenital abnormality of the lung, cystic fibrosis, or tuberculosis.

Bronchiolitis

This common condition is caused by a viral infection mainly RSV. Annual winter epidemics occur in babies aged 1–9 months and many will be hospitalized. The infection causes an inflammatory response, predominantly in the bronchioles; hence the name.

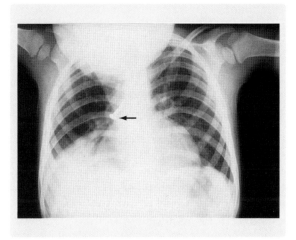

Fig. 14.4 CXR of an inhaled foreign object. Nail seen in the right intermediate bronchus with distal collapse of right middle and lower lobes.

- Bronchiolitis is a common and severe infection in infants in the winter months.
- Oxygen is the most important part of management of bronchiolitis. Little evidence exists for drug or nebulized therapy.

Clinical features

Coryzal symptoms are followed by a cough with increasing breathlessness and associated difficulty in breathing. Small infants may develop apneic episodes. Ex-preterm infants with chronic lung disease and infants with congenital heart disease are at particular risk of being severely affected. Examination reveals:

- Tachypnea.
- Subcostal and intercostal retraction.
- Chest hyperinflation.
- Bilateral fine crackles.
- Wheeze on auscultation.

Infants at high risk of developing severe disease complicated by apneic episodes or respiratory failure include:

- Preterm infants.
- Infants under 6 weeks of age.

Management of bronchiolitis	
Mild	Feeding well Respiratory rate <40/min Minimal intercostal retractions $SpO_2 > 92\%$ in air Manage at home—regular follow-up
Moderate	Difficulty with feeding Moderate tachypnea—rate >40/min Marked intercostal retractions $SpO_2 < 92\%$ on air Admit to hospital O_2 via nasal cannula or head box Fluids intravenously or nasogastrically
Severe	Tachypnea—rate >60/min Recurrent apnea Severe retractions or nasal flaring Hypoxia in air—saturation <92% Admit to ICU High inspired O_2 Intubation and assistive ventilation for respiratory failure or recurrent severe apnea IV fluids

Fig. 14.5 Management of bronchiolitis.

- Infants with chronic lung disease (e.g., cystic fibrosis, bronchopulmonary dysplasia).
- Infants with congenital heart disease.

Diagnosis

The CXR, if taken, usually shows hyperinflation of the lungs. The virus can be detected by immunofluorescence and cultured on a nasopharyngeal aspirate.

Management

Management is supportive with attention to treating hypoxia and maintaining hydration (Fig. 14.5). Breathing (apnea monitor), heart rate, and oxygen saturation (pulse oximeter) are monitored. Oxygen is the mainstay of treatment and is given via nasal cannulas or humidified via a head-box. Some infants may be well enough to continue oral feeds but most require fluids to be given either by nasogastric tube or intravenously. A minority of hospitalized infants require assisted ventilation (only 1–2%). Secondary bacterial infection may occur (<1%), in which case antibiotic therapy is appropriate.

For high-risk infants, a monoclonal antibody (palivizumab) can be given in the winter months to reduce severity.

Complications

Although most infants make a full recovery within 2 weeks, some—especially those hospitalized—have recurrent episodes of cough and wheeze over the subsequent few years. It is known that a subset of these infants will develop asthma.

Whooping cough (pertussis)

Whooping cough or pertussis is a highly contagious clinical syndrome caused by a number of pathogens, most commonly *Bordetella pertussis*. It is endemic, with epidemics occurring every 4 years. An effective vaccine exists and is a component of the routine triple vaccine containing diphtheria, tetanus, and pertussis (DTP).

Whooping cough is spread by droplet infection and has an incubation period of 7–10 days. A case is infectious from 7 days after exposure to 3 weeks after the onset of the paroxysmal cough.

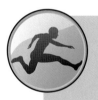

- Whooping cough is most dangerous to very young infants.
- Vaccination is given early to confer protection on this vulnerable group.

Clinical features

The clinical course can be divided into catarrhal, paroxysmal, and convalescent stages.

During a paroxysm of coughing (which is often worse at night) the child may go blue and vomit. The inspiratory whoop can be absent in infants. Nosebleeds and subconjunctival hemorrhage can occur after vigorous coughing. Symptoms can persist for 3 months (the "100-day" cough).

Complications

Complications, including pneumonia, convulsions, apnea, bronchiectasis, and death, are more common in infants under 6 months of age.

Diagnosis

A marked lymphocytosis ($>15.0 \times 10^9$/L) is characteristic, and the organism can be identified by direct fluorescent antibody (DFA) or cultured from a pernasal swab early in the disease.

Treatment

Erythromycin given early in the disease eradicates the organism and reduces infectivity but does not shorten the duration of the disease.

Asthma

Asthma is a chronic inflammatory disorder of the airways associated with widespread variable airflow obstruction and an increase in airways resistance in response to a variety of stimuli. The symptoms are reversible spontaneously or with treatment.

Asthma is the most common chronic respiratory disorder of childhood with a prevalence of 10–15% in the USA. It has increased in prevalence in the past decade and is twice as common in boys as girls. It is also more common among African-Americans and Latinos.

Etiology

Asthma is associated with a number of risk factors.
- Family history or coexistent atopy.
- Male sex.
- Parental smoking.
- Hospitalized for bronchiolitis in infancy.
- Preterm birth.

Pathophysiology

The pathophysiology of airway narrowing in asthma includes chronic inflammation of the bronchial mucosa associated with mucosal edema, secretions, and the constriction of airway smooth muscle (Fig. 14.6).

Diagnosis

A working practical definition is a child with recurrent cough and wheeze in a clinical setting where asthma is likely (e.g., atopy, family history of asthma) and in whom other—rarer—causes (e.g., suppurative lung disease) have been excluded. In most children, a careful history and examination should distinguish those with asthma. Evidence of brochial hyperreactivity by pulmonary function testing is difficult in young children, although children over 7 years may be able to perform spirometry, which can support a diagnosis of asthma.

Conditions that need to be distinguished from asthma are shown in Fig. 14.7.

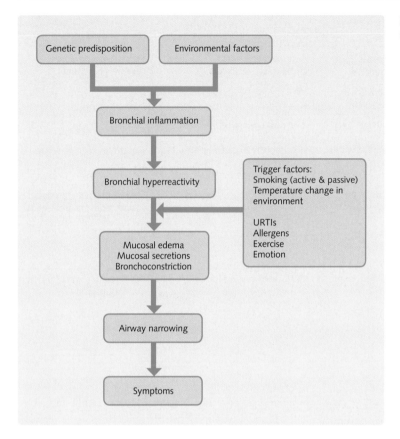

Fig. 14.6 Factors in the pathogenesis of asthma.

Fig. 14.7 Differential diagnosis of asthma.

Differential diagnosis of asthma	
	Clues
Cystic fibrosis	Failure to thrive, productive cough, and finger clubbing
Gastroesophageal reflux	Excessive vomiting
Central airways disease	Inspiratory stridor with wheeze
Laryngeal problems	Abnormal voice
Inhaled foreign body	Sudden onset
Postural wheeze	Recent respiratory infections in children <2 years old without risk factors

History

Inquiry should be made concerning the pattern of symptoms (episodic or persistent), a family history of asthma, trigger factors, and features that allow the clinical evaluation of severity (exercise tolerance, night-time disturbance, school absence). A full history should cover the differential diagnosis (e.g., growth, infections, gastrointestinal symptoms).

There are distinct patterns of asthma in childhood (Fig. 14.8).

Examination

Auscultation of the chest is usually normal between attacks. Chronic, severe asthma is associated with thoracic deformity:

- Hyperexpansion.
- Pigeon chest (pectus carinatum).

107

	Asthma: patterns		
Pattern	Infrequent episodic (mild intermittent)	Frequent episodic (moderate recurrent)	Persistent episodic (severe persistent)
Proportion affected	Most common: 75% of all asthmatics	20%	5%
Clinical features	Triggered by viral URTIs Normal lung function and examination	Exacerbations more severe but mild interval symptoms, especially exercise-induced Abnormal lung function when symptomatic	Daily symptoms and use of bronchodilators Abnormal lung function
Management step	Treat with intermittent bronchodilators and short course of oral steroids for severe exacerbations Step 1	Treat with inhaled steroids ± add-on therapy Steps 2–3	Treat with inhaled steroid with add-on therapy Need specialist advice Steps 4–5
Prognosis	40% remain symptomatic in adulthood	70% remain symptomatic in adulthood	90% remain symptomatic in adulthood

Fig. 14.8 Asthma: patterns.

Investigations

A plain CXR can be useful at initial presentation. In children aged over 5 years, the peak expiratory flow rate (PEFR) can aid diagnosis if the child can carry this out reliably. Significant diurnal variability or decrease after exercise suggests bronchial hyperreactivity. Spirometry in older children may demonstrate reversible airways obstruction. However, in the majority of children a diagnosis is made without lung function testing because this is too difficult to measure in young children; instead, an assessment of the child's response to a treatment is performed.

Allergy tests may indicate evidence of atopy, which is associated with asthma, but 50% of asthmatics are nonatopic.

Differential diagnosis

The differential diagnosis includes several important acute and chronic conditions. It must be remembered that "all that wheezes is not asthma." Alternative diagnoses are listed in Fig. 14.7.

Management

The aim of asthma treatment is to control symptoms and prevent exacerbations, optimize lung function, and keep the side effects of medication to a minimum. Important ways of achieving these goals are:

- An education and management plan for child and carers (The National Heart, Lung, and Blood Institue [NHLBI] guidelines are a useful source of information).
- Establishing the minimal effective dose of preventer medication, especially steroids.
- An age-appropriate delivery device.
- Accurate diagnosis and assessment of severity, with regular follow-up.
- Avoiding triggers.

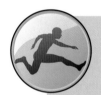

There is a color code for asthma drug inhaler devices:
- "Preventers" are mostly brown (e.g., inhaled steroid). Other colors are purple, green, and orange.
- "Relievers" are blue (e.g., inhaled albuterol, salbutamol).

Triggers of asthma

Although the evidence for allergy avoidance is poor, skin-prick testing or specific IgE may identify allergens and a trial of avoidance may be indicated. Simple measures include:

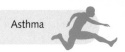

- House-dust mite: frequent vacuuming, damp dusting, and foam filling for duvets and pillows.
- Animals: remove pets from home.

Food allergy is uncommon as a trigger in asthma. Parental smoking should be discouraged.

Medication

The drugs used in the management of asthma in children can be classified into preventers and relievers.

A stepwise approach to treatment has been devised (NHLBI Guidelines for Asthma Management) and is summarized in Fig. 14.9. Patients should start treatment at the step most appropriate to the initial severity. Once control is achieved, treatment can be stepped down. A rescue course of oral prednisolone may be needed at any step (under 1 year old:

1–2 mg/kg/day; 1–5 years: 20 mg/day; maximum dose 40 mg/day). In children with marked seasonal variation in asthma severity, the treatment should be varied according to the season.

Inhalation therapy is central to most asthma treatment. The basic systems available are considered in Figs. 14.10 and 14.11.

The mode of action, indications for use and side effects of the most commonly used bronchodilator drugs are outlined in Fig. 14.12.

Steroid therapy in asthma

Glucocorticoids are key drugs in the management of asthma, both in prophylaxis and the treatment of acute attacks. They can be given:
- By inhalation.
- Orally.
- Intravenously: in acute asthma.

Stepwise management of chronic asthma in children	
Step 1	All asthmatic children should have an inhaled β_2 bronchodilator
Step 2 (if requiring 2–3 times daily inhaled β_2 agonists)	Add low-dose inhaled steroids
Step 3	Try adding long-acting or leukotriene receptor antagonists β_2 agonists before increasing inhaled steroid dose
Step 4 (if increasing steroid dose ineffective)	Consider: Leukotriene receptor antagonist Oral theophylline High-dose inhaled steroid
Step 5	Alternate day oral steroids

Fig. 14.9 Stepwise management of chronic asthma in children.

Administration of medication by inhalation		
	Advantages	**Disadvantages**
Metered-dose inhaler with spacer	Coordination not required Usable at all ages	Bulky
Dry powder inhaler (DPI)	Coordination unimportant Small and portable Easy to operate	Requires rapid inspiration Unsuitable for children <5 years old
Nebulizer	Coordination unimportant Usable at all ages Effective in severe attack	Expensive, noisy, cumbersome Treatment takes a long time: >5 min Frightens some infants

Fig. 14.10 Administration of medication by inhalation.

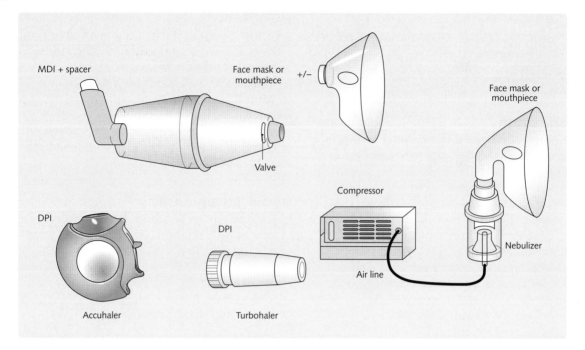

Fig. 14.11 Inhaler devices.

Asthma drug therapy: mode of action, indications, and side effects of bronchodilators			
Relievers (bronchodilators)	**Mode of action**	**Use**	**Side effects**
Short-acting β_2 agonists (e.g., albuterol, terbutaline)	Smooth muscle relaxation	Relief of bronchospasm	Tachycardia Hypokalemia Restlessness
Long-acting β_2 agonists (e.g., salmeterol)	Smooth muscle relaxation	Nocturnal asthma Exercise-induced asthma Trial alternative to high-dose steroids	
Theophylline	Phosphodiesterase inhibition	Oral theophylline for nocturnal asthma, IV aminophylline in acute severe asthma	Restlessness Diuresis Cardiac arrhythmias
Anticholinergics (e.g., ipratropium bromide)	Inhibit cholinergic bronchoconstriction	Add-on to β_2 agonists in acute attacks	Dry mouth Urinary retention

Fig. 14.12 Asthma drug therapy: mode of action, indications, and side effects of bronchodilators.

110

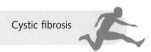

Which inhaler device for which patient?
- MDI: suitable only for competent older children (breath-activated MDIs are available and do not require such a high level of coordination).
- MDI and spacer: beneficial in all children and as effective as nebulizers if used correctly.
- DPI: children from age 5 years.

Inhaled steroids

Inhaled steroids are now the preventers of choice in the management of childhood asthma. The lowest dose that achieves control should be used. They are indicated in frequent interval symptoms, nocturnal asthma, poor lung function tests, and if using bronchodilator more than 3 times a week as rescue treatment. Inhaled steroids:
- Inhibit synthesis of inflammatory mediators (cytokines, leukotrienes, and prostaglandins).
- Reduce airway hyperresponsiveness.
- Reduce both the symptoms and frequency of attacks.
- Prevent irreversible airway narrowing.

Local side effects, such as oral thrush or dysphonia, are uncommon. Ninety percent of the dose is deposited in the mouth and pharynx, but this can be reduced by the use of a spacer (with metered-dose inhalers [MDIs]) and mouth washing (with dry powder inhalers [DPIs]). High doses are associated with decreased growth and adrenal suppression, and children taking inhaled steroids must have their height monitored closely.

Long-acting β_2 agonists

This class of drug can be used as an add-on therapy in children over 4 years of age if control is poor with low-dose inhaled steroids. New combination inhaled steroid and long-acting β_2 agonists are available.

Leukotriene receptor antagonists

This is a new class of drug and can be used as an add-on therapy from infancy.

Theophylline

This can be used in difficult to treat asthma but its use is limited by side effects.

Oral steroids

Prednisolone as a single daily dose is the drug of choice. Short courses (3–5 days) are indicated for acute exacerbations. Regular oral steroids are indicated only for the most severe asthma that cannot be controlled with high-dose inhaled steroids and regular bronchodilators. Alternative day dosage is preferred to reduce systemic side effects.

Acute severe asthma

This is considered in more detail in Chapter 26. Features of acute severe asthma include:
- Respiratory rate >50 breaths/min.
- Pulse >140 beats/min.
- Use of accessory muscles.
- Too breathless to talk.

Life-threatening features include:
- Cyanosis.
- Silent chest (insufficient airflow to generate wheeze).
- Exhaustion, poor respiratory effort.
- Agitation, diminished consciousness (indicate hypoxia).

Immediate management
- High-flow O_2 via facemask.
- Albuterol (2.5–5.0 mg) or terbutaline (5.0–10.0 mg) via MDI space or via an oxygen-driven nebulizer.
- Prednisolone orally or IV hydrocortisone.
- Pulse oximetry: O_2 saturation <92% in air indicates need for hospitalization.

In the presence of life-threatening features (or poor response):
- Intravenous aminophylline or intravenous albuterol.
- Intravenous hydrocortisone.
- Add ipratropium bromide to nebulized β_2-agonist.

Prognosis of asthma

Most children with asthma improve as they get older. Prognosis is better with earlier age at diagnosis. Children with poor pulmonary function testing and frequent wheezy episodes are associated with recurrent wheeze in adulthood.

Cystic fibrosis

Incidence and etiology

Cystic fibrosis (CF) is the most common lethal genetic disease in Caucasian people. It has a carrier rate of 1 : 25 and incidence of 1 : 2500 live births. CF is an autosomal recessive disease arising from mutations in a gene on chromosome 7 that encodes an ATP-binding cassette (ABC) transporter, the cystic fibrosis transmembrane regulator (CFTR) protein. The most common mutation is a three base-pair deletion that removes the phenylalanine at position 508 (ΔF508). This is found in 70% of disease chromosomes, but several hundred different mutations have now been identified.

The mutations in the CFTR result in defective chloride ion transport across epithelial cells and increased viscosity of secretions, especially in the respiratory tract and exocrine pancreas. This predisposes to recurrent chest infections and pancreatic insufficiency. In addition, abnormal transport in sweat gland epithelium results in high concentrations of sodium and chloride in sweat, which form the basis of the most useful diagnostic test, the sweat test.

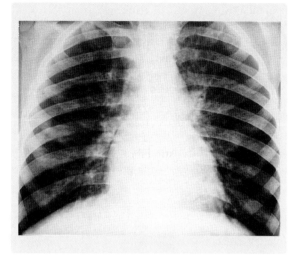

Fig. 14.13 Typical CXR of a child with cystic fibrosis, showing bilateral severe lung pathology: hyperinflated lungs with bronchial wall thickening.

Clinical features

Cystic fibrosis should be considered in any child with recurrent chest infection and failure to thrive. Viscid mucus in the small airways predisposes to infection with *Staphylococcus aureus*, *Haemophilus influenzae*, and *Pseudomonas* species. Repeated infection leads to bronchial wall damage with bronchiectasis and abscess formation.

There is a cough productive of purulent sputum and on examination there may be:

- Hyperinflation.
- Crepitations.
- Wheeze.
- Finger clubbing.

An example of typical chest x-ray changes is shown in Fig. 14.13.

In most children, deficiency of pancreatic enzymes (protease, amylase, and lipase) results in malabsorption, steatorrhea, and failure to thrive. Stools are pale, greasy, and offensive. About 10% of infants with CF present with "meconium ileus" in the neonatal period, in which inspissated meconium causes internal obstruction.

Diagnosis

The gold-standard diagnostic test is the sweat test, using pilocarpine iontophoresis. Failure of the normal reabsorption of sodium and chloride by the sweat duct epithelium leads to abnormally salty sweat:

Multisystem aspects of cystic fibrosis	
Nonpulmonary system	**Symptoms/signs**
Airway	Nasal polyps
Gastrointestinal	Distal ileal obstruction syndrome
Pancreas/endocrine	Cystic fibrosis and diabetes Poor growth Osteoporosis
Reproductive	Infertility in males from absent vas deferens
Joints	Arthropathy
Vascular	Vasculitis
Hepatic	Portal hypertension

Fig. 14.14 Multisystem aspects of cystic fibrosis.

chloride concentrations of 60–125 mmol/L are found (the normal value is <1 5 mmol/L). Two sweat tests showing a chloride of >60 mmol/L confirm CF.

A CF genotype using DNA analysis is also available for the more common mutations and can help confirm a diagnosis.

Management

Cystic fibrosis is a multisystem disease (Fig. 14.14) and management requires a multidisciplinary approach, which is delivered most effectively by a specialist center. The main aims are to:

- Prevent progression of lung disease.
- Promote adequate nutrition and growth.

A team approach is required, involving pediatricians with an interest in CF, physiotherapists, dieticians, CF nurses, community nurses, the primary care team, and last—but not least—the child's parents or caregivers. The Cystic Fibrosis Foundation plays an extremely important role in supporting families.

Cornerstones of CF treatment are:
- Aggressive treatment and prevention of infection.
- Effective mucociliary clearance.
- Nutritional support.
- Exercise.

Respiratory management

Physiotherapy (chest percussion with postural drainage, breathing exercises, positive expiratory pressure [PEP] masks and flutter devices) is the mainstay of respiratory management. Many centers recommend continuous prophylactic antibiotics with oral flucloxacillin in the first 2 years of life and, if children are colonized with *Pseudomonas*, antipseudomonal nebulized antibiotics. Acute exacerbations require vigorous treatment, with IV antibiotics directed against the common bacterial pathogens (*Haemophilus influenzae*, *Staphylococcus aureus*, and *Pseudomonas aeruginosa*) and guided by recent sputum culture results if available. Use of indwelling vascular devices (e.g., Port-A-Cath) aid regular intravenous antibiotic courses.

Mucolytics such as nebulized DNase or hypertonic saline to reduce sputum viscosity can help mucociliary clearance.

Nutritional management

The combined threats of malabsorption due to pancreatic insufficiency, poor appetite, increased metabolism due to chronic infection, and increased respiratory work render nutritional management of vital importance in CF. The following supplements can be given:

- A high-calorie diet with vitamin supplements, especially of fat-soluble vitamins A, D, E, and K.

- Pancreatic enzyme supplementation using enteric-coated microspheres in gelatin-coated capsules (e.g., Pancrease), which contain amylase, lipase and protease. This usually has a marked effect on steatorrhea and allows "catch-up" growth.

Prognosis

The median survival in the USA in the 1990s was 40 years, and this will hopefully improve further. Lung transplantation for some patients is an option but lack of donors mean its role is limited.

Genetic screening

Isolation of the CF gene and identification of the common mutations has made it technically possible to screen newborns for CF and the population in order to identify carriers. However, population screening has associated logistical, ethical, technical, and psychological problems that need to be solved before any national program can be introduced.

The CFTR protein:
- Acts as a cAMP-dependent chloride channel in the apical membranes of epithelial cells.
- Is composed of 1480 amino acid residues.
- Contains functional domains including membrane-spanning regions, ATP-binding domains, and a regulatory domain.
- Is an ATP-binding cassette (ABC) transporter.

Mutations in the CFTR gene:
- The ΔF508 mutation is found on 70% of CF chromosomes.
- A three base-pair deletion causes the loss of the phenylalanine (F) at residue number 508.
- 700 mutations have now been reported in the CFTR gene, but few of these occur at a worldwide frequency of more than 1%.

- How do upper respiratory tract infections present?
- What are the clinical features of acute otitis media?
- How can chronic otitis media with effusion affect child development?
- How is croup differentiated from epiglottitis?
- What are the clinical features of bronchiolitis? How is it different from asthma?
- Describe the management of bronchiolitis.
- What infants are at risk of severe RSV infections?
- How is asthma diagnosed?
- What are the patterns of asthma? How do they correlate with treatment strategy?
- What is the prognosis of asthma?
- Describe the common gene defect in cystic fibrosis.
- What nonrespiratory complications of CF exist?

Further reading

King VJ et al. Pharmacologic treatment of bronchiolitis in infants and children: a systematic review. *Archives of Pediatric and Adolescent Medicine* 2004; 158:127–137.

National Heart, Lung, and Blood Institute (NHLBI) guidelines on the management of asthma.

Spencer H, Jaffe A. Newer therapies for cystic fibrosis. *Current Paediatrics* 2003; 13:259–263.

15. Disorders of the Gastrointestinal System

Both medical and surgical disorders of the gastrointestinal tract are common in pediatric practice. At least 5 million young children die each year from diarrheal diseases.

The range of pathologic processes affecting the gastrointestinal tract is broad. It includes:
- Congenital abnormalities.
- Infection.
- Immune-mediated allergy or inflammation.

Infantile colic

This is a common syndrome characterized by recurrent inconsolable crying or screaming accompanied by drawing up of the legs during the first few months of life. It can occur several times a day, particularly in the evening.

Diagnosis
The differential diagnosis of inconsolable screaming includes some important conditions. Occasionally "colic" may be due to cow's milk protein intolerance or gastroesophageal reflux.

With inconsolable crying in an infant, consider:
- Colic.
- Otitis media.
- Incarcerated hernia.
- Urinary tract infection.
- Anal fissure.
- Intussusception.

Treatment and prognosis
The condition is benign and has a good prognosis, although it may provoke nonaccidental injury in infants at risk. Sympathetic counseling is important. There is no evidence that any medical intervention is effective.

Gastroesophageal reflux

The involuntary passage of gastric contents into the esophagus is a common problem, especially in babies during the first year of life. Functional immaturity of the lower esophageal sphincter, liquid milk rather than solid feeds and a supine posture are all contributory factors. It is a physiologic finding in infancy.

Clinical features
Symptoms are usually mild (regurgitation/spit-up), and no treatment is required. In a minority, however, symptoms are severe and complications such as failure to thrive, esophagitis, or recurrent aspiration pneumonia may occur.

Infants at risk of severe gastroesophageal reflux include:
- Preterm infants: especially those with chronic lung disease (bronchopulmonary dysplasia).
- Children with cerebral palsy.
- Infants with congenital esophageal anomalies (e.g., after repair of a tracheoesophageal fistula).

The main symptom is recurrent regurgitation or vomiting. About 10% of infants with symptomatic reflux develop complications. Esophagitis may be manifested by:
- Irritability.
- Features of pain after feeding.
- Blood in the vomit.
- Iron-deficiency anemia.

Reflux can cause recurrent aspiration pneumonia, failure to thrive, cough, bronchospasm (with wheezing), and exacerbation of chronic lung diseases such as cystic fibrosis or bronchopulmonary dysplasia.

Diagnosis
Most reflux can be diagnosed clinically but several techniques are available for confirming the diagnosis and assessing the severity:

- 24-hour ambulatory esophageal pH monitoring: gold standard in older children but less useful in infants and neonates.
- Barium studies: may be required to exclude underlying anatomic abnormalities.
- Endoscopy: indicated in patients with suspected esophagitis.
- Nuclear medicine milk scan.

In the majority of mildly affected infants, reassurance and the early introduction of solids at 3 months are all that is required and 95% will resolve by the age of 18 months. Nursing the baby in a 30° prone position after feeds can help. Thickening the feed with inert carob-based agents may help some cases.

The following drugs can be used in more severe reflux:

- Prokinetic drugs such as domperidone: these speed gastric emptying and increase lower esophageal sphincter pressure.
- Drugs to reduce gastric acid secretion (H_2 antagonists or proton pump inhibitors): especially if there is evidence of esophagitis.

Surgery is required for very severe cases with complications. The most commonly used procedure is Nissen fundoplication, in which the fundus of the stomach is wrapped around the lower esophagus. This is commonly combined with a gastrostomy for feeding.

Gastroenteritis

Gastroenteritis is an infection of the gastrointestinal tract, usually viral, which presents with a combination of diarrhea and vomiting (D&V).

Incidence and etiology

In developed countries it is usually mild and self-limiting (affecting 1 in 10 children under the age of 2 years), but in the developing world approximately 5 million children under 5 years old die from gastroenteritis each year.

Rotavirus is the most common pathogen in the USA, but gastroenteritis can also be caused by:

- Bacteria, including *Shigellae*, *Salmonellae*, and *Campylobacter* species, and *Escherichia coli*.
- Three parasites: *Entamoeba histolytica*, *Giardia lamblia*, and *Cryptosporidium* species.

Clinical features

Viral infection can cause a prodromal illness followed by vomiting and diarrhea:

- The vomiting may precede diarrhea and is not usually stained with bile or blood.
- Abdominal pain and blood or mucus in the stool suggests an invasive bacterial pathogen.
- The severity of diarrhea can be underestimated if it pools in the large bowel or if a very watery stool is mistaken for urine in the diaper.

On examination, the most important physical signs relate to the presence and severity of dehydration (Fig. 15.1). The high surface area to bodyweight ratio in babies and infants renders them susceptible to rapid derangement of fluid and electrolyte balance.

Diagnosis

The differential diagnosis includes at least two important surgical conditions:

- In young infants, especially boys (aged 2–12 weeks), vomiting may be due to pyloric stenosis. Stool output is reduced and visible peristalsis with a palpable pyloric mass may be evident.
- In older infants and toddlers (aged 1–2 years) intussusception presents with vomiting. Paroxysmal abdominal pain and the eventual passage of "redcurrant jelly" stools should raise suspicion of this condition, which is lethal if overlooked.

Investigations should include:

- Measurement of the BUN and electrolytes if dehydrated.
- Stool culture and microscopy.
- Stool viral antigen detection.

Dehydration can be further classified according to whether the plasma sodium concentration is normal, low (hyponatremia), or high (hypernatremia). This has a bearing on the fluids used for rehydration (see below).

Management
Rehydration

The key to management is rehydration with correction of the fluid and electrolyte imbalance. The strategy depends on the severity of dehydration.

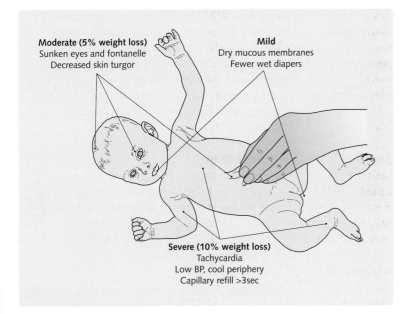

Fig. 15.1 Clinical features of dehydration.

Moderate (5% weight loss)
Sunken eyes and fontanelle
Decreased skin turgor

Mild
Dry mucous membranes
Fewer wet diapers

Severe (10% weight loss)
Tachycardia
Low BP, cool periphery
Capillary refill >3sec

Mild dehydration

Oral rehydration solutions (ORS; e.g., Pedialyte) are used. These contain dextrose to stimulate sodium and water reabsorption across the bowel wall.

Moderate to severe dehydration

Oral rehydration is still indicated if tolerated. IV rehydration should be reserved for those with vomiting or severe dehydration.

 Early refeeding reduces duration of diarrheal illness caused by gastrointestinal infections. IV therapy is overused.

If there are signs of circulatory failure, immediate resuscitation is achieved by intravenous administration of 10–20 mL/kg of 0.9% NaCl (normal saline). Further rehydration can usually be achieved satisfactorily with 5% dextrose/0.45% saline with KCl added at a concentration of 20–40 mmol/L.

The volume required in 24 hours is calculated from estimated deficit, maintenance, and ongoing losses:

Deficit = % dehydration × bodyweight in kg
(1 kg = 1000 mL).

Maintenance.
- 100 mL/kg/24 h for 0–10 kg bodyweight.
- 50 mL/kg/24 h for 10–20 kg bodyweight.
- 20 mL/kg/24 h for >20 kg bodyweight.

Ongoing losses. Estimate the volume of vomit and diarrhea. Calculate the volume required as shown in the following example of a child weighing 10 kg with estimated 10% dehydration:
- Deficit = 10% of 10 kg = 1 kg = 1000 mL.
- Maintenance in 24 h = 100 mL/kg = 1000 mL.
- Total required in 24 h = 2000 mL.

1. Give IV 0.9% NaCl 20 mL/kg over 30 min = 200 mL.
2. Give 1800 mL 5% dextrose/0.18% NaCl over 24 h (i.e., IV infusion at 75 mL/hr).

Medication

There is no role for antiemetic or antidiarrheal medication in gastroenteritis. Antibiotics are rarely indicated except for specific bacterial infections, such as invasive salmonellosis or severe *Campylobacter* infection, and amebiasis or giardiasis.

Pyloric stenosis

Pyloric stenosis is due to hypertrophy of the smooth muscle of the pylorus and is an important cause of vomiting in babies.

117

Incidence

Pyloric stenosis is five times more common in boys and is familial with multifactorial inheritance.

The incidence of pyloric stenosis is 1–5 per 1000 live births:
- It is more common in boys.
- It causes a metabolic alkalosis.
- Surgical treatment is by pylorotomy.

Clinical features

It presents with persistent, projectile nonbilious vomiting between 2 and 6 weeks of age (it does not occur in the newborn or beyond 3 months of age). The infant remains hungry and eager to feed after vomiting. Weight loss, constipation, mild jaundice, and dehydration develop after a few days (Fig. 15.2).

Diagnosis

Diagnosis is clinical and made by palpation of the hypertrophied pylorus during a test feed. Peristaltic waves may be visible.

Ultrasound of the abdomen can confirm diagnosis, demonstrating the hypertrophied pylorus. In addition, a characteristic electrolyte disturbance develops with a hypochloremic metabolic alkalosis (serum HCO_3^- elevated to 25–35 mEq/L). This is due to the loss of acidic gastric contents and the kidneys excreting hydrogen ions to maintain potassium.

Management

The definitive treatment is pylorotomy, in which the hypertrophied pyloric musculature is divided. This is not an emergency procedure, and it is vital to correct the dehydration and biochemical abnormality with IV fluid therapy before anesthesia and surgery are undertaken.

Intussusception

Intussusception is a condition in which one segment of bowel telescopes into an adjacent distal part of the bowel. It most commonly begins just proximal to the ileocecal valve (ileum invaginates into cecum-ileocolic). The peak age is between 6 and 9 months, when the lead point is believed to be Peyer's patches that have been enlarged by a preceding viral infection. An anatomical lead point,

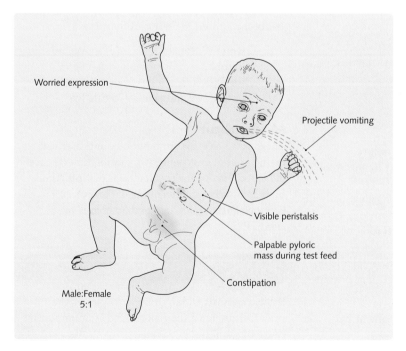

Fig. 15.2 Clinical features of pyloric stenosis.

Worried expression

Projectile vomiting

Visible peristalsis

Palpable pyloric mass during test feed

Constipation

Male:Female 5:1

such as a Meckel's diverticulum or polyp, is more likely to be present in an older child.

Clinical features

The classic presenting triad is:
- Colicky abdominal pain.
- Vomiting.
- An abdominal mass.

The typical history is of episodes of screaming during which the infant draws up the legs and becomes pale. Vomiting occurs and the vomit may be bile-stained. As the blood supply to the bowel becomes progressively compromised, the characteristic "redcurrant jelly" stool will be passed; this is a late sign.

Suspect intussusception if there is:
- An infant aged 6–9 months.
- Paroxysmal colicky abdominal pain.
- Vomiting.
- "Redcurrant jelly" stool.
- A "sausage-shaped" mass in right upper quadrant.

Examination may reveal a "sausage-shaped" mass formed by the intussusceptum, which is usually palpable in the right upper quadrant. Signs of intestinal obstruction and shock develop over 24–48 hours. Ultrasound is the imaging modality of choice.

Management

Intussusception is a life-threatening condition and can easily be misdiagnosed as gastroenteritis or colic by the unwary. If suspected, an immediate diagnostic enema using air or contrast material (barium or gastrograffin) should be carried out.

In most cases, reduction by air enema is possible, however if this is unsuccessful, operative reduction is necessary.

Enema and attempts at hydrostatic reduction are contraindicated if the history is long (24–48 hours) or if there are signs of intestinal obstruction, peritonitis, or shock.

Meckel's diverticulum

This remnant of the fetal vitello-intestinal duct occurs in 2% of the population. It is usually 2 inches (5 cm) long and found 2 feet (60 cm) proximal to the ileocecal valve (the rule of 2s). It contains ectopic gastric mucosa. Diagnosis is by a technetium scan. The majority are asymptomatic but the most typical presentation is painless, severe rectal bleeding due to peptic ulceration. Treatment is surgical.

Acute appendicitis

This important cause of acute abdominal pain occurs when the appendix becomes obstructed (usually by a fecolith) or inflamed by lymphatic hyperplasia. It occurs at any age, although it is rare in infants when the lumen of the appendix is wider and well drained.

Clinical features

The classic symptoms are a central abdominal pain that moves to the right iliac fossa (RIF) over a period of hours. The pain is of increasing severity and aggravated by movement (as the peritoneum is exquisitely pain sensitive).

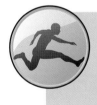

Atypical presentations with poorly localized pain are common in young children (<5 years) or when the inflamed appendix is retrocecal or pelvic.

Anorexia is usual and often associated with nausea and vomiting. Constipation may be a feature. Clinical signs include:
- Mild fever.
- Tachycardia.
- Dehydration.
- RIF tenderness.
- Guarding in a toxic child.

The differential diagnosis is shown in Fig. 15.3.

The differential diagnosis of acute abdominal pain	
Surgical	**Medical**
Appendicitis	Mesenteric adenitis
Intussusception	Gastroenteritis
Meckel's diverticulum	UTI
Strangulated hernia	Lower lobe pneumonia
Ovarian torsion	Diabetic ketoacidosis
	Henoch–Schönlein purpura
	Sickle-cell crisis

Fig. 15.3 The differential diagnosis of acute abdominal pain.

Diagnosis

The diagnosis is usually made clinically. If there is diagnostic uncertainty, useful investigations include:
- Urine: microscopy and culture.
- Complete blood count (CBC).
- Chest x-ray (CXR): pneumonia can mimic appendicitis.
- Abdominal ultrasound.

Management

A short period of observation can be undertaken before appendectomy when there is uncertainty, although progression to peritonitis can occur within a few hours in young children.

Other complications include septicemia, appendix abscess, and appendix mass. An abscess requires surgical drainage. Conservative management is given for an appendix mass with elective appendectomy carried out 6 weeks later.

Mesenteric adenitis

This nonspecific inflammation of mesenteric lymph nodes is thought to provoke a peritoneal reaction causing acute abdominal pain that mimics appendicitis.

Clinical features

It occurs commonly in children and is often associated with other systemic symptoms and signs including fever, headache, pharyngitis, and cervical lymphadenopathy. It is likely to be viral in origin.

Diagnosis and management

Observation in hospital is often required due to the difficult diagnosis. Management is conservative, as the symptoms are self-limiting, although persisting right iliac fossa tenderness warrants surgical exploration to identify appendicitis.

Celiac disease

Incidence and etiology

Celiac disease arises from malabsorption caused by gluten-mediated immunological damage to the mucosa of the proximal small intestine with subsequent atrophy of the villi and loss of the absorptive surface. The incidence varies between 1 in 250 and 1 in 4000 live births, and appears to be increasing in some areas of the world.

There is a familial predisposition with 10% of first-degree relatives affected. There appear to be associations with HLA DQ2.

Clinical features

A few children present with failure to thrive following weaning when gluten-containing foods are introduced to the diet. Malabsorption of fat (steatorrhoea) occurs first, with bulky, light-colored, offensive stools. On examination, there is:
- Poor weight gain.
- Abdominal distention.
- Buttock wasting.

The majority of cases present with more subtle problems such as:
- Diarrhea.
- Transient poor weight gain.
- Irritability.
- Growth failure.
- Ataxia.
- Anemia due to iron or folate deficiency: this is the most common symptom.

Diagnosis

Specific IgA antigliadin or antiendomysial antibodies are useful as a screening test. Definitive diagnosis requires the demonstration of a flat mucosa on jejunal biopsy followed by clinical improvement on dietary gluten withdrawal. A third biopsy on gluten challenge should be then taken to confirm the diagnosis.

Management

A diet free of gluten-containing products should be adhered to for life. Dietary supervision is required. Manufacturers use a special sign on packaging to indicate that food is gluten-free.

Celiac disease is associated with a variety of autoimmune disorders, including thyroid disease and pernicious anemia, and the risk of small bowel malignancy (especially lymphoma) is increased 20-fold. A strict gluten-free diet may protect against this risk of malignancy and decrease the risk of autoimmune disease.

Food intolerance

Adverse reactions to specific foods or food ingredients are not uncommon and can be transitory or permanent. The majority are immune-mediated reactions, usually to proteins, and are properly referred to as food allergies. However, non-immune-mediated intolerance also occurs, e.g. lactose intolerance due to intestinal disaccharidase deficiency.

Transient dietary protein intolerances

These are more common in infants with a strong family history of atopy or IgA deficiency. They are most commonly manifested by protracted diarrhea with or without vomiting and failure to thrive. However, allergy to specific proteins may also play a role in eczema and migraine and, occasionally, can cause acute anaphylaxis.

Intolerance to the following foods has been described:
- Cow's milk.
- Soy.
- Wheat.
- Fish, egg, chicken, and rice.
- Nuts.

Diagnosis

Diagnosis is made when the symptoms are relieved by removal of specific foods or food constituents, and recur on reintroduction.

Management

Cow's milk protein intolerance, if severe, can cause a protein-losing enteropathy and blood loss. It is best managed with a casein-hydrolysate-based formula as up to 30% of infants will also be, or will become,

intolerant to soy. Most patients grow out of their intolerance by the age of 2 years, which is therefore an appropriate time to conduct a dietary challenge.

Lactose intolerance

Lactose is the predominant disaccharide in milk and requires the intestinal brush-border enzyme lactase for its digestion. Lactase deficiency is most commonly encountered as a secondary and transient phenomenon after gastroenteritis. Congenital lactase deficiency is rare; hereditary late-onset lactose intolerance is predominantly seen in African-American and Asian people.

Clinical features

Accumulation of intestinal sugar results in watery diarrhea and bacterial production of organic acids, which lowers stool pH and causes excoriation of the perianal region.

Diagnosis

Lactose is a reducing sugar and may therefore be detected in the stool by the Clinitest method.

Treatment

Treatment is with a diet free of products containing lactose and milk.

Inflammatory bowel disease

Up to one-quarter of cases of inflammatory bowel disease have their onset during childhood or adolescence.

Crohn's disease

Crohn's disease, or regional enteritis, is a transmural and focal inflammatory process that can affect any portion of the gastrointestinal tract from the mouth to the anus; the distal ileum or the colon are most frequently involved. The cause is unknown, although there is a clear genetic predisposition. Affected intestine is thickened and noncaseating epithelioid cell granulomata are found on histology.

Ulcerative colitis

Ulcerative colitis is a chronic, recurrent inflammatory disease involving the mucous membrane of the colon. The disease process is restricted to the mucosa and begins in the rectum, extending proximally.

Clinical features of inflammatory bowel disease

It presents with:

- Cramping lower abdominal pain.
- Bloody diarrhea.
- Weight loss/failure to thrive.

Extraintestinal features may be present, including growth retardation, delayed puberty, arthritis, spondylitis, and erythema nodosum.

Management

Crohn's disease is managed initially by dietary measures with steroids for active relapse. Elemental diets are as effective as steroids but without the side effects. Immunosuppressives are the next line, and new therapies such as anti-TNF antibodies are used routinely. Surgery remains an option for failure of medical treatment.

Ulcerative colitis is treated with the aminosalicylates with steroids reserved for active disease. Surgery is curative but requires a colectomy. The role of probiotics is under study.

Hirschsprung's disease (congenital aganglionic megacolon)

This is a rare genetic disorder of bowel innervation. There is an absence of ganglion cells in the myenteric and submucosal plexuses for a variable segment of bowel extending from the anus to the colon. The aganglionic segment is narrow and contracted. It ends proximally in a normally innervated and dilated colon. It is more common in males.

Clinical features

Infants with the disease usually present in the neonatal period with:

- Delayed passage of meconium (>48 hours of life).
- Subsequent intestinal obstruction with bilious vomiting and abdominal distention.

Enterocolitis is a severe, life-threatening complication.

Older children present with:

- Chronic, severe constipation present from birth.
- Abdominal distention.
- An absence of feces in the narrow rectum.

Diagnosis and management

A unprepped barium enema may demonstrate a transition zone where the bowel lumen changes in diameter. Confirmation of the diagnosis is made by demonstrating the absence of ganglion cells on a suction biopsy of the rectum. Surgical resection of the involved colon is required. An initial colostomy is usually followed by a definitive pull-through procedure to anastomose normally innervated bowel to the anus.

Bile duct obstruction

Obstruction of bile flow due to biliary atresia or a choledochal cyst are rare, but treatable, causes of persistent neonatal jaundice. Early recognition and diagnosis of these liver diseases is important.

Biliary atresia

This is a rare disorder of unknown etiology in which there is either destruction or absence of the extrahepatic biliary tree. It represents a rare but important cause of persistent neonatal jaundice (Fig. 15.4).

Clinical features

The jaundice persists from the second day after birth and is distinguished by being due to a predominantly conjugated hyperbilirubinemia accompanied by dark urine and pale stools. As the disease progresses there is failure to thrive due to:

- Malabsorption.
- Enlargement of the liver and spleen.

A bleeding tendency may develop due to vitamin K deficiency.

Diagnosis

Abdominal ultrasound, liver biopsy, and intraoperative cholangiography may be required to clarify the diagnosis.

Treatment

Treatment consists of the Kasai procedure (hepatoportoenterostomy), which should ideally be carried out before the age of 6 weeks. Liver transplantation is needed if this fails or if presentation is late. Even with treatment, prognosis is poor.

Liver disease presenting in the newborn period: causes of unconjugated hyperbilirubinemia	
Bile duct obstruction	Biliary atresia Choledochal cyst
Neonatal hepatitis	Congenital infection Inborn errors: α_1 antitrypsin deficiency Galactosemia

Fig. 15.4 Liver disease presenting in the newborn period: causes of conjugated hyperbilirubinemia.

Constipation

Functional constipation is an increasingly common condition and presents as infrequency in stooling, difficulty in bowel movements, and stool retention. It is important to distinguish this from Hirschprung's disease in that vomiting is unusual, it occurs during toilet training, stool palpable in rectal vault, and soiling commonly occurring.

Note that functional constipation is not associated with abdominal pain and treatment is often prolonged with stool softeners and stimulant laxatives. Psychological help is often sought for difficult cases.

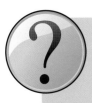

- How is gastroenteritis treated?
- What investigations are useful in gastroesophageal reflux?
- How do you manage a child with colic?
- What are the diagnostic features of pyloric stenosis?
- Describe the classic features of intussusception.
- What is the differential diagnosis of acute appendicitis?
- How is Hirschprung's disease differentiated from simple constipation?
- What are the long-term complications of celiac disease and how are they managed?
- How is inflammatory bowel disease treated?

Further reading

King AL, Ciclitira PJ. Celiac disease. *Current Opinion in Gastroenterology* 2000; 16:102–106.

16. Renal and Genitourinary Disorders

Structural abnormalities of the kidney and urinary tract are common and many are now identified on antenatal ultrasound screening. The most common disease encountered in this system is urinary tract infection, which has special significance because of its potential to damage the growing kidneys, leading to hypertension and chronic renal failure.

Presentation of urinary tract anomalies:
- Urinary tract infection.
- Recurrent abdominal pain.
- Palpable mass.
- Hematuria.
- Failure to thrive.

Urinary tract anomalies

Congenital abnormalities of the kidneys and urinary tract can be identified in about 1 in 400 fetuses. They may be detected on antenatal ultrasound screening or present with a variety of symptoms and signs in infancy or later childhood.

Congenital anomalies of the urinary tract include:
- Renal anomalies.
- Obstructive lesions of the urinary tract.
- Vesicoureteral reflux.

Renal anomalies

Absence of both kidneys (renal agenesis) results in Potter syndrome in which oligohydramnios (caused by lack of fetal urine) is associated with lung hypoplasia and postural deformities. Other anomalies include:
- Abnormalities of ascent and rotation.
- Duplex kidney (Fig. 16.1).
- Horseshoe kidney (Fig. 16.1).
- Cystic disease of the kidney.
- Renal dysplasia.

Ectopia of the kidney is common, and pain arising from an ectopic kidney can be misleading on account of its site.

Duplex systems are commonly associated with other abnormalities such as renal dysplasia and vesicoureteral reflux. The upper pole ureter may be ectopic (draining into the urethra or vagina) and the lower pole ureter often refluxes.

There are many conditions associated with cystic kidneys, including:
- Autosomal recessive infantile polycystic kidney disease.
- Autosomal dominant adult-type polycystic kidney disease.
- Tuberous sclerosis.

Obstructive lesions of the urinary tract

The site of obstruction may be at the pelvic-ureteral (PU) junction, the vesicoureteral (VU) junction, the bladder, or the urethra (Fig. 16.2). If undetected before birth, the patient can present with:
- A urinary tract infection.
- Abdominal or groin pain.
- Hematuria.
- A palpable bladder or kidney.

Pelvic-ureteral obstruction (congenital hydronephrosis)

Obstruction is caused by a narrow lumen or compression by a fibrous band or blood vessel, and can vary in degree from partial to almost complete obstruction (with gross hydronephrosis and minimal remaining renal tissue).

Mild degrees of obstruction can resolve spontaneously but severe obstruction requires surgical treatment with conservation of renal tissue wherever possible.

Antenatal hydronephrosis is commonly seen and often resolves after birth, but urgent investigation is indicated if hydronephrosis is bilateral because it may indicate urethral obstruction.

125

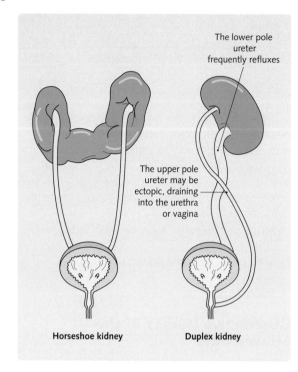

Fig. 16.1 Urinary tract anomalies.

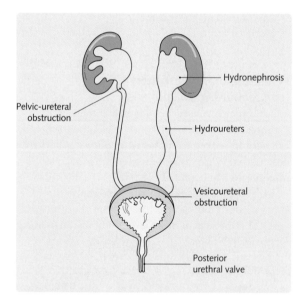

Fig. 16.2 Sites of urinary tract obstruction and dilatation.

Vesicoureteral obstruction

Obstruction can be due to stenosis and kinking or dilatation of the lower part of the ureter (ureterocele) and can be unilateral or bilateral. There is a combination of hydroureter and hydronephrosis.

Posterior urethral valves

These are abnormal folds of the urethral mucous membrane, which occur in males in the region of the verumontanum. They impede the flow of urine with back-pressure on the bladder, ureters, and kidneys. The degree of obstruction varies from the very severe (with death in utero from renal failure or after birth from Potter syndrome) to the less severe (which usually presents with urinary tract infection, poor urinary stream and renal insufficiency in a male).

Vesicoureteral reflux

Primary vesicoureteral reflux (VUR) is caused by a developmental anomaly of the vesicoureteral junction. The ureters enter directly into the bladder, rather than at an angle and the segment of ureter within the bladder wall is abnormally short. Urine refluxes up the ureter during voiding, predisposing to infection and exposing the kidneys to bacteria and high pressure. There is a spectrum of severity which is graded I–V (Fig. 16.3).

Clinical features

VUR is often associated with other genitourinary anomalies and may be secondary to bladder pathology (e.g., neuropathic bladder). The important consequences of VUR include:
- Predisposition to urinary tract infection.
- Urinary tract infection and pyelonephritis.
- Reflux nephropathy: this is destruction of renal tissue with scarring due to infection and back-pressure. If severe, it may result in high blood pressure and chronic renal failure.

Diagnosis

VUR is diagnosed by a voiding cystourethrogram (VCUG).

Management

Mild VUR resolves spontaneously (10% each year) but prophylactic antibiotics (e.g., trimethoprim) are given to prevent infection until the child:

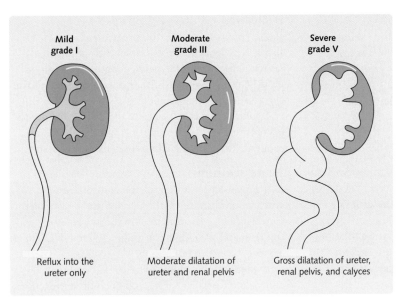

Fig. 16.3 Grades of vesicoureteral reflux.

Mild grade I	Moderate grade III	Severe grade V
Reflux into the ureter only	Moderate dilatation of ureter and renal pelvis	Gross dilatation of ureter, renal pelvis, and calyces

- Is free of infection.
- Has regained normal bladder control.
- Is older than 5 years.

Surgery is indicated if prophylaxis fails and the VUR is in grades IV or V. The siblings of children should be investigated.

Genitalia

Inguinoscrotal disorders
Inguinoscrotal disorders include:
- Undescended testis.
- Inguinal hernia and hydrocele.
- Acute scrotum.

Undescended testis
The testes develop intra-abdominally and migrate through the inguinal canal to the scrotum in the third trimester. The testes are therefore normally in the scrotum in term newborns but are frequently undescended in preterm infants.

Clinical features and examination
A testis that has not reached the scrotum (undescended testis) may be:
- Incompletely descended: lying along normal pathway (the minority, 20%).
- Maldescended or ectopic: deviated from the normal path after emerging from the superficial inguinal ring (the majority, 80%).

An undescended testis must be distinguished from a "retractile" testis that can be coaxed down into the scrotum. (Examination should be undertaken in a warm room with warm hands.)

The testes are examined during routine surveillance in the newborn, at 6 weeks, and at each well-child visit. Referral to a surgeon should be made if either testis is impalpable or an ectopic testis is found at the 6-week check.

Further investigations are helpful if one or both testes are impalpable to determine their existence and location. These can include:
- Ultrasound.
- Magnetic resonance imaging.
- Laparoscopy.
- Endocrine investigations.

The testes may be absent in cases of intersex.

Management
Treatment is by orchidopexy and this is best performed between the age of 1 and 2 years. Potential, but unproven, benefits include:
- Reduced risk of torsion.
- Psychological and cosmetic benefits.
- Reduced risk of malignancy.
- Improved fertility.

Orchidectomy is indicated for a unilateral intra-abdominal testis that is not amenable to orchidopexy.

127

Inguinal hernias and hydroceles

The testis descends into the scrotum, taking with it a connecting fold of peritoneum (the processus vaginalis), which normally becomes obliterated at or around birth. Failure of the processus vaginalis to close results in an inguinal hernia or a hydrocoele (Fig. 16.4).

Inguinal hernias

Inguinal hernias are more common in boys, premature babies, and infants, with a positive family history. A minority are bilateral. The parents notice an intermittent swelling in the groin or scrotum.

The main concern is the risk of strangulation, which is higher in young infants. Referral for prompt surgery is indicated. Danger signs in the initially irreducible hernia are:
- Hardness.
- Tenderness.
- Vomiting.

These suggest entrapment of bowel within the sac and compromise of its vascular supply (strangulation). Urgent referral is imperative.

Sedation, analgesia, and expert manipulation allow reduction, which is followed by surgical repair.

Hydroceles

If the connection with the processus vaginalis is small, a hydrocele forms rather than an inguinal hernia. The swelling is painless and, being full of fluid, it transilluminates. It is possible to get above the swelling, which cannot be reduced.

Spontaneous resolution by the age of 12 months is common and treatment during infancy is not required unless the hydrocele is extremely large.

Acute scrotum

Acute pain and swelling of the scrotum are an emergency because of the possibility of testicular torsion. Acute scrotum occurs most frequently in the neonatal period and at puberty but can occur at any age.

Inadequate fixation to the tunica vaginalis allows the testis to rotate and occlude its vascular supply. Doppler studies can assist in diagnosis.

Surgical exploration must not be delayed, as the testis may become nonviable. The defect is often bilateral, so the contralateral testis should also be fixed at surgery.

The differential diagnosis includes:
- Tosion of the testicular appendix (hydatid of Morgagni).
- Epididymo-orchitis.
- Idiopathic scrotal edema.

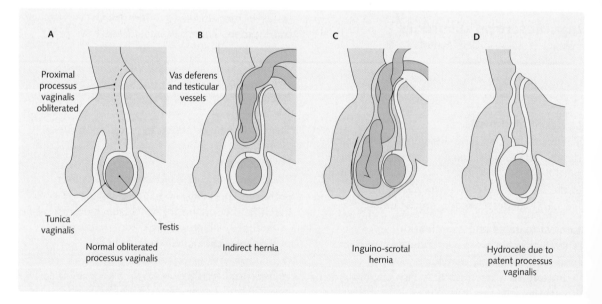

Fig. 16.4 (A) The normal testis. Following normal testicular descent, the processus vaginalis, an evagination of the parietal peritoneum between the internal inguinal ring and testis, disappears leaving only the tunica vaginalis around the testis. Persistence of the processus vaginalis results in an inguinal hernia (B, C), or a hydrocele (D).

Penile abnormalities

Penile abnormalities include:
- Hypospadias.
- Phimosis.

Hypospadias

A spectrum of congenital abnormalities of the position of the urethral meatus occurs. Severe forms are associated with chordee, a ventral curvature of the penis.

Phimosis

This refers to adhesion of the foreskin to the glans penis after the age of 3 years. Mild degrees can be managed with periodic, gentle retraction. Paraphimosis is irreducible retraction of the foreskin beyond the coronal sulcus.

Circumcision

Nonretractility of the foreskin and preputial adhesions are normal in small boys and forcible attempts to retract the foreskin are ill-advised because this may result in scarring and phimosis.

Ballooning of the prepuce during urination is not uncommon and usually resolves as the prepuce becomes more retractile.

Balanitis xerotica obliterans (lichen sclerosus) causes a thickened, scarred, white prepuce that is fixed to the glans. This, recurrent balanitis (infection of the glans), and sometimes recurrent urinary tract infection (UTI) are the only medical indications for circumcision. Most circumcisions are performed for religious reasons.

Complications of circumcision
- Hemorrhage.
- Infection.
- Damage to the glans.

The procedure should not be undertaken lightly. An infant with hypospadias must *not* be circumcised because the foreskin is used at surgical correction.

Vulvovaginitis

Inflammation of the vulva and vaginal discharge is a common gynecologic complaint in prepubertal girls. Poor hygiene and tight-fitting clothes have *not* been shown to be predisposing factors. A vulval swab may detect a yeast or streptococcal infection, which can be treated with the appropriate topical or oral therapy. It is important to think of foreign bodies if a persistent discharge is seen. Rarely, vulvovaginitis results from sexual abuse.

Urinary tract infection

Infection of the urinary tract is common in children. About 3–5% of girls and 1–2% of boys will have a symptomatic UTI during childhood; boys outnumber girls until 3 months of age.

In children, most infections are caused by *Escherichia coli* originating from the bowel flora. Other pathogens include *Proteus* (especially in boys), *Klebsiella*, *Pseudomonas*, and *Enterococcus* species. The most common host factor predisposing to UTI is urinary stasis. Important causes of urinary stasis include:
- Vesicoureteral reflux (VUR).
- Obstructive uropathy (e.g., ureterocoele, urethral valve).
- Neuropathic bladder (e.g., spina bifida).
- Habitual infrequent voiding and constipation.

UTIs occur:
- Predominantly in boys up to age of 3 months.
- Equally in boys and girls from 3 to 12 months.
- Increasingly in girls rather than boys after age 1 year.
- UTI presents with nonspecific features in infants.
- UTI must be suspected in any febrile infant with no obvious clinical source.

Clinical features

The clinical features vary markedly with age:
- In neonates and very young infants: jaundice may occur and septicemia can develop, rapidly leading to shock and hypotension.
- In infants: UTI can occur, with or without fever, and symptoms are nonspecific; vomiting, diarrhea, irritability, failure to thrive.
- Between 1 and 5 years of age: fever, malaise, abdominal discomfort, urinary frequency, and nocturnal enuresis are the presenting features. In this age group, dysuria may also be due to balanitis or vulvovaginitis.

- Over 5 years of age: the classic presenting features of cystitis (frequency, dysuria, fever, and enuresis) or pyelonephritis (fever and groin pain) occur. Asymptomatic bacteriuria is common in school-age girls. This does not need treatment.

Diagnosis

Confirmation of diagnosis requires culture of a pure growth of a single pathogen of at least 10^8 colony-forming units per liter of urine. However, obtaining an uncontaminated urine sample from infants and children is not always easy (Fig. 16.5). Specimens should be chilled without delay to 4°C (i.e., refrigerate) to prevent bacterial multiplication.

A positive nitrite and leucocyte esterase stick test is a reliable test for coliform infection, but false negatives occur if the urine has been in the bladder for less than an hour or the organism does not convert nitrate (e.g., enterococci).

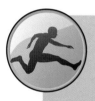

A urine sample should be cultured from:
- An infant with a fever and no obvious clinical source.
- Any child with recurrent or prolonged fever.
- Any child with unexplained abdominal pain.
- Any child with dysuria or frequency, enuresis, or hematuria.

Treatment of the acute infection

Prompt treatment with antibiotics is indicated to reduce the risk of renal scarring. This should be initiated as soon as a urine sample has been taken for culture. Treatment can be modified when urine culture results are available and stopped if the culture is negative.

Antibiotic choice

- Oral trimethoprim is a suitable initial choice for uncomplicated UTI in an older child but increasing microbial resistance is becoming a problem.
- Parenteral antibiotics (e.g., ampicillin plus gentamicin or cefuroxime) should be given to neonates, any systemically unwell older child, and to children with signs of acute pyelonephritis or a known urinary tract abnormality.
- Prophylactic antibiotics should be given in low dose after treatment of the acute infection, until investigation of the urinary tract is complete.

Further investigation

All children require further imaging of their urinary tract after a first confirmed UTI. The aim of this is to identify:

- Any predisposing underlying anatomic or functional abnormality of the urinary tract such as vesicoureteral reflux.
- Renal scars.

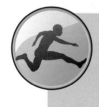

All children require further investigation after a first confirmed UTI to identify anatomic or functional abnormalities and renal scars.

Collecting a urine sample	
Method	Indication
Suprapubic aspirate	All babies under 6 months if an urgent or reliable sample is required
Bag or pad sample	Nonurgent samples or outpatient use
Clean catch	Older, more cooperative children
Catheter	Only fresh samples valid for infection

Fig. 16.5 Collecting a urine sample.

Although the outcome for the majority of infants and children with UTI is benign, a small minority are at risk of renal damage, especially those with recurrent infection associated with vesicoureteral reflux.

The exact scheme depends on the age of the child. No single imaging investigation provides a full assessment.

An initial ultrasound of the kidneys and urinary tract is performed on all infants and young children. A renal ultrasound scan is valuable for:

- Demonstrating the presence of two kidneys.
- Identifying obstruction with urinary tract dilatation.

It is not reliable for detecting renal scars or vesicoureteral reflux.

Infants aged under 1 year

In addition to ultrasonography, recommendations include:

- Voiding cystourethrogram (VCUG), to identify vesicoureteral reflux.
- Static radioisotope scan (DMSA), to identify renal scars.

These investigations are deferred until 3 months after the acute infection to avoid detecting transient abnormalities. Prophylactic antibiotics should be given in the interim.

Children aged between 1 and 5 years

Ultrasonography and a radioisotope scan are recommended. VCUG can be reserved for:

- Children in whom the radioisotope scan shows an abnormality.
- Children with recurrent infection.
- Children with a family history of reflux or reflux nephropathy.

The risk of developing renal scarring becomes less with increasing age and is uncommon with infection in children over 5 years of age.

Simple advice should be given concerning measures, which can reduce recurrence risk, including:

- High fluid intake.
- Regular unhurried voiding.
- Lactobacilli, cranberry juice.
- Good perineal hygiene.

Children with recurrent UTI or scarring require regular follow-up with a repeat urine culture, blood pressure monitoring, and further renal imaging to check for new scar formation and resolution of vesicoureteral reflux.

Acute nephritis

Acute nephritis is a clinical condition caused by inflammatory changes in the glomeruli. It is characterized by:

- Fluid retention (edema, hypertension).
- Hypertension.
- Hematuria.
- Proteinuria.

The majority of cases are postinfectious and follow a streptococcal throat or skin infection with group A β-hemolytic streptococci. Less common causes include:

- Henoch–Schönlein purpura.
- IgA nephropathy.
- Systemic lupus erythematosus (SLE).
- Mesangiocapillary glomerulonephritis.

Clinical features

The presenting history will be of discolored "smoky" urine. Physical examination reveals signs of fluid overload such as edema and raised blood pressure.

Diagnosis

The urine is positive for blood and protein, and microscopy may reveal red cells and casts. Renal function should be evaluated by measuring plasma urea, electrolytes, and creatinine.

An abdominal x-ray and ultrasound may be required to exclude other causes of hematuria.

The etiology is pursued with a throat swab, anti-DNAase B, complement C3 levels, and biopsy if severe.

Management

Management centers on:

- Control of fluid and electrolyte balance by monitoring intake and output.
- Use of diuretics and antihypertensives as required.

The prognosis of poststreptococcal nephritis is good. However, rarely, a rapidly progressive glomerulonephritis with renal failure occurs, especially in nephritis from other causes. No evidence that treatment of the preceding infection prevents renal complications.

Nephrotic syndrome

The nephrotic syndrome is a clinical condition characterized by heavy proteinuria, edema, and a low plasma albumin.

It is best classified into steroid-sensitive (90%) or steroid-resistant (10%) as this is predictor of outcome.

Clinical features

The usual presenting feature is edema, which manifests as:

- Puffiness around the eyes.
- Swelling of the feet and legs.
- In severe cases, gross scrotal edema, ascites, and pleural effusions.

Diagnosis

Diagnosis is confirmed by documentation of proteinuria and hypoalbuminemia, usually less than 25 g/L (normal range 35–40 g/L). Additional investigations should include biochemical renal function tests (urea, electrolytes, creatinine), urine microscopy, C3, C4, anti-DNAse B, and hepatitis serology.

The following features should prompt consideration of renal biopsy to identify rarer causes such as focal segmental glomerulosclerosis or membranoproliferative glomerulonephritis, which are usually steroid-resistant:

- Age: <1 year or >12 years.
- Presence of macroscopic hematuria.
- Low C3.
- Failure to respond to 4 weeks of steroid therapy.
- Persistent hypertension.
- Evidence of renal failure.

Management

If the clinical features are consistent with classic steroid-sensitive nephrotic syndrome, treatment is begun with oral steroids (prednisolone, 60 mg/m²/day). Remission usually occurs within 10 days and the doses tapered. Steroid resistance is defined as no remission after 4 weeks. These cases are often resistant to other drugs and associated with chronic renal failure.

Fluid balance must be closely monitored with daily weighing and salt restriction.

Several serious complications may occur, including:

- Hypovolemia (manifested by a high PCV, hypotension and peripheral vasoconstriction).
- Thrombosis.
- Secondary infection.
- Hyperlipidemia is not usually problematic in children.

Penicillin prophylaxis is given in the acute phase to prevent secondary infection.

Subsequent relapses may occur, which, if frequent, will require the use of additional immunosuppressive agents such as cyclophosphamide, levamisole, or cyclosporin A.

Hemolytic uremic syndrome

This is the most common cause of pediatric acute renal failure and is associated with diarrhea from *E. coli* 0157, which produces a verocytotoxin. This toxin is released from the gastrointestinal tract and results in fragmentation of the red blood cells, microangiopathic hemolytic anemia, and thrombocytopenia. The kidney vasculature becomes thrombosed and infarcted.

Management is supportive, and most (90%) children recover full renal function. Antibiotics are contraindicated.

- What is the significance of antenatal hydronephrosis?
- What happens to most antenatal hydronephrosis?
- Urinary tract infections need investigation. Why?
- What is the management of vesicoureteral reflux?
- Why is inguinal hernia operated on early in children?
- What are the differences between nephritis and nephritic syndrome?
- When would a renal biopsy be indicated in nephritic syndrome?

Further reading

Eddy AA, Symons JM. Neprotic syndrome in childhood. *Lancet* 2003; 362:629–639.

Larcombe J. Clinical evidence: urinary tract infection in children. *British Medical Journal* 1999; 319:1173–1175.

17. Neurologic Disorders

The developing nervous system is susceptible to damage by a host of diverse pathologic processes: inherited and acquired. Malformations, infections, trauma, genetic diseases, and tumors all affect the nervous system. Several important conditions affecting the nervous system are considered elsewhere:

- Neonatal hypoxic ischemia (see Chapter 25).
- Head injury (see Chapter 26).
- Coma (see Chapter 26).
- Brain tumors (see Chapter 20).
- Neural tube defects (see Chapter 9).

Malformations of the central nervous system

If severe, these cause fetal loss or early death. They encompass such important conditions as:

- Hydrocephalus.
- Craniosynostosis.
- Neural tube defects.

Hydrocephalus

Hydrocephalus is enlargement of the cerebral ventricles due to excessive accumulation of cerebrospinal fluid (CSF). This condition is the most frequent cause of an enlarged and rapidly expanding head in newborn infants.

Suspect hydrocephalus in an infant with a rapidly enlarging head circumference.

The causes include a variety of acquired pathological mechanisms as well as malformations (Fig. 17.1). Hydrocephalus is classified according to whether or not the ventricles communicate with the subarachnoid space:

- In noncommunicating hydrocephalus the obstruction is intraventricular.
- In communicating hydrocephalus the obstruction is extraventricular.

Clinical features

The presenting clinical features vary with age. Dilated ventricles can be detected on antenatal ultrasound. In infants:

- The head circumference is disproportionately large and its rate of growth is excessive.
- The pressure on the anterior fontanelle is increased, sutures become separated and scalp veins are prominent. If untreated, the eyes deviate downward (setting-sun sign).

In older children, the clinical features are those of raised intracranial pressure:

- Headache.
- Vomiting.
- Lethargy.
- Irritability.
- Papilledema.

Diagnosis

Diagnosis is confirmed by imaging. If the anterior fontanelle is still open, ultrasound can be used to assess ventricular dilatation. A computed tomography scan (CT) or magnetic resonance imaging (MRI) will establish the diagnosis, evaluate the cause, and is useful for monitoring treatment and detecting complications.

Treatment

The mainstay of treatment is insertion of a ventriculoperitoneal shunt. Complications of shunts include obstruction and infection.

Craniosynostosis

This is premature fusion of the cranial sutures. Most affected infants present soon after birth with an abnormal skull; the shape of this depends on which sutures have fused. The sagittal suture is most commonly involved, causing a long, narrow skull.

Generalized craniosynostosis is a cause of microcephaly.

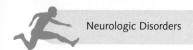

Causes of hydrocephalus
Noncommunicating (intraventricular obstruction) Congenital malformation: • Aqueduct stenosis • Dandy–Walker syndrome Intraventricular hemorrhage Ventriculitis Brain tumor
Communicating (extraventricular obstruction) Subarachnoid hemorrhage Tuberculous meningitis Arnold–Chiari malformation

Fig. 17.1 Causes of hydrocephalus.

Acute meningitis: common pathogens

Bacterial
Neisseria meningitidis
Streptococcus pneumoniae
Haemophilus influenzae type B
During the neonatal period:
   Group B streptococci
   E. coli
   Listeria monocytogenes

Viral Mumps Enteroviruses Epstein–Barr virus

Fig. 17.2 Meningitis: common pathogens.

Neural tube defects

These used to be the most common congenital defects of the CNS and are considered in detail in Chapter 9. The birth prevalence has fallen because of antenatal screening as well as the use of prenatal vitamin folate. There has also been a natural decline, the cause of which is uncertain. A range of lesions occur:

- Spina bifida occulta: the vertebral arch fails to fuse; seen in 5% of all children.
- Meningocele: meninges herniate through a vertebral defect. Usually minimal neurologic defects.
- Myelomeningocele: meninges and spinal cord herniated—the most severe form of spinal defect.
- Encephalocoele: extrusion of the brain and meninges through a midline skull defect.
- Anencephaly: the cranium and brain fail to develop (detected on antenatal ultrasound and termination of pregnancy is usually performed).

Infections of the CNS

Meningitis

A range of bacteria and viruses (Fig. 17.2) can cause acute meningitis. Rare causes include tuberculosis, fungal infections, and malignant infiltration. The serious and potentially lethal nature of bacterial meningitis renders it most important. Although more common, viral meningitis is a relatively benign and self-limiting disease.

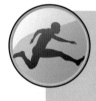 Early signs of meningitis in infants are nonspecific. Immediate treatment with parenteral penicillin is indicated for suspected meningococcal septicemia.

Bacterial meningitis

The peak age of incidence is younger than 5 years old and 80% of all cases occur in children under 16 years. Meningococcal meningitis accounts for over half of all cases; group B is the most common variety. Pneumococcal meningitis is uncommon but affects younger children and is associated with higher fatality and neurologic sequelae. Since the introduction of Hib vaccination, meningitis due to *H. influenzae* type B has become rare.

The pathogens are carried in the nasal passages and invade the meninges via the bloodstream. In the early stages, symptoms and signs are nonspecific, making diagnosis difficult, especially in infants.

Clinical features

There may be irritability, poor feeding, vomiting, fever, and drowsiness. More specific signs develop later, including:

- A bulging fontanelle in infants.
- Neck stiffness and photophobia in the older child.
- Seizures: beware the child diagnosed with benign febrile seizures.

Meningococcal infection can present with petechia, a characteristic nonblanching purpuric rash, if septicemia is present.

Diagnosis

Lumbar puncture (LP) and examination of the cerebrospinal fluid (CSF) are diagnostic. A high index of suspicion is necessary in young children in whom signs and symptoms of meningitis are nonspecific.

Treatment should be started and LP performed if there is no contraindication. Contraindications to LP include signs of raised intracranial pressure (depressed conscious state, papilledema, and/or focal neurologic signs), coagulopathy, and septic shock. A CT scan does not exclude raised intracranial pressure.

Rapid diagnostic tests are available (see Chapter 30). Blood cultures should also be taken prior to antibiotic therapy.

Treatment

Broad-spectrum intravenous antibiotic treatment is initiated using a third-generation cephalosporin (e.g., ceftriaxone). A febrile child with a petechial rash (i.e., suspected meningococcal sepsis) should be treated immediately with benzylpenicillin (IM or IV) and transferred urgently to hospital. Meningococcal septicemia can kill within hours and early antibiotic treatment significantly reduces fatality rates.

There is evidence that a component of the tissue damage in meningitis is caused by the host's inflammatory response. Attempts have been made to suppress this with steroids: dexamethasone has been shown to reduce the incidence of some neurologic sequelae in nonneonatal meningitis caused by *H. influenzae* and *S. pneumoniae*.

Complications

Acute complications of meningitis include:
- Subdural effusion.
- Cerebral edema.
- Seizures.
- SIADH.

Neurologic sequelae include sensorineural deafness: all children should have their hearing tested following meningitis. Rifampin, ciprofloxacin, or ceftriaxone should be given to all household contacts following infection with meningococcus to eradicate nasopharyngeal carriage.

Encephalitis

In encephalitis there is inflammation of the brain substance. Acute encephalitis is usually viral. The most common causes are:
- Herpes simplex virus 1 and 2.
- Enteroviruses.
- Varicella.

The common viral exanthems (measles, rubella, mumps, and varicella) can all cause encephalitis by direct viral invasion of the brain or can be complicated by an immune-mediated postinfectious encephalomyelitis (see below).

Clinical features

The clinical features include early nonspecific symptoms and signs such as fever, headache, and vomiting, followed by the abrupt development of an encephalopathic illness characterized by altered consciousness and personality and seizures.

Diagnosis and management

High-dose acyclovir should be given in all cases to cover herpes simplex until results of investigations awaited.

Diagnosis is difficult acutely, but EEG and MRI may show evidence of the characteristic temporal lobe abnormalities.

Supportive management for severe encephalitis requires:
- Admission to an intensive care unit if there are concerns about airway, breathing, or circulation.
- Seizure control and monitoring for raised intracranial pressure.

Postinfectious syndromes

These can affect the brain or peripheral nervous system:
- Postinfectious encephalomyelitis: delayed brain swelling caused by an immune-mediated inflammatory reaction to viral infection. It may follow any of the common viral exanthems.
- Varicella zoster typically causes an acute cerebellitis.

Acute postinfectious polyneuropathy (Guillain–Barré syndrome)

This demyelinating polyneuropathy follows 2–3 weeks after a viral infection with, for example, cytomegalovirus or Epstein–Barr virus, or infection with *Mycoplasma pneumoniae* or *Campylobacter jejuni*.

Clinical features

Guillain–Barré syndrome usually begins with fleeting sensory symptoms in the toes and fingers and progresses to a symmetrical, ascending paralysis with early loss of tendon reflexes. Autonomic involvement may occur, with dysrhythmias, and bulbar involvement can cause respiratory failure. The disease can progress over several weeks. The CSF protein is characteristically markedly raised without an increase in white cell count.

Management

Supportive care including assisted ventilation may be required. Respiratory function must be monitored closely. Specific therapy includes immunoglobulin infusion and plasma exchange. There may be residual neurological problems but in children a full recovery is expected.

Cerebral palsy

Cerebral palsy (CP) is a disorder of motor function due to a nonprogressive lesion of the developing brain. It is useful to remember that:

- Although the lesion is nonprogressive, the clinical manifestations evolve as the nervous system develops.
- Children with cerebral palsy often have problems in addition to disorders of movement and posture, reflecting more widespread damage to the brain.

The cause is unknown in many patients but identified risk factors can be categorized into antenatal, intrapartum, and postnatal (Fig. 17.3). It is important to be aware that perinatal asphyxia is an uncommon cause (3–21%) of CP.

Clinical features

There may be a history of risk factors and motor delay. CP can present with:

- Delayed motor milestones.
- Abnormal tone and posturing in infancy.
- Feeding difficulties due to lack of oromotor coordination.
- Speech and language delay.

Diagnosis

The diagnosis is made on clinical examination, which may show abnormalities of:

Causes of cerebral palsy

Antenatal (80%)
Congenital infections:
- Rubella
- CMV
- Toxoplasmosis

Intrapartum (10%)
Birth asphyxia

Postnatal (10%)
Preterm birth
- Hypoxic–ischemic enephalopathy
- Intraventricular hemorrhage
Hyperbilirubinemia
Hypoglycemia
Head injury
Intracranial infection:
- Meningitis
- Encephalitis

Fig. 17.3 Causes of cerebral palsy.

- Tone (e.g., hypertonia or hypotonia).
- Power (e.g., hemiparesis).
- Reflexes (e.g., brisk tendon reflexes or abnormal absence [or persistence] of primitive reflexes).
- Abnormal movements (e.g., athetosis or chorea).
- Abnormal posture or gait.

Problems associated with cerebral palsy:
- Mental retardation and learning difficulty
- Ophthalmic and auditory abnormalities
- Seizures
- Gastroesophageal reflux
- Feeding problems and failure to thrive
- Recurrent pneumonia

Classification

Cerebral palsy is classified according to the anatomical distribution of the lesion and the main functional abnormalities (Fig. 17.4).

Spastic cerebral palsy

Damage to the pyramidal pathways causes increased limb tone (spasticity) with brisk deep-

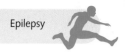

Classification of cerebral palsy
Spastic (70%)
Hemiplegic
Diplegic
Quadriplegic
Ataxic (10%)
Hypotonic
Dyskinetic (10%)
Athetoid
Dystonic
Mixed (10%)

Fig. 17.4 Classification of cerebral palsy.

tendon reflexes and extensor plantar responses. Hypotonia may precede spasticity. The distribution of affected limbs allows further classification:

- Hemiparesis: an arm may be affected more than leg or vice versa.
- Diplegia: all four limbs are affected, but legs more than arms. This is the characteristic CP of the preterm infant.
- Quadriplegia: all four limbs are affected, but arms worse than legs. There is often truncal involvement, with seizures and intellectual impairment. This is the most severe form and is the characteristic CP of severe birth asphyxia.

Ataxic cerebral palsy

Caused by damage to the cerebellum or its pathways. Features include early hypotonia with poor balance, uncoordinated movements, and delayed motor development.

Dyskinetic cerebral palsy

Caused by damage to the basal ganglia or extrapyramidal pathways (e.g., in kernicterus). The clinical presentation is often with hypotonia and delayed motor development. Abnormal involuntary movements, which include chorea (abrupt, jerky movements), athetosis (slow writhing continuous movements), or dystonia (sustained abnormal postures) may appear later.

Management

Management of CP requires a multidisciplinary approach. Accurate diagnosis and prognosis must be given to the parents. Prognosis in early infancy can be uncertain. A program of physiotherapy may be indicated, and orthopedic intervention is often beneficial (braces, surgery, special shoes). Attention must be paid to associated problems:

- Mental retardation and learning difficulty.
- Ophthalmic and auditory abnormalities.
- Seizures (experienced by 25–50% of all children with CP).
- Gastroesophageal reflux disease.
- Feeding problems and failure to thrive.
- Recurrent pneumonia.

New therapies include botulinum toxin for hypertonia.

Epilepsy

Epilepsy is common, affecting 5 out of 1000 school-age children. It is useful to distinguish between an "epileptic seizure," which is a transient event, and epilepsy, which is a disease or syndrome:

- An epileptic seizure is a transient episode of abnormal and excessive neuronal activity in the brain that is apparent either to the subject or an observer.
- Epilepsy is a chronic disorder of the brain characterized by recurrent epileptic seizures.

Several important features of these definitions require emphasis. With epileptic seizures:

- The abnormal neuronal activity during an epileptic seizure can be manifested as a motor, sensory, autonomic, cognitive, or psychic disturbance. The neurophysiologic basis is inferred on clinical grounds.
- A convulsion is a subtype of seizure in which motor activity occurs.
- An electrophysiologic disturbance unaccompanied by any clinical change is *not* classified as an epileptic seizure.
- Many paroxysmal disturbances ("funny turns") mimic epileptic seizures (see Chapter 5).

A diagnosis of epilepsy is made in a patient in whom epileptic seizures recur spontaneously. However, it is important to recognize that an "epileptic seizure" can be provoked in individuals who do *not* have epilepsy (examples of provoking insults include fever, hypoglycemia, trauma, and hypoxia).

Partial seizures are further classified into:
- Simple, in which consciousness is retained.
- Complex, in which consciousness is impaired or lost.

A partial seizure can become secondarily generalized.

Classification of epilepsies and epilepsy syndromes

The initial division is according to the seizure type (Fig. 17.6):
- Generalized epilepsies and syndromes.
- Localization: related epilepsies and syndromes.

An additional category is provided for those in which it is undetermined whether seizures are focal or generalized, either because the seizure type is uncertain or because both focal and generalized seizures occur.

Further subdivision is according to etiology into:

> Diagnosis of epilepsy rests in a good history from a witness, not on investigations.
> - Epilepsy affects 5 per 1000 school-age children.
> - Up to 75% of childhood epilepsy will have no identifiable cause.
> - Children with partial seizures require brain imaging.

Classification and terminology

The International League Against Epilepsy has devised a useful classification system for epileptic seizures and for epilepsies and epilepsy syndromes. In any patient, an attempt should be made to:
- Identify the types of seizure occurring.
- Diagnose the epilepsy or epilepsy syndrome present.

Classification of epileptic seizures

The initial division is into (Fig. 17.5):
- Generalized seizures: in which the first clinical change indicates initial involvement of both cerebral hemispheres.
- Partial seizures: in which there is initial activation of part of one cerebral hemisphere.

Classification of epileptic seizures

Generalized
Absence seizures
Myoclonic seizures
Clonic seizures
Tonic seizures
Tonic–clonic seizures
Atonic seizures

Partial
Simple (consciousness not impaired)
- With motor symptoms (Jacksonian)
- With somatosensory or special sensory symptoms
- With autonomic symptoms
- With psychic symptoms
Complex (with impairment of consciousness)
- Beginning as simple partial seizure
- With impairment of consciousness only
- With automatisms
Partial seizure with secondary generalization

Fig. 17.5 Classification of epileptic seizures.

Classification of epilepsy

Generalized seizures and epilepsy syndromes
Idiopathic generalized seizures; defined syndromes include:
- Benign familial neonatal seizures
- Childhood absence seizure
- Juvenile absence seizure
- Juvenile myoclonic seizure
Symptomatic generalized seizures; defined syndromes include:
- Infantile spasms (West syndrome)
- Lennox-Gastault syndrome
- Cerebral malformation
- Progressive myoclonic seizures, including:
     Inborn errors of metabolism
     Neurodegenerative diseases

Localization-related seizures and epilepsy syndromes
Idiopathic partial seizures; defined syndromes include:
- Benign childhood seizure with centrotemporal spikes (benign rolandic epilepsy)
Symptomtatic partial seizure; defined syndromes include:
- Epilepsy caused by local lesions of the brain associated with:
     Cortical dysgenesis
     CNS infection
     Head injury
     AV malformations
     Brain tumors

Fig. 17.6 Classification of epilepsy.

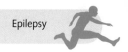

- Idiopathic (or primary): in which there is no apparent cause except perhaps for genetic predisposition.
- Symptomatic: in which the cause is known or suspected.

Causes of epilepsy

Epilepsy can result from a very diverse group of pathologic processes, but it is important to realize that in about 50% of children no cause will be identified, even after extensive evaluation. It can be assumed that the etiology in these cases of so-called idiopathic or primary epilepsy is genetic. A specific cause (Fig. 17.7) is more likely to be identifiable in patients with partial or intractable epilepsy.

Diagnosis

A careful and complete history is the mainstay of diagnosis. A detailed description is required of the events before, during and after a suspected seizure (a video recording is a potentially useful adjunct). The first aim is to distinguish true epileptic seizures from the many paroxysmal disturbances (see Chapter 5) that can mimic them:

- Breath-holding attacks.
- Reflex anoxic seizures.
- Vasovagal syncope (simple faints).
- Cardiac dysrhythmias.

Inquire about possible predisposing events (head injury, intracranial infection) and any family history of epilepsy.

Causes of "symptomatic" epilepsy
Cortical dysgenesis
Cerebral malformations
Genetic diseases:
• Neurocutaneous syndromes
• Down syndrome
• Fragile X syndrome
• Neurodegenerative disorders
• Inborn errors of metabolism
Cerebral tumors
Cerebral damage due to:
• Head trauma
• Birth asphyxia, hypoxia–ischemia
• Intracranial infection (meningitis, encephalitis)

Fig. 17.7 Causes of "symptomatic" epilepsy.

Physical examination in a child with uncomplicated epilepsy is frequently normal. Careful attention should be paid to the skin to identify the stigmata of neurocutaneous syndromes (including Wood's light examination) and to the fundi because retinal changes can provide a clue to etiology.

Always examine the skin completely in children with recurrent seizures.

Investigations
EEG

This may be useful as an aid to diagnosis, in identifying a particular epilepsy syndrome, or in identifying an underlying anatomical lesion or neurodegenerative disorder. However, it must be kept in mind that a single interictal EEG will be normal in up to 50% of children with epilepsy, and nonspecific or even so-called "epileptiform" abnormalities can be found in 2–3% of normal asymptomatic children. A routine interictal EEG does not therefore prove or disprove a diagnosis of epilepsy. Additional information can be obtained from ambulatory EEG monitoring, telemetry with simultaneous video recording or recordings during sleep or after sleep deprivation.

Neuroimaging

Not all children with epilepsy require a brain scan. Indications for neuroimaging include:
- Partial seizures.
- Intractable, difficult to control seizures.
- A focal neurologic deficit.
- Evidence of a neurocutaneous syndrome or of neurodegeneration.

CT is more readily available and quicker to perform. However, new modalities of MRI offer greater sensitivity in the detection of small lesions, e.g. in temporal lobe or subtle cortical dysgeneses.

Other investigations

Additional specific investigations, which may be appropriate if there is clinical suspicion of an underlying neurometabolic disorder, include:

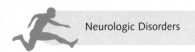
- Plasma and urine amino acids.
- Biopsy of skin or muscle.
- Measurement of white blood cell enzymes.
- DNA analysis.

Some important epilepsy syndromes

Infantile spasms (West syndrome)

This is a sinister but happily uncommon variety of epilepsy with peak onset between 4 and 6 months of age. Myoclonic seizures occur, often as "salaam attacks"—violent flexor spasms of head, trunk, and limbs followed by extension of the arms. They are often multiple and can be misdiagnosed as colic. The EEG shows hypsarrhythmia, a chaotic pattern of large-amplitude slow waves with spikes and sharp waves. Seventy percent of the patients have the symptomatic form, and important causes include tuberous sclerosis and perinatal hypoxic–ischemic encephalopathy. The prognosis is poor but can be improved by early treatment. Treatment is with adrenocorticotrophic hormone (ACTH) or antiepileptic medications.

Childhood absence seizures

This relatively common variety of epilepsy has a peak onset at 6–7 years of age (range 4–12 years). The absence seizures present with transient unawareness (blank spells). They typically last for 5–15 seconds but can be very frequent, with up to several hundred daily. Episodes can be induced by hyperventilation. The ictal EEG is characterized by generalized, bilaterally synchronous three-per-second spike-wave discharges (Fig. 17.8). The prognosis is good with spontaneous remission in adolescence in the majority of children. Valproic acid is the drug of first choice, although medication is not required for infrequent absences.

Management of epilepsy

Effective management of a child with seizures involves far more than the prescription of antiepilepsy drugs (AEDs). Both the child and parents need to be educated about the condition, the prognosis, and the nature of the particular epilepsy or epilepsy syndrome.

Children with seizures should be encouraged to participate in and enjoy a full social life. Certain activities, however, do require special precautions:

- Swimming: a competent adult swimmer should be present to provide supervision.
- Domestic bathing: patients should be supervised in the bath.
- Cycling: a helmet must be worn and traffic avoided.
- Climbing: climbing trees and rocks is best avoided.

It is important to consider the psychological and educational implications. Overprotection by the parents should be sympathetically discouraged. Behavioral and emotional difficulties can occur in the teenage years, with loss of self-esteem, anxiety, or depression. The diagnosis should be discussed with school staff. Learning difficulties are present

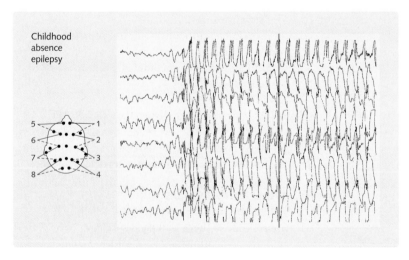

Childhood absence epilepsy

Fig. 17.8 EEG in a typical absence seizure. There is 3/s spike and wave discharge, which is bilaterally synchronous.

in a proportion of children with epilepsy, but only a minority require special schooling.

Antiepilepsy drugs (AEDs)

Not all children with seizures require drug treatment. Many clinicians would not start treatment after a single brief generalized tonic–clonic seizure or for infrequent myoclonic or absence seizures. Commonly used AEDs are valproic acid and carbamazepine. The currently recommended first-line treatment is:

- Valproic acid for generalized epilepsy.
- Carbamazepine for partial epilepsy.

Monotherapy will achieve total seizure control in 70% of children. Blood level monitoring reflects compliance and not efficacy. A number of newer AEDs are now available, including lamotrigine and other antiepileptic medication. The latter is particularly effective in treating infantile spasms but is associated with permanent visual field defects.

Febrile seizures

A febrile seizure is a seizure associated with fever in a child between 6 months and 6 years of age in the absence of intracranial infection or an identifiable neurologic disorder.

Febrile seizures are the most common cause of seizures in childhood and occur in about 3% of children. There may be a familial predisposition. The seizures usually occur when body temperature rises rapidly. They are typically brief (1–2 min), generalized, tonic–clonic seizures.

The underlying infection causing the fever may be a viral illness or a bacterial infection such as otitis media, tonsillitis, pneumonia, or urinary tract infection.

Clinical features

Most children are well after the seizure but meningitis can present with seizures and fever, so it is very important to exclude this diagnosis. This often requires a lumbar puncture in young children (under 18 months) presenting with a first febrile seizure in whom specific signs of meningitis may be absent. Prognosis is very good and, despite a 30% chance of recurrence, a normal neurologic outcome is expected.

Management

Management includes:

- Identification and treatment of underlying infection: this may be apparent on clinical examination but additional investigations to consider include CXR, CBC, blood culture, urine microscopy and culture, and lumbar puncture.
- Keeping the patient cool with regular antipyretics and tepid sponging.
- Termination of a prolonged convulsion (i.e., for longer than 5–10 minutes) with rectal diazepam.
- Parental education (Fig. 17.9).

Neurocutaneous syndromes

It is no surprise that skin and CNS disease are associated as both organs develop from the endoderm.

Neurofibromatosis type 1 (von Recklinghausen disease)

This is an autosomal dominant disorder affecting about 1 in 4000 live births. About 50% of cases result from new mutations and have no family history. The important clinical features include:

- Café-au-lait patches on the skin: at least 6 must be present because 50% of normal individuals have at least one.
- Lisch nodule (pigmented hamartomas on the eye): usually seen after 5 years of age.
- Neurofibromas, which may be palpable, on the peripheral nerves: these manifest after 8 years of age.

Neurofibromatosis type 2 (NF2)

Also known as central neurofibromatosis, NF2 is a distinct disease due to mutations in a different gene on chromosome 22. It is much rarer than type 1 (affecting 1 in 40,000 people) and is characterized by bilateral acoustic neuroma and other CNS tumors.

Tuberous sclerosis

This is an autosomal dominant disorder affecting 1 in 7000 live births. Up to 75% of cases represent new mutations. It is genetically heterogeneous with one disease gene on chromosome 9 and a second gene on chromosome 16.

Information for parents about febrile seizures	
Will it happen again?	About one-third of children have recurrent febrile seizures Recurrence is more likely if the first seizure occurs before the age of 18 months or if there is a family history
Can I prevent further episodes?	During febrile illnesses, the child should be kept cool with antipyretics, removal of clothing, and tepid sponging
What should I do if a convulsion occurs?	Place the child in recovery position on his or her side Parents of children at risk of frequent or prolonged seizures can be supplied with rectal diazepam to administer if a seizure lasts longer than 10 minutes
Is it epilepsy?	Febrile seizures are not classified as epilepsy About 3% of children with febrile seizures develop afebrile recurrent seizures (i.e., epilepsy) in later childhood Risk factors for epilepsy include: • Seizures that are focal, prolonged (>15 min), or recur in the same illness • First-degree relative with epilepsy • Neurologic abnormality

Fig. 17.9 Information for parents about febrile seizures.

Classically it presents with seizures, mental retardation, and facial angiofibromas (adenoma sebaceum). Examination reveals hypopigmented macules, which can be seen only on examination with a Wood's light.

It is a multisystem disease, affecting not only the skin and brain but also the heart, kidneys, and lungs.

Sturge–Weber syndrome

This sporadic disorder is characterized by
• Unilateral facial nevus (port-wine stain) in the distribution of the trigeminal nerve.
• Leptomeningeal vessels in the brain leading to seizures.
• Hemangiomas in the spinal cord.

There are abnormal blood vessels over the surface of the brain, which may be associated with seizures, hemiplegia, and learning difficulties. Ocular involvement can result in glaucoma.

A CT scan of the brain typically shows unilateral intracranial calcification with a double contour like a railway line and cortical atrophy.

Neurodegenerative disorders of childhood

A large number of individually rare but important inherited diseases are associated with progressive neurodegeneration in childhood. Most are autosomal recessively inherited and genetic and biochemical defects have been established at a molecular level in many cases.

Clinical features

The clinical hallmark is a progressive, worsening deficit. Features include:
• Progressive dementia.
• Epilepsy.
• Visual loss.
• Ataxia.
• Alterations in tone and reflexes (depending on the precise pattern of nervous system involvement).

Parental consanguinity increases the risk of such disorders (Fig. 17.10).

Neuromuscular disorders

These are best considered according to their anatomic site in the lower motor pathway (Fig. 17.11). Genetic, infective, inflammatory, and toxic factors can cause this group of diseases.

Clinical features

The hallmark of these disorders is weakness. They can present with:

Inherited neurodegenerative diseases—some examples

Lysosomal storage diseases
- Sphingolipidosis (e.g., Tay–Sachs disease)
- Mucopolysaccharidosis (e.g., Hurler syndrome [MPS1])

Perioxosmal disorders
- Adrenoleukodystrophy

Trace metal metabolism
- Wilson's disease
- Menke's syndrome

Fig. 17.10 Inherited neurodegenerative diseases—some examples.

Neuromuscular disorders

Anterior horn cell
- Spinal muscular atrophy
- Poliomyelitis

Peripheral nerve
- Hereditary neuropathy
- Guillain–Barrè syndrome
- Bell's palsy

Neuromuscular junction
- Myasthenia gravis

Muscle
- Muscular dystrophies
- Myotonia
- Congenital myopathies

Fig. 17.11 Neuromuscular disorders.

- Floppiness (hypotonia).
- Delayed motor milestones.
- Weakness, fatiguability.
- Abnormal gait.

Clinical features on examination include hypotonia, muscle weakness or wasting, abnormal gait, and reduced tendon reflexes.

Diagnosis
Special investigations useful in the diagnosis of neuromuscular diseases include:
- Muscle enzymes: serum creatine kinase is elevated in Duchenne and Becker dystrophies.
- Electrophysiology: nerve conduction studies and electromyography.

- Biopsy: muscle or nerve may be biopsied.
- DNA analysis: direct mutational analysis of disease genes in certain disorders.
- Imaging: ultrasound, CT, or MRI of muscle.
- Edrophonium test: for myasthenia gravis.

Muscular dystrophies
This group of inherited disorders is characterized by progressive degeneration of muscle and absence of abnormal storage material. The most common and important is Duchenne muscular dystrophy.

Duchenne muscular dystrophy
This X-linked recessive disease affects 1 in 4000 male infants. About one-third of cases are new mutations. The disease gene is very large and encodes dystrophin, a sarcolemmal membrane protein.

Affected boys usually develop symptoms between 2 and 4 years of age. Independent walking tends to be delayed and affected children never run normally. Patients are wheelchair bound by 12 years of age and die from congestive heart failure or pneumonia by 25 years of age.

Clinical features
Associated clinical features include:
- Pseudohypertrophy of calf muscles and proximal muscle weakness.
- Positive Gower's sign (evident at 3–5 years): the hands are used to push up on the legs to achieve an upright posture, indicating weakness of the lower back and pelvic girdle muscles.
- Scoliosis and contractures.
- Dilated cardiomyopathy.
- Mild learning difficulties.

Diagnosis
Investigations to confirm the diagnosis include:
- Serum creatine kinase level (10–20 times normal).
- Muscle biopsy and EMG.
- DNA analysis (identification of mutations in the dystrophin gene): positive in 65%.

Management
Treatment is supportive. Walking can be prolonged by provision of orthoses, and scoliosis can be helped by a truncal brace or molded seat. Early diagnosis is important to allow identification of female carriers and genetic counseling. Respiratory

143

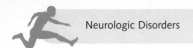

symptoms can be helped with noninvasive
respiratory ventilation in certain cases.

Becker muscular dystrophy

This disease is milder than Duchenne muscular
dystrophy but is caused by a mutation in the same
gene. The average age of onset is much later (in the
second decade of life) with prolonged survival.

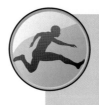

Loss of acquired skills is the
hallmark of a neurodegenerative
disorder. Most are genetic but
acquired forms do occur, such
as prion disease and subacute
sclerosing panencephalitis.

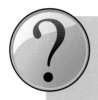

- What are the differential diagnoses of seizures?
- Describe the different types of cerebral palsy.
- What skin conditions are associated with seizures?
- What are the serious infections that can affect the brain?
- How do neurocutaneous disorders present?
- What are the management problems in children with neuromuscular disease?
- What are the complications associated with cerebral palsy?
- How do you distinguish febrile seizures from other seizure disorders?

Disorders of the hip and knee

Developmental dysplasia of the hip

This term has replaced the previous name of "congenital dislocation" of the hip. Perinatal hip instability results in progressive malformation of the hip joint; it occurs in 1.5 in 1000 births.

Developmental dysplasia of the hip (DDH) represents a spectrum of hip instability ranging from a dislocated hip to hips with various degrees of acetabular dysplasia (in which the femoral head is in position but the acetabulum is shallow). It was previously thought to be entirely congenital, but is now known to also occur after birth in previously normal hips. There are two types:
1. Typical, which affects normal infants.
2. Tetralogic, which occur in neurologic and genetic conditions. Tetralogic DDH requires specialized management.

All babies are screened clinically, but 40% will be missed. The use of universal ultrasound screening remains controversial, but ultrasound screening may be indicated for female infants with breech delivery. Ninety percent will spontaneously resolve without treatment.

Clinical features

The cause is unknown but risk factors for DDH include:
- Congenital muscular torticollis.
- Congenital foot abnormalities.
- Breech or cesarean delivery.
- Family history.
- Neuromuscular disorders.
- Female sex.

Babies are screened at birth and at the 6-week check using the Barlow and Ortolani maneuvers. With increasing age, contractures form and these tests are then unhelpful. Warning signs may be:
- Delayed walking.
- A painless limp.
- A waddling gait.

Asymmetrical skin creases are found in 30% of all infants and are an unreliable guide; 10% of all babies have hip clicks and this is normal.

Diagnosis

Typically, on examination there is limited abduction (a supine child should be able to abduct fully the flexed hip up until the age of 2 years). The femur may be shortened (Allis sign). Ultrasound scanning is diagnostic. Hip x-rays are not useful until after 4–5 months of age when the femoral head has ossified (Fig. 18.1).

Management

Note that clinical examination will miss many hip dislocations and ultrasound of high-risk babies is indicated.

This involves:
- Fixing the hip in abduction with a Pavlik or Von Rosen harness. This is effective in children under 8 months of age.
- Important to note the harness must be adjusted every 2 weeks for growth and be kept on at all times.

For children in whom the diagnosis has been delayed, open reduction and derotation femoral osteotomy needs to be performed. In these cases, accelerated degenerative changes may necessitate total hip replacement in early adult life.

Legg–Calvé–Perthes disease

This idiopathic disorder results in osteonecrosis of the femoral head prior to skeletal maturity. It results in growth disturbance associated with temporary ischemia of the upper femoral epiphysis. This leads to a cycle of avascular necrosis with flattening and fragmentation of the femoral head. Revascularization and reossification occurs with the resumption of growth (which may not be normal);

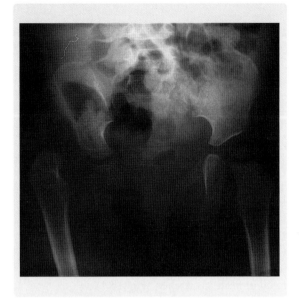

Fig. 18.1 X-ray of congenital dislocation of the right hip in an older child.

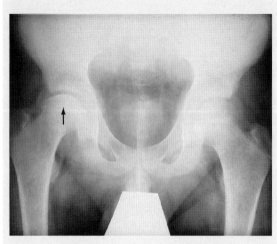

Fig. 18.2 Perthe's disease. Increased density in the right femoral head, which is reduced in height.

the whole cycle takes 3–4 years. Risk factors include:

- A previous family history.
- Male sex: it is five times more common in boys.

The incidence is 1 in 2000.

Clinical features

There is an insidious onset of limp between the ages of 3 and 12 years (the majority occur between 5 and 7 years). Pain, which may be intermittent, can be felt in the hip, thigh, or knee. Between 10 and 20% of cases are bilateral. Abduction and rotation is limited on examination.

Diagnosis

Hip x-rays are diagnostic (Fig. 18.2). If there is doubt then serial films or MRI may be necessary.

Management

The prognosis in most children is good, especially in those under 6 years of age or if less than half of the femoral head is involved. In younger children only analgesia and mild activity restriction with bracing is needed.

In older children, and those in whom more than half of the epiphysis is involved, permanent

deformity of the femoral head occurs in over 40%, resulting in earlier degenerative arthritis. In severe disease, the hip needs to be fixed in abduction allowing the femoral head to be covered and moulded by the acetabulum as it grows. Plaster, calipers, or femoral or pelvic osteotomy may achieve fixation.

Transient synovitis (irritable hip)

This common self-limiting condition occurs in children between 2 and 12 years of age often following a viral infection. Typical features are:

- Sudden onset of hip pain.
- Limp.
- Refusal to bear weight on the affected side.

There is no pain at rest. Examination reveals limited passive abduction and rotation in an otherwise well and afebrile child. The critical differential diagnosis is septic arthritis, in which the child is febrile, unwell with pain at rest, and refusal to move the affected joint.

Diagnosis

This is a diagnosis of exclusion, and it is important to distinguish transient synovitis from septic arthritis:

- Acute-phase reactants: white blood cell count (WBC), C-reative protein (CRP), and erythrocyte sedimentation rate (ESR).
- Blood cultures.

Hip x-ray does not enable differentiation and is therefore not useful. If there is doubt, antibiotics should be given and the joint aspirated for culture.

Irritable hip is a diagnosis of exclusion. Septic arthritis must always be considered.

Management

Treatment is supportive (bed rest and analgesia) because the condition spontaneously resolves in 2 weeks.

Slipped capital femoral epiphysis (SCFE)

In this relatively uncommon condition of unknown etiology, there is progressive posterior and medial translation of the femoral head on the femoral neck through the epiphysis. SCFE occurs during the adolescent growth spurt and:

- Is most common in boys (obese white or tall thin black).
- Is associated with delayed skeletal maturation and endocrine disorders.
- Typically presents between 10 and 15 years of age.
- Presents with limp or with hip or referred knee pain.

Thirty percent have a family history and 20% are bilateral, although not necessarily synchronous. Diagnosis is by plain radiographs and unstable hips are an orthopedic emergency. Complications are avascular necrosis and premature fusion of the epiphysis. Management is by pinning the femoral head or osteotomy. Nonsurgical treatment is ineffective.

Disorders of the spine

Back pain

Back pain is uncommon before adolescence. In infants and young children it is usually associated

with significant pathology such as connective tissue disorders. Referral is warranted.

In adolescence back pain may be caused by:

- Muscle spasm or soft tissue pain: this is usually a sports-related injury.
- Scheuermann's disease: this is osteochondritis (idiopathic avascular necrosis of an ossification centre) of the lower thoracic vertebrae causing localized pain, tenderness, and kyphosis.
- Spondylolysis and spondylolisthesis: there is a defect in the pars interarticularis of (usually) L4 or L5 (spondylolysis). If there is anterior shift of the vertebral body—graded according to severity—there is lower back pain exacerbated by bending backwards (spondylolisthesis).
- Vertebral osteomyelitis or discitis: this presents with severe pain on weight bearing and walking associated with local tenderness.
- Tumors: these can be benign or malignant and may cause cord or root compression.
- Idiopathic: this is a diagnosis of exclusion but pain may be exacerbated by stress and poor posture.

Think of malignancy in bone pain. Suggestive features include:
- Nonarticular bone pain.
- Back pain.
- Pain out of proportion to swelling or at night.

Scoliosis

This is lateral curvature of the spine associated with a rotational deformity and affects 4% of children. It is classified according to cause:

- Vertebral abnormalities (e.g., hemivertebra, osteogenesis imperfecta).
- Neuromuscular (e.g., polio, cerebral palsy).
- Miscellaneous (e.g., idiopathic [most common], dysmorphic syndromes).

Idiopathic scoliosis

As well as lateral curvature, there is rotation of the thoracic region, which can be demonstrated as the child bends forwards and a rib hump is noted (Fig. 18.3). More than 85% cases occur in adolescence. It is most common in girls and often there is a

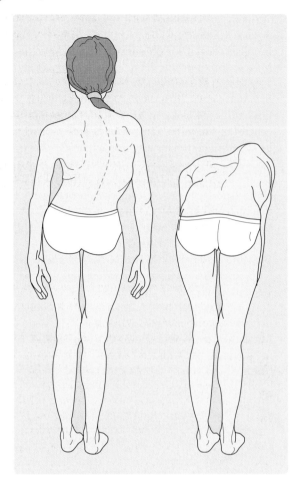

Fig. 18.3 Idiopathic adolescent scoliosis showing vertebral rotation (rib hump) when bending forward.

family history. Pain is not a typical feature. The scoliosis is monitored clinically, radiologically, and chronologically:

- Mild curves are not treated.
- Moderate curves are braced (23 hours a day until growing has stopped).
- Severe curves (>40°) require surgery that fuses the spine and therefore terminates further growth. Untreated severe curves result in later degenerative changes, pain, and unwanted cosmetic appearance.

Torticollis

Acute torticollis (wry neck) is a relatively common and self-limiting condition in young children, often associated with an upper respiratory tract infection.

The most common cause of torticollis in infants is a sternomastoid tumor. A mobile nontender nodule within the sternomastoid muscle is noticed in the first few weeks of life. The cause is unknown. It usually resolves by 1 year and is managed conservatively by passive stretching. Surgery is reserved for persistent cases.

Bone and joint infections

Osteomyelitis

Early recognition and aggressive treatment are essential for a favorable outcome in bone infections. The infection is usually hematogenous in origin or may be secondary to an infected wound. It typically starts in the metaphysis, where there is relative stasis of blood. Two-thirds of cases occur in the femur and tibia. The peak incidence is bimodal, occurring in the neonatal period and in older children (9–11 years).

In all age groups, the most common pathogen is *Staphylococcus aureus*, although group B streptococci and *E. coli* occur in neonates.

Children with sickle-cell disease have increased susceptibility to salmonella osteomyelitis. *M. tuberculosis* should also be considered.

Bacterial bone and joint infections: *Staphylococcus aureus* is the most common pathogen in all age groups.

Clinical features

Infants present with fever and refusal to move the affected limb. Older children will localize the pain and are also systemically unwell. Examination reveals exquisite tenderness over the affected bone usually with warmth and erythema. Pain limits movement.

Diagnosis

The acute-phase reactants (WBC, CRP, and ESR) are usually significantly elevated. Blood cultures are positive in more than half of the cases and aspiration of the bone is therefore necessary to identify the organism and its sensitivity. Bone scans are more sensitive in the early phase of the illness (24–48 hours) compared with x-rays, which tend to be normal in the first 10 days. Periosteal elevation or radiolucent necrotic areas can usually be demonstrated between 2 and 3 weeks.

Treatment
Early treatment with intravenous antibiotics is imperative until there is clinical improvement and normalizing of the acute-phase reactants. Several weeks of oral antibiotics follow. Failure to respond to medical treatment is an indication for surgical drainage.

Complications include:
- Chronic osteomyelitis.
- Septic arthritis.
- Growth disturbance and limb deformity (occurs if the infection affects the epiphyseal plate).

Septic arthritis
Purulent infection of a joint space is more common than osteomyelitis and can result in bone destruction and considerable disability. The incidence is highest in children younger than 3 years of age and is usually hematogenous in origin. Other causes include:
- Osteomyelitis.
- Infected skin lesions.
- Puncture wounds.

In infants, the hip is the most common site (the knee is the most common site in older children). *Staphylococcus aureus* is the most common pathogen in all age groups. The organisms are similar to those found in osteomyelitis and the conditions may occur together.

Clinical features
The typical presentation is a painful joint with:
- Fever.
- Irritability.
- Refusal to bear weight.

Infants often hold the limb rigid (pseudoparalysis) and cry if it is moved. There is tenderness and a variable degree of warmth and swelling on examination.

Investigation
The acute-phase reactants are usually elevated. Aspiration of the joint space may reveal organisms and the presence of white cells. The aspirate can then be cultured.

Ultrasound can identify effusions, but x-rays are often initially normal or show a nonspecific, widened joint space.

Management
Early and prolonged intravenous antibiotics are necessary. Surgical drainage is indicated only if the infection recurrent or if it affects the hip.

Rheumatic disorders

These include:
- Juvenile idiopathic arthritis (JIA).
- Dermatomyositis.
- Systemic lupus erythematosus.

Juvenile idiopathic arthritis
Juvenile idiopathic arthritis has replaced the terms "juvenile chronic arthritis" and "juvenile rheumatoid arthritis." It is diagnosed after arthritis in one or more joints for 6 weeks after excluding other causes in a child. It occurs in 1 : 1000 children. There are eight groups and three are discussed in detail below; classification is by mode of onset over the first 6 months (Fig. 18.4). Blood investigations for antinuclear antibodies (ANA) and rheumatoid factor (RF) are helpful in classification but not diagnostic.

Systemic (previously Still's disease)
This mainly affects children under 5 years. The arthritis primarily affects the knees, wrist, ankles, and tarsal bones. Other features include:
- High daily spiking fever.
- A salmon-pink rash.
- Lymphadenopathy and hepatosplenomagaly.
- Arthralgia, malaise and myalgia.
- Inflammation of pleura and serosal membranes.

There is often no arthritis at presentation. One-third will have a progressive course and the worst prognosis occurs in the younger age.

Polyarticular
Rheumatoid factor (RF)-negative
This affects all ages and all joints but spares metacarpophalangeal joints (MCPs). Limitation of the motion of the neck and temporomandibular joints is seen. It has a good prognosis but disease may be prolonged.

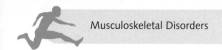

Classification of juvenile idiopathic arthritis			
	Systemic	Polyarticular	Oligoarticular
Number of joints involved	Variable	Greater than 4	4 or less
Joints involved	Knees Wrist Ankle and tarsal	Any joint	Knees Ankles Elbows Hips spared
Pattern	Symmetrical	Symmetrical	Asymmetrical
Rheumatoid factor	Negative	Positive or negative	Negative
Eye involvement	No	No	Yes in 30%
Clinical course	Poor in one-third	Good if rheumatoid factor-negative	Good

Fig. 18.4 Classification of juvenile idiopathic arthritis.

Rheumatoid factor (RF) positive

This mainly affects females over 8 years and causes arthritis of the small joints of the hand and feet. Hip and knee joints are affected early and rheumatoid nodules are seen over pressure points. There may be a systemic vasculitis; functional prognosis is poor.

Oligoarticular (pauciarticular)

Early onset is the most common subtype and typically occurs in young girls under 6 years with asymmetric arthritis involving knees, ankles, and elbows. Antinuclear antibodies are nearly always present and one-third will develop chronic iridocyclitis (inflammation of the iris and ciliary body, which comprise the anterior uveal tract: anterior uveitis). The definition "oligoarticular" requires that the disease affects four or fewer joints, and it has a good prognosis, but eye involvement is independent of the joints. There is a subclass called "extended oligoarticular," in which more than four joints are affected after 6 months; this has a poorer prognosis.

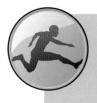 Ophthalmologic screening with a slit lamp to detect anterior uveitis is especially important in children with oligoarticular JIA.

Diagnosis

Useful tests for the evaluation of JIA include:
- CBC: anemia occurs in systemic disease.
- Acute-phase reactants: elevated.
- RF: negative in the majority.
- ANA.
- X-rays: soft tissue swelling in early stages. Bony erosion and loss of joint space later.

Management

A multidisciplinary team approach is required. This will encompass:
- Physiotherapy: to optimize joint mobility, prevent deformity, and increase muscle strength.
- Medication: pain control and suppression of inflammation are provided by nonsteroidal anti-inflammatory agents (NSAIDs), such as ibuprofen or naproxen. Systemic steroids are indicated for severe systemic disease or severe uveitis. The early use of methotrexate is indicated to reduce joint damage, and local steroid injections. Biologics, which target specific parts of the inflammatory pathway, are used in severe cases.

Genetic skeletal dysplasias

Achondroplasia

See Chapter 25.

Osteogenesis imperfecta (brittle bone disease)

Osteogenesis imperfecta is a heterogeneous group of disorders:

- Caused by mutations in type I collagen genes.
- Characterized by fragile bones and frequent fractures.

There are four forms:

- Type I (the most common form) is an autosomal dominant disorder. Affected children have recurrent fractures, blue sclerae, and conductive hearing loss.

- Type II is a severe, lethal form with multiple fractures present before birth. Many affected infants are stillborn. Inheritance is usually autosomal recessive.
- Type III causes severe bone fragility but the sclerae are not blue in later life. Survival to adulthood is uncommon. This is autosomal recessive.
- Type IV is mild with a variable age of onset and only bone fragility without the other features of type I.

Management is by aggressive orthopedic treatment of fractures to correct deformities and genetic counseling of the parents.

- Describe the types of osteogenesis imperfecta.
- What are the different types of juvenile arthritis?
- How would you diagnose septic arthritis?
- How do the different types of hip pain differ with age?
- How would you manage juvenile idiopathic arthritis?
- Why is screening for developmental dysplasia of the hip important?

Further reading

Kocher MS, Zurakowski D, Kasser JR. Differentiating between septic arthritis and transient synovitis of the hip in children: an evidence-based clinical prediction algorithm. *Journal of Bone and Joint Surgery* 1999; 81(12):1662–1170.

Petty RE, Southwood TR, Baum J et al. Revision of the proposed classification criteria for juvenile idiopathic arthritis: Durban, 1997. *Journal of Rheumatology* 1998; 25:1991–1994.

19. Hematologic Disorders

These encompass defects in the cellular elements of the blood or in those soluble elements involved in hemostasis. Neoplastic diseases of the white cells or lymphatic system are considered separately (see Chapter 20). The most common problem encountered is iron deficiency anemia.

Normal developmental variations are important in the interpretation of changes in the blood in infancy and childhood.

Hematopoiesis

Early prenatal hematopoiesis occurs in the liver, spleen, and lymph nodes. It commences in the bone marrow at about the fourth or fifth month of gestation. At birth, hematopoietic activity is present in most of the bones, especially long bones.

Cells in the peripheral blood have a relatively short life span. Continuous replenishment in massive amounts from the bone marrow is required to maintain adequate blood counts.

Life span of peripheral blood cells:
- Red cells: 120 days.
- Platelets: 10 days.
- Neutrophils: 6–7 hours.

Normal developmental changes in hemoglobin

The hemoglobin (Hb) concentration and hematocrit are relatively high in the term newborn infant because of the low oxygen tension prevailing in utero. The wide range encountered, 14–20 g/dL, is accounted for by:
- Variation in how rapidly the umbilical cord is clamped.
- The infant's position after delivery.

If cord clamping is delayed and the baby is held lower than its placenta, hemoglobin and blood volume are both increased by a placental transfusion. These values subsequently decline, reaching a nadir at:
- About 7 weeks in preterm infants.
- 2–3 months for term infants.

The lower limit of normal for this "physiologic" anemia is 9.0 g/dL. During this period, there is erythroid hypoplasia of the marrow and a change from fetal to adult hemoglobin.

The hemoglobin concentration:
- Is high at birth: 14–20 g/dL.
- Falls to a nadir of 9–13 g/dL at 2–3 months in term infants.
- HbF values decline postnatally to 2% of total at 9–12 months.

Anemia

Anemia is a decrease of the hemoglobin concentration in the blood to below normal. Dietary iron deficiency is the most common cause but there are many others. In clinical practice, anemia can be classified initially according to the red cell:
- Color intensity (normochromic/ hypochromic).
- Size (microcytic/normocytic/macrocytic).

Important causes based on this classification are shown in Fig. 19.1.

Iron deficiency anemia (IDA)

This is the most common cause of anemia in childhood. It usually results from inadequate dietary intake rather than loss of iron through hemorrhage.

Classification and causes of anemia

Microcytic hypochromic anemia
Defects of heme system
  • Iron deficiency
  • Chronic inflammation/disease
Defects of globin synthesis
  • Thalassemia

Normocytic normochromic anemia
Hemolytic anemias
  • Intrinsic red cell defects
    Membrane deficits: spherocytosis
    Hemoglobinopathies: sickle-cell disease
    Enzymopathies: G6PD deficiency
  • Extrinsic disorders
    Immune-mediated: Rh incompatibility
    Microangiopathy
    Hypersplenism
Hemorrhage (acute or chronic)
  • Hookworm infestation
  • Meckel's diverticulum
  • Menstruation
Hypoproduction disorders
  • Red cell aplasia (e.g., renal disease)
  • Pancytopenia (e.g., marrow aplasia, leukemia)

Macrocytic anemia
Bone marrow megaloblastic
  • Vitamin B_{12} deficiency
  • Folic acid deficiency
Bone marrow not megaloblastic
  • Hypothyroidism
  • Fanconi anemia

Fig. 19.1 Classification and causes of anemia.

Iron requirements

The fetus absorbs iron from the mother across the placenta.
- Term infants have adequate reserves for the first 4 months of life.
- Preterm infants have limited iron stores and because of their higher rate of growth, they outstrip their reserves by 8 weeks of age.

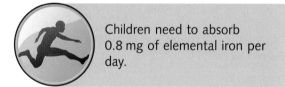

Children need to absorb 0.8 mg of elemental iron per day.

Both breast milk and unmodified cow's milk are low in iron concentration (0.05–0.10 mg/100 mL). However, 50% of the iron is absorbed from breast milk, in comparison to just 10% from cow's

Dietary iron deficiency	

Infants	Preterm infants require iron supplements from 6–8 weeks of age
	Term infants will develop iron deficiency after 4 months of age if:
	  • Mixed feeding is unduly delayed
	  • Unmodified cow's milk is introduced early

Children	Poor diet associated with low socioeconomic status or strict vegetarian diets

Fig. 19.2 Dietary iron deficiency.

milk. Most formula milks are fortified with iron and contain 10 times the concentration in breast milk (1.0 mg/100 mL); however, only 4% is absorbed.

Dietary sources of iron include red meat, fortified breakfast cereals, dark green vegetables, and bread. About 10–15% of dietary iron is absorbed. Absorption is:
- Enhanced by ascorbic acid (vitamin C).
- Reduced by tannin in tea.

Iron requirements increase during adolescence, especially for girls who lose iron through menstruation.

Concerning iron in milk:
- Breast and unmodified cow's milk are low in iron.
- Iron is better absorbed from breast milk (50%) than cow's milk (10%).
- Formula milks are fortified with iron.

Causes of iron deficiency

Nutritional deficiency is common in certain at-risk groups (Fig. 19.2). Malabsorption can be complicated by iron deficiency. Blood loss is a less common cause but may occur with:
- Menstruation.
- Hookworm infestation.
- Repeated blood draw in babies.
- Meckel's diverticulum.
- Recurrent epistaxis.

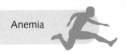

Clinical features

Mild iron deficiency is asymptomatic. As it becomes more severe there may be:
- Irritability.
- Lethargy.
- Fatigue.
- Anorexia.

On examination, the only signs may be pallor of the skin and mucous membranes.

Severe anemia can cause congestive cardiac failure. IDA in infancy and early childhood is associated with developmental delay and poor growth, which is reversible by long-term oral iron treatment.

Diagnosis

Diagnosis is confirmed by the blood count and smear, supplemented by investigations of iron status. If dietary deficiency is likely, the latter can be omitted and diagnosis confirmed by a positive response to a therapeutic trial of iron.

Management

Primary prevention in infants can be achieved by the:
- Avoidance of unmodified cow's milk.
- Use of iron-supplemented formulas.

Mild to moderate anemia is treated with dietary counseling and oral iron, using, for example, ferrous sulfate. Therapy should be continued for 3 months to allow replenishment of tissue iron stores.

Severe anemia with cardiac decompensation may require transfusion. Investigation for occult gastrointestinal tract bleeding is indicated if there is a failure of response to treatment or recurrence despite an adequate intake.

Reference nutrient intakes of iron are:
- 6 months: 4 mg/day.
- 12 months: 8 mg/day.
- Adult male: 9 mg/day.
- Adult female: 15 mg/day.

Thalassemias

The thalassemias are a group of hereditary anemias caused by defects of globin polypeptide chain synthesis. They are classified into:
- α-thalassemia: reduced synthesis of α-globin polypeptide chains.
- β-thalassemia: reduced synthesis of β-globin polypeptide chains.

Mutations in the globin genes lead to a reduction or absence of the corresponding globin chains. Excess unpaired globin chains produce insoluble tetramers that precipitate causing membrane damage and either:
- Cell death within the bone marrow (ineffective erythropoiesis).

or
- Premature removal by the spleen (resulting in hemolytic anemia).

β-thalassemia

This occurs most frequently in people from the Mediterranean and Middle East. Over 150 million people carry β-thalassemia mutations. There are two main types:
1. Homozygous β-thalassemia (β-thalassemia major, Cooley's anemia).
2. Heterozygous β-thalassemia (β-thalassemia minor, β-thalassemia trait).

β-thalassemia major

There is usually a complete absence of β-globin chain production (genotype β^0/β^0), although some mutations allow partial synthesis (genotype β^+/β^+); hemoglobin A (HbA) cannot be synthesized.

Clinical features. Affected infants usually present at 6 months with severe hemolytic anemia, jaundice, failure to thrive, and hepatosplenomegaly. If untreated, bone marrow hyperplasia occurs with development of the classical facies:
- Maxillary hypertrophy.
- Skull bossing.

Diagnosis Hemoglobin electrophoresis reveals a markedly reduced or absent HbA with increased hemoglobin F (HbF) (30–90%) (see Chapter 30).

Treatment. The mainstay of treatment is regular blood transfusion, aiming to maintain the hemoglobin concentration above 10 g/dL. Unfortunately, chronic transfusion therapy is complicated by iron overload. Iron accumulates in

155

parenchymal organs including the heart, liver, pancreas, gonads, and skin.

Chelation therapy with subcutaneous desferrioxamine, given regularly overnight, is used to promote iron removal but negative iron balance is rarely achieved. Many patients succumb to congestive heart failure due to cardiomyopathy in their second or third decade.

Splenectomy is useful in selected patients and bone marrow transplantation can restore hematopoietic function. In the future, the developments of bone marrow transplantation, oral chelating agents, and gene therapy hold promise.

β-thalassemia minor (β-thalassemia trait)

The only abnormality is a mild, hypochromic, microcytic anemia. Most are asymptomatic. β-thalassemia trait can be misdiagnosed as iron deficiency anemia. The important diagnostic feature is the raised HbA_2 and about 50% have a mild elevation of HbF (1–3%) on electrophoresis.

α-thalassemia

This is caused by absence or reduced synthesis of α-globin genes. Most result from gene deletion. The manifestations and severity depend on the number of genes deleted (Fig. 19.3).

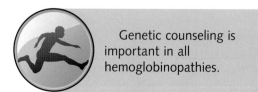

Genetic counseling is important in all hemoglobinopathies.

Hemolytic anemia

Hemolytic anemia occurs when the life span of the red blood cell is shorter than the normal 120 days. Hemolytic anemia can be caused by:

- Intrinsic red cell defects (e.g., spherocytosis, sickle-cell disease, glucose-6-phosphate dehydrogenase [G6PD] deficiency).
- Extrinsic defects (e.g., Rhesus [Rh] incompatibility, microangiopathy, and hypersplenism).

It is characterized by:

- Anemia.
- Reticulocytosis.
- Increased erythropoiesis in the bone marrow.
- Unconjugated hyperbilirubinemia.

Hereditary spherocytosis

This is an autosomal dominant disorder caused by abnormalities in spectrin, a major supporting component of the red blood cell membrane. About 25% of cases are sporadic with no family history and are due to new mutations. As the name suggests the red cell shape is spherical and the life span is reduced by early destruction in the spleen.

Clinical features

The clinical features are highly variable and include:

- Mild anemia: 9–11 g/dL.
- Jaundice: hyperbilirubinemia.
- Splenomegaly: mild to moderate.

Complications

These include:

- Aplastic crises secondary to parvovirus B_{19} infection.

Clinical manifestations of α-thalassemia variants			
Variant	**Number of genes deleted**	**Hb pattern**	**Clinical features**
α-thalassemia major	Four	4F (Hb Bart)	Hyrdops fatalis/death in utero
Hemoglobin H disease	Three	B4A (Hb H) (beyond early infancy)	Severe anemia, persists throughout life
α-thalassemia minor	Two	Normal	Mild anemia
Silent carrier	One	Normal	No anemia Normal RBC indices

Fig. 19.3 Clinical manifestations of α-thalassemia variants.

- Gallstones: caused by increased bilirubin excretion.

Diagnosis

Spherocytes are seen on peripheral blood film. Diagnosis is confirmed by the osmotic fragility test (spherocytes already have maximum surface area to volume and rupture more easily than biconcave red cells in hypotonic solutions).

Management

Mild disease requires no treatment other than folic acid to meet the increased demands of the marrow.

Splenectomy is indicated for more severe disease, but should be deferred until school age because of the subsequent risk of overwhelming infection. The child should receive:

- Hib, meningococcal, and pneumococcal vaccines before splenectomy.
- Prophylactic penicillin for life afterwards.

Sickle-cell disease

This chronic hemolytic anemia occurs in patients homozygous for a mutation in the β-globin gene (which causes substitution of valine for glutamine in the sixth amino acid position of the β-globin chain). This causes a solubility problem in the deoxygenated state: hemoglobin S (HbS) aggregates into long polymers that distort the red cells into a sickle shape.

The heterozygous state (sickle-cell trait) confers resistance to falciparum malaria; this "heterozygote advantage" explains the high incidence of the mutation in populations originating in malarious areas such as tropical Africa, the Mediterranean, the Middle East, and parts of India.

Sickled red cells have a reduced life span and are trapped in the microcirculation, causing ischemia.

Clinical features

The synthesis of HbF during the first few months affords protection until the age of 4–6 months. Progressive anemia with jaundice and splenomegaly then develops, and the infant may present with an episode of dactylitis or overwhelming infection. The subsequent course of the disease is punctuated by crises, of which vaso-occlusive events are by far the most common.

Vaso-occlusive crises

These episodes are often precipitated by infection, dehydration, chilling, or vascular stasis. The clinical features depend on the tissue involved but episodes most commonly manifest as a "painful" crisis, with pain in the long bones or spine. Cerebral or pulmonary infarction are less common but more serious. The latter may present as "acute chest syndrome," which is characterized by:

- Fever.
- Crepitous.
- Chest pain.
- Pulmonary shadowing on chest x-ray arising from a combination of infarction and infection.

In infancy, patients with sickle-cell disease have a functional hyposplenism despite splenomegaly. Repeated vaso-occlusive episodes lead to infarction and fibrosis so that the spleen is no longer palpable from 5 years of age (so-called "autosplenectomy"). These patients are, therefore, at risk of overwhelming infection with encapsulated organisms (*Haemophilus influenzae*, *Streptococcus pneumoniae*). There is an increased risk of osteomyelitis due to *Salmonella* and other organisms.

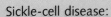

Sickle-cell disease:
- HbS differs from HbA by the substitution of valine for glutamine at position 6 in the β-globin chain.
- HbS forms insoluble polymers in the deoxygenated state.
- The heterozygous state confers some protection against malaria.

The spleen in sickle-cell disease:
- In infancy, there is splenomegaly.
- Recurrent infarction and "autosplenectomy" cause the spleen to regress and become impalpable after age 5 years.
- Splenic hypofunction renders patients susceptible to encapsulated organisms.

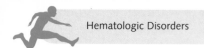

The long-term consequences of sickle-cell disease include:

- Myocardial damage and heart failure.
- Aseptic necrosis of long bones.
- Leg ulcers.
- Gallstones.
- Renal papillary necrosis.

Management

Antenatal screening is available and this allows initiation of antibiotic prophylaxis early in life. Prophylactic penicillin should be taken to prevent pneumococcal infection. Daily folic acid supplements help to meet the demands of increased red cell breakdown. Pneumococcal and meningococcal vaccine should be given as well as the standard course of Hib vaccine. Hydroxyurea reduces vaso-occlusive crisis.

The treatment of a vaso-occlusive crisis includes:

- Analgesia: opioids for severe pain.
- Oxygenation.
- Hyperhydration with IV fluids.

Exchange transfusion, designed to reduce the proportion of sickle cells, is indicated for brain or lung infarction and priapism. Transfusion with packed red cells may be required if a sudden fall in hemoglobin occurs during an aplastic sequestration or hemolytic crisis.

Sickle-cell trait

The heterozygote with sickle-cell trait (HbAS) is asymptomatic unless subjected to hypoxic stress (e.g., general anesthesia). Sickle cells are not seen on peripheral smear and diagnosis requires a solubility test (e.g., sodium metabisulfate slide test) or Hb electrophoresis. The trait is worth detecting to allow genetic counseling and precautions to be taken against hypoxemia during flying and general anesthesia.

Red cell enzyme deficiencies

These include glucose-6-phosphate dehydrogenase (G6PD) deficiency and the much rarer pyruvate kinase deficiency.

G6PD deficiency

This is an X-linked recessive disorder with variable clinical severity. Over 100 million people are affected worldwide, particularly in the Mediterranean, Middle Eastern, Asian, and Afro-Caribbean populations. G6PD-deficient red cells do not generate enough glutathione to protect the cell from oxidant agents. Males are more severely affected, but females can manifest the phenotype.

Clinical features

G6PD deficiency can manifest with:

- Neonatal jaundice: worldwide it is the most common cause of neonatal jaundice requiring exchange transfusion.
- Hemolytic episode: induced by infection, oxidant drugs, or fava beans. Intravascular hemolysis occurs with fever, malaise, and the passage of dark urine (hemoglobinuria).

Pyruvate kinase deficiency

This is an autosomal recessive condition and is characterized by infection associated (parvovirus) hemolysis and tolerance of low hemoglobin levels. Management by splenectomy is sometimes useful.

Bleeding disorders

Normal hemostasis requires a complex interaction between three factors:

- Blood vessels.
- Platelets (thrombocytes).
- Coagulation factors.

A bleeding diathesis can result from a deficiency or disorder of any of these elements. Clinical presentation of a generalized bleeding diathesis may include:

- Petechiae or purpura.
- Prolonged bleeding after dental extraction, surgery, or trauma.
- Recurrent bleeding into muscles or joints.

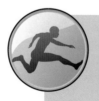

It is unlikely that inherited bleeding disorders are present if the child has had a major hemostatic challenge (e.g., major surgery) without complications.

Disorders of blood vessels

Injury to blood vessels provokes two responses that limit bleeding:

- Vasoconstriction.
- Activation of platelets and coagulation factors by subendothelial collagen.

Rare inherited disorders include Ehlers–Danlos syndrome associated with excessive capillary fragility and hereditary hemorrhagic telangiectasia.

Acquired disorders include vitamin C deficiency (scurvy) and Henoch–Schönlein purpura.

Henoch–Schönlein purpura

This is a multisystem vasculitis involving the small blood vessels. It commonly follows an upper respiratory tract infection or exposure to a drug or allergen, and is assumed to be immune-mediated with IgA playing a major role.

It is more common in boys and 75% of affected children are under 10 years old.

Clinical features

The condition affects skin, joints, gastrointestinal tract, and kidneys. Clinical features are described in Fig. 19.4.

Diagnosis and management

Diagnosis is clinical. Normal platelet count and coagulation studies exclude other causes of purpura.

Treatment is symptomatic and supportive. Steroids may be of benefit in severe gastrointestinal disease. The prognosis is excellent.

Most children recover within 4–6 weeks, although, rarely, chronic renal disease can develop.

Disorders of platelets

These may be quantitative or qualitative, with the former (thrombocytopenia) being most common.

Thrombocytopenia

A decreased number of platelets (from the normal count of $150–450 \times 10^9/L$) is the most common cause of abnormal bleeding. Purpura usually occurs when the count is below $20 \times 10^9/L$. The cause may be decreased platelet production or reduced platelet survival (Fig. 19.5).

Idiopathic thrombocytopenic purpura (ITP)

This is the most common cause of thrombocytopenia in childhood and refers to an immune-mediated thrombocytopenia for which an exogenous cause is not apparent. The platelets are destroyed within the reticuloendothelial system, mainly in the spleen.

Clinical features

ITP mainly affects children between 2 and 10 years of age. Presentation is with purpura and superficial bleeding, which may be accompanied by bleeding from mucosal surfaces (e.g., epistaxis). The spleen is palpable in a minority of cases.

Diagnosis

The differential diagnosis includes:

- Acute leukemia.
- Nonaccidental injury.
- Henoch–Schönlein purpura.

Clinical features of Henoch–Schönlein purpura	
Skin	A purpuric rash typically affects the legs and buttocks
GI tract	Colicky abdominal pain accompanied by gross or occult bleeding Intussusception may occur
Joints	Pain and swelling of the large joints (e.g., knees and ankles)
Kidneys	Glomerulonephritis manifested by microscopic hematuria; rarely severe and progressive

Fig. 19.4 Clinical features of Henoch–Schönlein purpura.

Causes of thrombocytopenia

Decreased production
Bone marrow failure
- Aplastic anemia
- Leukemia
Wiskott–Aldrich syndrome

Decreased survival
Immune-mediated thrombocytopenia
- Idiopathic thrombocytopenic purpura (most common)
- Secondary to viral infections, drugs
Hypersplenism
Giant hemangioma
Disseminated intravascular coagulation

Fig. 19.5 Causes of thrombocytopenia.

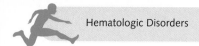

A complete blood count reveals thrombocytopenia but not pancytopenia. Bone marrow aspiration to exclude marrow infiltration, or aplasia, is advocated by some. This should be done if there is doubt about the diagnosis or steroid therapy is contemplated (see below). An increase in megakaryocytes (platelet precursors) is characteristic.

Treatment

In most children, the disease is acute, benign, and self-limiting, and no therapy is required. Even platelet levels $<10 \times 10^9$ are well tolerated. Serious bleeding is extremely rare as the platelets function more efficiently. Platelet infusions are rapidly destroyed and have no role except in life-threatening emergencies. Intravenous gammaglobulin infusions cause a rise in the platelet count and may be indicated in severe cases.

A short course of oral steroids is an alternative. These act by reducing capillary fragility and inhibiting platelet destruction. Bone marrow should be examined to exclude leukemia before starting steroids.

Teenage girls have a higher risk of chronic disease (greater than 1 year) and splenectomy may have to be used if medical therapy fails.

Coagulation disorders

Hemophilia A and B and von Willebrand disease account for the majority of inherited coagulation disorders.

Hemophilia A (factor VIII deficiency)

This is an X-linked recessive disorder due to reduced or absent factor VIII. The incidence is 1 in 5000–10,000 males. It is the result of a new mutation in one-third of cases. The factor VIII molecule is a complex of two proteins:

- VIII:C: small molecular weight unit, antihemophiliac factor.
- VIII:R: large molecular weight unit, von Willebrand factor.

Clinical features

Hemophilia A results from deficiency of VIII:C. Clinical severity varies greatly and depends on the factor VIII levels (Fig. 19.6). The characteristic

Factor VIII levels in hemophilia A	
Mild	5–25% of normal
Moderate	1–4% of normal
Severe	No detectable factor VIII activity

Fig. 19.6 Factor VIII levels in hemophilia A.

clinical feature is spontaneous or traumatic bleeding, which can be:

- Subcutaneous.
- Intramuscular.
- Intra-articular.

Mild hemophilia may remain undetected until excessive bleeding occurs (e.g., after dental extraction). Even severely affected boys often have few problems in the first year of life (unless circumcision is performed, but early bruising and abnormal bleeding is noted from the time they begin to walk and fall over.

In later life, recurrent soft tissue, muscle, and joint bleeding are the main problems. Hemarthroses cause pain and swelling of the affected joint and repeated hemorrhage may result in chronic joint disease. Life-threatening internal hemorrhage (e.g., intracranial) can follow trauma.

Diagnosis

Diagnostic evaluation reveals a prolonged activated partial thromboplastin time (APTT), indicating a defect in the intrinsic pathway; factor VIII assay confirms the diagnosis.

Management

Bleeding is treated by replacement of the missing clotting factor with intravenous infusion of factor VIII concentrate. The amount required depends on the site and severity of the bleed. Prompt and adequate therapy is important to avoid chronic arthropathy; home therapy can avoid delay and minimize inconvenience.

Recombinant DNA technology is now used to produce factor VIII that is safer than the blood products previously used. In the past, infection with hepatitis B and C, and with HIV, occurred from contaminated blood products. Antibodies to factor VIII can develop.

Mild hemophilia can be managed with infusion of desmopressin that releases factor VIII from tissue stores.

Hemophilia B (factor IX deficiency, Christmas disease)

This is an X-linked recessive disorder caused by deficiency of factor IX. It is clinically similar to hemophilia A, but much less common. Investigation reveals a prolonged APTT and reduced factor IX activity. Treatment is with prothrombin complex concentrate.

von Willebrand disease

This is due to a deficiency of von Willebrand factor (VWF; VIII:R), which has two major roles:
- Carrier protein for factor VIII:C (preventing it from breakdown).
- Facilitates platelet adhesion.

Around 1% of the population is known to be affected. Inheritance is usually autosomal dominant with variable penetrance. The clinical hallmark is bleeding into the skin and mucous membranes (gums and nose).

Disseminated intravascular coagulation (DIC)

Intravascular activation of the coagulation cascade may be secondary to various disease processes:
- Damage to vascular endothelium: sepsis, renal disease.
- Thromboplastic substances in the circulation (e.g., in acute leukemia).
- Impaired clearance of activated clotting factors (e.g., in liver disease).

There is fibrin deposition in small blood vessels with tissue ischemia, consumption of labile clotting factors, and activation of the fibrinolytic system.

Clinical features

Clinical features are:
- A diffuse bleeding diathesis, with oozing from venepuncture sites.
- Bleeding from the lungs.
- Bleeding from the gastrointestinal tract.

Diagnosis and treatment

Investigations reveal:
- Prolonged prothrombin type (INR), activated partial thromboplastin time (PTT), and thrombin time (TT).
- Thrombocytopenia and microangiopathic red cell morphology.
- Decreased fibrinogen.
- Elevated fibrin degradation products.

Supportive treatment includes treating the underlying cause and replacement of platelets and fresh frozen plasma.

Thrombotic disorders in childhood

Recognition of thrombotic disorders in children is increasing. Although thrombosis is usually rare in children, certain genetic conditions predispose to it:
- Factor V Leiden: caused by an abnormal factor V protein that is resistant to activated protein C.
- Protein C deficiency: protein C factor V and VIII and it stimulated fibrinolosis.
- Protein S deficiency: protein S is a cofactor to protein C.
- Antithrombin III deficiency.

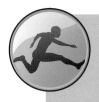

Thromboembolic diseases are rare in children because thrombin is inhibited more than it is in adults and is generated less readily.

- How does the composition of hemoglobin change in the first year of life?
- What are the different types of anemias?
- What are the complications of sickle-cell anemia?
- How would you manage iron deficiency anemia?
- What is the treatment of immune thrombocytopenic purpura?

20. Malignant Disease

Cancer in childhood is uncommon. Approximately 1 out of 600 children between the ages of 1 and 15 years will develop cancer. Despite the dramatic increases in survival rate due to new treatments, it remains an important cause of death in childhood. The spectrum of cancer in childhood is very different from that in adults (Fig. 20.1). Leukemia accounts for over one-third of cases.

The etiology, clinical features, investigation, and management of malignant disease in childhood are considered first before the individual diseases are described.

Etiology

Most childhood cancers are of uncertain cause and occur sporadically in otherwise healthy children. Risk is increased by a combination of:
- Genetic predisposition: genetic factors are often more evident in childhood than adult malignancy.
- Environmental factors.

Malignant cells proliferate and develop abnormally because they have escaped normal control mechanisms. In younger children in particular, the malignant cells may be immature precursor cells that fail to mature into normal, differentiated functional cells.

Important causative factors in childhood malignancy include:
- Genetic.
- Infectious.
- Environmental.

Genetic causes of childhood cancer

During periods of rapid proliferation, a normal cell may undergo a genetic alteration that transforms it into a malignant cell. Two important mechanisms of transformation are:
- Activation of oncogenes.
- Loss of tumor suppressor genes.

Examples of childhood cancer with an identifiable genetic etiology are shown in Fig. 20.2.

Infections

Two viruses that infect the cells of the human immune system are associated with malignancy:
- Epstein–Barr virus: the virus transforms human B cells. If not limited by an effective immune response, a translocation disrupts the *c-myc* oncogene on chromosome 8 leading to malignant change, e.g., Burkitt's lymphoma.
- Human immunodeficiency virus (HIV): this retrovirus targets the human helper T cells. Children who develop AIDS are susceptible to lymphoid malignancies.

Environmental

Carcinogens and toxins are less often a cause of childhood cancer. One important risk factor, sadly, is previous treatment of malignancy in a child.

Clinical features

Cancer in childhood presents in a limited number of ways, some of which are nonspecific (Fig. 20.3). Classification systems employ numerical staging for solid tumors based on the extent of dissemination:
- Stage I: localized.
- Stages II and III: advanced, localized disease.
- Stage IV: disseminated disease with metastases.

Investigations

Histologic confirmation is the cornerstone of diagnosis. This is provided by biopsy (although initial biopsy is not possible at some sites, such as brain tumors) or bone marrow aspiration.

Imaging is a vital aid, and all modalities can be useful: ultrasound, x-ray, computed tomography (CT), and magnetic resonance imaging (MRI) scans.

Tumor markers are useful in certain tumors (e.g., α-fetoprotein in liver tumors, urinary catecholamines in neuroblastoma).

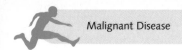

Relative frequencies of childhood cancer	
Type	% of childhood cancer
Leukemia	35
CNS tumors	23
Lymphomas	12
Wilms' tumor	7
Neuroblastoma	7
Bone tumors	6
Others	10

Fig. 20.1 Relative frequencies of childhood cancer.

Genetic childhood cancer syndromes	
Genetic cancer syndromes	Gene defect
Retinoblastoma	Chromosome13—deletion of tumor suppressor gene
Li-Fraumeni	p53 mutation
Ataxia-telangiectasia	DNA repair defect
Down syndrome	Trisomy 21

Fig. 20.2 Genetic childhood cancer syndromes.

Childhood cancer—clinical features at presentation	
Clinical feature	Type of cancer
Constitutional symptoms: fever, weight loss, night sweats	Lymphomas
Localized mass in: • Abdomen • Thorax • Soft tissue	Wilms' tumor, neuroblastoma Non-Hodgkin's lymphoma Rhabdomyosarcoma
Lymph node enlargement	Lymophomas
Bone marrow failure, e.g. anemic infections	Acute leukemia
Bone pain	Leukemia, bone tumor
Signs of increased ICP	Primary CNS tumors

Fig. 20.3 Childhood cancer—clinical features at presentation.

Management

The main therapeutic strategies available are:
- Surgery: required for biopsy, total or partial removal of solid tumors (debulking), or for removal of residual disease after chemotherapy or radiotherapy.
- Radiotherapy: has an important role in specific circumstances (e.g., brain tumors).
- Chemotherapy: has a prominent role. A number of highly effective antineoplastic agents have been developed in the past four decades. Their use is based on a number of principles. Most children are enrolled into clinical trials on diagnosis.

Chemotherapy may be used as:
- Primary therapy for disseminated malignancy (e.g., the leukemias).
- To shrink bulky primary or metastatic disease before local treatment.
- Adjunctive treatment for micrometastases.

Bone marrow toxicity is the limiting factor for many therapeutic regimens. This can be circumvented by using bone marrow transplantation to "rescue" patients after administering potentially lethal, but possibly curative, doses of chemotherapy or radiation.

Supportive care

Treatment produces many predictable and often severe side effects in many systems. Supportive care is a vital part of treatment (Fig. 20.4).

Supportive care in the treatment of cancer	
Problem	Supportive care
Anemia and thrombocytopenia	Blood and platelet transfusions
Nausea and vomiting	Antiemetics and steroids
Pain control	Use of appropriate analgesia
Long-term vascular access	Surgically implanted venous access

Fig. 20.4 Supportive care in the treatment of cancer.

Long-term problems in survivors of childhood cancer	
Secondary tumors	Leukemia and lymphoma
Reduced fertility	From alkylating chemotherapy
Cognitive and psychosocial difficulties	Associated with methotrexate
Reduced growth and endocrine problems	From irradiated glands
Auditory	From platinum-containing drugs
Cardiac	From doxorubicin

Fig. 20.5 Long-term problems in survivors of childhood cancer.

Indwelling central venous catheters allow pain-free blood sampling and injections.

Psychosocial support is very important. Diagnosis of a potentially fatal illness provokes enormous anxiety, guilt, fear, and sadness. Children and their siblings need an explanation of the illness tailored to their age. The severe stress may give rise to relationship problems between the parents and behavioral difficulties in siblings. Help with practical difficulties such as transport and finances may be required.

For some children, a time comes when further treatment represents postponement of inevitable death rather than prolongation of life. A definite decision to concentrate on palliative care is then appropriate. For survivors, long-term follow-up is required to detect and manage long-term sequelae (Fig. 20.5).

Chemotherapy in childhood cancer:
- Chemotherapy is most likely to effect a cure when the malignant cell burden is small.
- Adverse effects are produced on rapidly dividing normal cells (e.g., those of the bone marrow, gastrointestinal tract, and hair follicles).
- Most children with leukemia are enrolled into clinical trials.

The leukemias

Leukemia is a disease characterized by proliferation of immature white cells and is the most common malignancy of childhood. Acute leukemias account for the majority (97%) of cases. Note that chronic myeloid leukemia is rare and that chronic lymphocytic leukemia is confined to adults. The malignant cells are termed "blasts."

The leukemias are classified according to the white blood cell line involved:
- Acute lymphocytic (lymphoblastic) leukemia (ALL): cells of lymphoid lineage.
- Acute myeloid leukemia: cells of granulocytic or monocytic lineage.

It is of note that prognosis continues to improve with reductions in treatment-related mortality and matching of therapies to different prognostic groups.

Clinical features

In most children with acute leukemia, there is an insidious onset of symptoms and signs arising from infiltration of the bone marrow or other organs with leukemic blast cells. Most will have one or more of the following:
- Pallor and malaise: anemia.
- Hemorrhagic diathesis: purpura, easy bruising, epistaxis due to thrombocytopenia.
- Hepatosplenomegaly, lymphadenopathy: reticuloendothelial cell infiltration.
- Bone pain: due to expansion of marrow cavity.
- Infection: due to neutropenia.

Investigations

Peripheral blood investigations reveal:

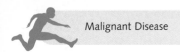

- Anemia: normocytic, normochromic.
- Thrombocytopenia.
- Neutropenia: total WBC may be low, normal or high.
- Blast cells.

Bone marrow examination reveals replacement of normal elements by leukemic cells.

A diagnosis of leukemia should always be confirmed by bone marrow aspiration.

Acute lymphocytic leukemia (ALL)

This accounts for 80% of childhood leukemia and has a peak incidence between the ages of 3 and 6 years. It is slightly more common in boys than girls. Lymphoblasts in these children do not successfully complete the rearrangement of immunoglobulin and T cell receptor genes necessary for full maturation. Coupled with genetic alterations, which permit them to survive and proliferate, the lymphoblasts remain "frozen" at an early stage of development.

ALL can be classified according to cell-surface antigens (immunophenotype) into:

- Non-T, non-B cell (common) ALL: 80% are mostly early B cell clone.
- T cell ALL: 15%.
- B cell ALL: 1%.

Clinical features

Prognosis and clinical presentation vary with subtype. T cell ALL tends to occur in older children and teenagers, with a high peripheral white cell count and mediastinal mass. The prognosis is related to tumor load and can be defined according to certain clinical and laboratory features (Fig. 20.6).

Management

Overall, at least 65% of patients with ALL can now expect to be cured. Children with null cell (common) ALL have the best prognosis:

- 75% will go into remission.
- 75% survive beyond 5 years.

A typical treatment regimen can be divided into six phases:

1. Induction: an intensive regimen of between three and five drugs with the aim of reducing tumor load.
2. Early CNS-directed therapy.
3. Consolidation: continued systemic therapy after remission.
4. CNS prophylaxis without irradiation.
5. Intensification of therapy depending on risk of relapse.
6. Maintenance: chemotherapy continues for 2 years from diagnosis.

Initial preparation involves:

- Blood transfusion.
- Treatment of infection.
- Allopurinol to protect the kidneys against the effects of rapid cell lysis.

Relapses can occur in bone marrow, CNS, or testes. The prognosis in these cases is poor and high-dose chemotherapy with total body irradiation and bone marrow transplantation may be necessary for survival. In ALL, bone marrow transplant is used only for high-risk groups because the benefits are counterbalanced by the risks of transplant-related mortality.

Prognostic groups in acute lymphocytic leukemia		
Factors	Good >70% cure (all factors required)	Poor <70% cure (any factor sufficient)
Age	2–9 years	<1 year
WBC	$<50 \times 10^9$ g/L	$>50 \times 10^9$ g/L
Lineage	Non-T, non-B cell	T cell or B cell

Fig. 20.6 Prognostic groups in acute lymphocytic leukemia.

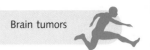

Acute myeloid leukemia

This is classified into seven subtypes; 80% are associated with chromosomal abnormalities and the treatment is more intensive than ALL and carries a worse prognosis. Treatment approach is similar to that of ALL. Bone marrow transplant is used in high-risk groups only because of the mortality associated with the procedure and because studies in good- and intermediate-risk groups have shown no overall benefit.

Lymphomas

These can be classified into:
- Non-Hodgkin's lymphoma (NHL): more common in young children.
- Hodgkin's disease: more common in adolescents and young adults.

Non-Hodgkin's lymphoma (NHL)

NHLs are a heterogeneous group of lymphomas with different characteristics and cells of origin. NHLs cause about 7% of all childhood cancer. They can develop in immunocompromised children with HIV infection, severe combined immunodeficiency, or other severe inherited immunodeficiencies.

Clinical features

NHLs tend to be aggressive and rapidly growing and may present with:
- Peripheral lymph node enlargement: usually B cell origin.
- Intrathoracic mass: usually T cell origin.
- Mediastinal mass or pleural effusion.
- Abdominal mass: usually advanced B cell disease.
- Gut or lymph node masses.

Subtypes of ALL and NHL may represent a continuation of the same disease.

Treatment

Chemotherapy is the mainstay of treatment but extensive surgical debulking may be required for abdominal tumors. Localized disease has a 90% survival at 5 years. Complications in the acute setting are superior vena cava syndrome and tumor lysis syndrome.

Hodgkin's disease

This is characterized histologically by the Reed–Sternberg cell. It is relatively uncommon in prepubertal children and usually presents in adolescence or young adulthood, with a slight preponderance in females.

Clinical features

The usual presentation is with painless cervical or supraclavicular lymphadenopathy. Systemic symptoms are uncommon. Metastatic disease occurs in the lungs, liver, and bone marrow.

Diagnosis

Diagnosis is confirmed by histological examination of a lymph node biopsy. Classification based on histopathology identifies four subtypes of different prognosis:
1. Lymphocyte predominance: best prognosis.
2. Mixed cellularity.
3. Nodular sclerosing: most common in children and adolescents.
4. Lymphocyte depletion: least common, worst prognosis.

Treatment

The disease is staged, to determine treatment, using imaging of chest, mediastinum, and abdomen. Treatment is combination chemotherapy for all except patients with localized disease, who can be treated with radiotherapy. The overall prognosis is good and 80% of patients are cured overall.

Brain tumors

Brain tumors are the second most common form of childhood cancer and the most common solid tumor of childhood. Most are located infratentorially and present with signs and symptoms of raised intracranial pressure and cerebellar dysfunction. Metastasis is rare and diagnosis is often difficult and delayed.

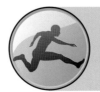

Brain tumors are the most common solid tumor of children. Two-thirds arise below the tentorium.

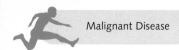
Classification of brain tumors in childhood

Astrocytic tumors
High-grade astrocytomas
• Supratentorial
Low-grade astrocytomas
• Cerebellar
Brainstem gliomas

Neuroepithelial tumors
Primitive neuroendocrine tumors (PNET) (includes
cerebellar medulloblastomas)

Fig. 20.7 Classification of brain tumors in childhood.

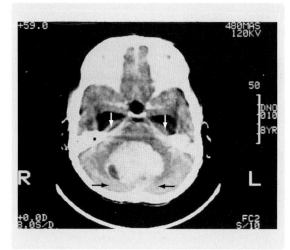

Fig. 20.8 CT of an enhancing posterior fossa tumor (black arrows) with hydrocephalus demonstrated by dilated temporal horns (white arrows).

A classification based on histology is shown in Fig. 20.7. An example of a posterior fossa tumor with hydrocephalus is shown in Fig. 20.8.

Astrocytomas (40%)
Cerebellar astrocytomas are usually low-grade, slow-growing, cystic gliomas occurring between the ages of 6 and 9 years. Presentation may be with:
• Headache and vomiting: caused by obstructive hydrocephalus; papilloedema may be present.
• Cerebellar signs: ataxia, nystagmus, and uncoordination.
• Diplopia, squint: sixth nerve palsy.

Supratentorial astrocytomas and gliomas are less common and present with focal neurologic signs and seizures.

Brainstem gliomas (6%) present with cranial nerve palsies, ataxia and pyramidal tract signs.

Diagnosis is usually based on clinical findings and MR imaging as biopsy is hazardous. Prognosis is poor, with median survival of less than 1 year from diagnosis despite radiotherapy.

Primitive neuroectodermal tumors (medulloblastomas) (20%)
These are the most common malignant brain tumors of childhood, with a peak incidence between the ages of 2 and 6 years, and a preponderance in boys. They usually arise in the midline and invade the fourth ventricle and cerebellar hemispheres. Unlike other CNS tumors they seed through the CNS and up to 20% have spinal metastases at diagnosis.

Presentation is usually with headache, vomiting, and ataxia.

Treatment is surgical removal and whole CNS irradiation (5-year survival rates are 50%). Adjuvant chemotherapy may be added for children with higher than average risk of recurrence.

Craniopharyngioma (4%)
These arise from the squamous remnant of Rathke's pouch and are locally invasive. They present with:
• Visual field loss: due to compression of the optic chiasm.
• Pituitary dysfunction: growth failure, diabetes insipidus.

Most are calcified and are visible on skull radiographs. Treatment is surgical excision and/or radiotherapy. Prognosis is good but sequelae include visual impairment and endocrine deficiency.

Neuroblastoma

Neuroblastoma is a malignancy of neural crest cells that normally give rise to the paraspinal sympathetic ganglia and the adrenal medulla. It is the second most common solid tumor of childhood, occurring predominantly in infants and preschool children with a median age at diagnosis of 2 years. It is unusual in that it can regress spontaneously in very young children (stage IV-S).

Clinical features

The clinical features depend on the location and may include:

- Abdominal mass: a firm, nontender abdominal mass is the most common mode of presentation.
- Systemic signs: pallor, weight loss, bone pain from disseminated disease.
- Hepatomegaly or lymph node enlargement.
- Unilateral proptosis: periorbital swelling and ecchymosis from metastasis to the eye.
- Opsoclonus–myoclonus: "dancing-eye" syndrome caused by an immune response.
- Watery diarrhea due to secretion of vasoactive intestinal peptide.
- Mediastinal mass on CXR.

Diagnosis

Diagnosis is usually made from the characteristic clinical and radiologic features.

- Raised urinary catecholamines (vanillylmandelic acid, homovanillic acid) are useful in diagnosis and monitoring response to therapy.
- Confirmatory biopsy is usually possible and scanning using MIBG (meta-iodobenzyl guanidine), a radiolabeled tumor-specific agent, is useful to measure disease extent.

Treatment

Treatment of neuroblastoma includes:

- Surgical resection.
- Chemotherapy.
- Irradiation.

Prognosis is worse for older children and those with metastatic disease. Overexpression of the *N-myc* oncogene in tumor material is associated with a poor prognosis.

Wilms' tumor (nephroblastoma)

Wilms' tumor arises from embryonal renal cells of the metanephros. It is predominantly a tumor of the first 5 years of life with a median age of presentation of 3 years of age. Sporadic and familial forms occur. Most tumors are unilateral.

Clinical features

The most common clinical presentation is an asymptomatic abdominal mass that does not cross the midline. Other features may include:

- Abdominal pain: due to hemorrhage into the tumor.
- Hematuria.
- Hypertension: in 25% of cases. This can be caused by compression of the renal artery or renin production by tumor cells.

A Wilms' tumor susceptibility gene has been recognized from the rare association of Wilms' tumor, sporadic aniridia and deletions of part of chromosome 11. Associated abnormalities found in some children include:

- Hemihypertrophy.
- Genitourinary tract abnormalities.
- Mental retardation.
- Aniridia.

Wilms' tumor:
- Arises from embryonic renal cells.
- Usually presents as an abdominal mass in a child under 5 years old.
- Is bilateral in 5% of cases.
- Is associated with aniridia (absent iris).

Diagnosis

Diagnosis is normally made from the characteristic appearance on CT (Fig. 20.9), which shows an *intrinsic* renal mass with mixed solid and cystic densities, and from biopsy. A search for distant metastases, which are most common in lungs and liver, should be made.

Treatment

Treatment involves surgical resection of the primary tumor, chemotherapy tailored to the stage and histology, and radiotherapy for those with advanced disease. Overall, the prognosis is good, with an 80% chance of cure if there is no metastasis, although this falls to 30% if metastases are present.

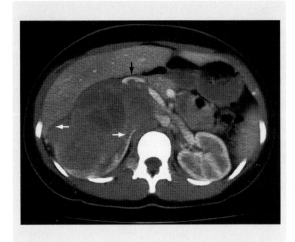

Fig. 20.9 CT scan of nephroblastoma. Wilms' tumor mass arising out of right kidney (white arrows) displacing the inferior vena cava (black arrow).

Soft tissue sarcomas

These arise from primitive mesenchyme. The most important is rhabdomyosarcoma, but even rarer forms include fibrosarcomas and liposarcomas.

Bone tumors

Primary malignant bone tumors account for 4% of childhood cancer. They are uncommon before puberty and are most common in adolescents with a preponderence in boys. The two main types are:
- Osteogenic sarcoma: older children, most common.
- Ewing's sarcoma: younger children, less common.

Osteogenic sarcoma

This is a malignant tumor of the bone-producing mesenchyme and is twice as common in males as females.

Clinical features

The usual presenting feature is local pain and swelling. Persistent bone pain precedes the detection of a mass. Half of all cases occur around the knee joint in the metaphysis of the distal femur or proximal tibia. Systemic symptoms are rare. Metastases are mainly to the lungs and are often asymptomatic.

Diagnosis

Bone x-ray shows destruction and a characteristic "sunburst" appearance as the tumor breaks through the cortex and spicules of new bone are formed.

Treatment

Treatment involves surgery of primary and metastatic deposits. En bloc resection may allow amputation to be avoided. Aggressive neoadjuvant chemotherapy is important to treat micrometastatic disease. Survival has improved and is greater than 50%.

Ewing's sarcoma

This is less common than osteogenic sarcoma. It is an undifferentiated sarcoma of uncertain tissue of origin that arises primarily in bone, but occasionally in soft tissues.

It most commonly affects the long bones, especially the mid- to proximal femur, but can also affect flat bones such as the pelvis.

Clinical features and diagnosis

Pain and localized swelling are the usual presenting complaints. X-ray demonstrates a destructive lesion with periosteal elevation or a soft tissue mass (so-called "onion skin" appearance). Metastases occur to the lungs and other bones.

Treatment

Radiotherapy to the primary tumor is combined with chemotherapy for the prevention or treatment of metastases.

Bone tumors:
- Are most common in adolescence.
- Are more common in boys.
- Most commonly affect the long bones.

Retinoblastoma

This is a cause of an absent red reflex in the neonate. It is associated with deletion of a tumor suppressor gene on chromosome 13 and is bilateral in 40%.

Langerhans cell histiocytosis

Formerly called histiocytosis X, this disease encompasses a group of relatively rare diseases characterized by the clonal proliferation of Langerhans cells (components of the bone-marrow-derived mononuclear phagocytic system). It is now not considered a true malignancy but the potentially aggressive course and response to chemotherapy brings it within this sphere of clinical practice.

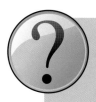

- Describe the approach to treatment in leukemia.
- What acute complications occur as a result of chemotherapy?
- What are the long-term complications in childhood oncology survivors?
- How would you diagnose brain tumors?
- What are the complications of chemotherapy for cancer?

Further reading

Will A. Recent advances in the management of leukemia. *Current Paediatrics* 2003; 13:201–216.

21. Endocrine and Metabolic Disorders

The most common and important of this group of disorders is insulin-dependent diabetes mellitus (IDDM), also known as type 1 diabetes mellitus. Although less common, a host of other childhood endocrine and metabolic diseases exist and affect such vital processes as growth, sexual maturation, and calcium metabolism. Finally, there are several hundred inborn errors of metabolism that are individually rare but important to recognize as many are treatable and genetic counseling for parents is often required.

Disorders of carbohydrate metabolism

The three most important disorders of carbohydrate metabolism are:
- Diabetes mellitus.
- Hypoglycemia (not associated with diabetes mellitus).
- Ketotic hypoglycemia.

Diabetes mellitus

This is a heterogeneous group of disorders, characterized by hyperglycemia and caused by reduced or absent insulin secretion or action. Type 1 diabetes (formerly called insulin-dependent diabetes) is the most common form of childhood diabetes, although other varieties may be encountered. Type 2 diabetes is characterized by insulin resistance, and its increasing incidence has been associated with childhood obesity; however, the discussion below refers to type 1.

Etiology

There is good evidence that type 1 diabetes results from T-cell-mediated autoimmune destruction of β cells in the pancreatic islets of Langerhans, perhaps triggered by environmental factors (e.g., viruses) in people with a genetic predisposition (Fig. 21.1). The incidence of the disorder is increasing in the USA.

Pathophysiology

The pathophysiologic pathways are described in Fig. 21.2. Key features include:
- Insulin deficiency becomes clinically significant when 90% of the β cells are destroyed.
- Osmotic diuresis ensues when blood glucose concentration exceeds renal threshold.
- Ketoacidosis develops when insulin deficiency is severe.

Clinical features

Although type 1 diabetes can present at any age, the most common age of onset is between 7 and 15 years of age. Increasingly, type 1 diabetes is diagnosed at an early stage, when the principal features are:
- Polyuria: increased frequency of urination (possibly enuresis).
- Polydipsia: increased thirst.
- Weight loss.

Always check for glycosuria in a child with a history of polyuria and polydipsia. Never ascribe increased frequency of micturition to urinary tract infection without checking for glycosuria and culturing urine.

Diabetic ketoacidosis supervenes at a late stage over a short period and is characterized by abdominal pain, vomiting, features of severe dehydration, and ketoacidosis. Younger children develop more severe complications of ketoacidosis.

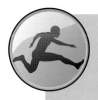
Traps for the unwary regarding diabetic ketoacidosis include mistaking the abdominal pain for acute appendicitis and mistaking the hyperventilation for pneumonia.

Etiology of insulin-dependent mellitus (IDDM)

Genetic factors
Inherited susceptibility is demonstrated by increased incidence of IDDM in first-degree relatives: 2–5% in siblings and offspring. Concordance for identical twins is 30%. There is an 8–10 times risk for IDDM in people who are HLA-DR3, HLA-DR4, or both

Autoimmune factors
Autoimmune basis is supported by:
- Anti-islet cell antibodies
- Lymphocyte infiltration of pancreas
- Association with other autoimmune disorders (e.g., thyroiditis, Addison disease)

Environmental factors
Triggers may include viruses and dietary proteins

Fig. 21.1 Etiology of insulin-dependent diabetes mellitus.

Diagnosis

Diagnosis is confirmed in a symptomatic child by documenting hyperglycemia—a random plasma glucose level >200 mg/L (11.1 mmol/L). If there is doubt, as may occur very early in the disease process, a fasting plasma glucose >125 mg/dL (7 mmol/L) or a raised glycosylated hemoglobin level will clarify the situation. Oral glucose tolerance tests are rarely needed in children.

Management

The discovery of insulin in 1922 transformed type 1 diabetes mellitus from a fatal disease into a treatable one. Initial management depends on the child's clinical condition. Long-term management of this life-long condition rests on:

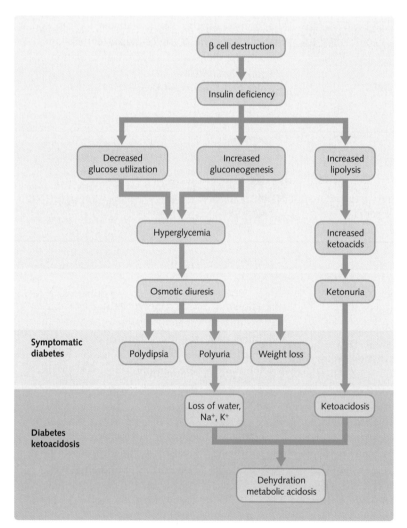

Fig. 21.2 Pathophysiology of insulin-dependent diabetes mellitus.

- Insulin replacement.
- Diet.
- Exercise.
- Monitoring.
- Education and psychological support.
- Management of complications: hypoglycemia and diabetic ketoacidosis.

These are considered in turn.

Insulin replacement

The important features of insulin replacement are:

- Average requirement is 1.0 unit/kg/day. During the "honeymoon" or remission phase, which can last for weeks or months after presentation, residual islet cell function causes a reduction in insulin requirements temporarily.
- The total daily dose is divided in a 1 : 3 proportion between short-acting (regular, soluble) insulin and medium-acting (isophane) insulin. Two-thirds is usually given before breakfast and one-third before the evening meal, so two injections per day are administered.
- Ultra-rapid acting insulins are becoming common as their convenience leads to improved glucose control.
- Injections are given subcutaneously and can be given in upper arms, outer thighs, or abdomen. The site must be rotated to avoid local complications such as fat atrophy.
- During puberty, insulin requirements increase. More frequent insulin injections are often required as they offer greater flexibility in glycemic control.

Diet and exercise

Food intake needs to match the time course of insulin absorption and be adjusted for heavy exercise. Dietary management therefore encompasses:

- High fiber, complex carbohydrates: this provides sustained release of glucose and avoids rapid swings in blood glucose generated by refined carbohydrates (e.g., sweets or ice cream).
- Food intake is divided between the three main meals and intervening snacks.
- Food intake is increased before or after heavy exercise to avoid hypoglycemia.

Monitoring

Monitoring of blood glucose concentrations is necessary to evaluate the management and control. This is performed using finger-prick samples, which are convenient and easy to take. Readings are recorded in a diary so changes to insulin regimens can be appropriately made. Twenty-four-hour profiles are more useful than single daily records. Urine testing is more indirect, does not detect unacceptably low levels of glucose, and is often less popular, especially with teenagers. However, urine testing for ketones is important if ketoacidosis is suspected.

The measurement of glycosylated hemoglobin (HbA1c) reflects glycemic control over the past 6–8 weeks and allows long-term glucose control to be optimized. A higher level of HbA1c is accepted in children compared to adults because hypoglycemia has potential for greater morbidity in children and compliance with complex regimens is more likely to be poor.

Urine testing to monitor glucose control is inaccurate and should not be done.

Education and psychological support

Children and their families require an educational program that covers:

- A basic understanding of diabetes in lay language.
- The influence of diet and exercise on blood glucose levels.
- Practical aspects of insulin injection and blood glucose monitoring.
- Recognition and treatment of hypoglycemia.
- Adjustments for intercurrent illness, significance of ketonuria.
- The importance of good control.

The diagnosis of type 1 diabetes provokes strong emotional responses in the child and family, including anger, guilt, resentment, and fear. Adjustment to these normal responses is facilitated by open discussion. Voluntary groups (e.g., the American Diabetes Association) are important sources of support.

Adolescence and diabetes mellitus:
- Adolescence is often a difficult time for the diabetic.
- There may be conflict at home and with health care professionals.
- Problems occur with self-image, self-esteem, and desire for independence.
- Denial or indifference can lead to poor compliance.
- "Feeling well" is equated with good control and long-term risks are often ignored.
- Helpful strategies include: a united team approach, clear guidelines plus short-term goals, and peer group pressure.

Management of complications

These can be divided into immediate complications, which include hypoglycemia and diabetic ketoacidosis, and late complications.

Hypoglycemia

The concentration of glucose in the blood can fall when there is a mismatch between insulin dose, time of administration, carbohydrate intake, and exercise. Many young children are not aware of hypoglycemic episodes, and repeated hypoglycemic episodes increase this lack of awareness.

Symptoms usually occur at blood glucose levels below 40 mg/dL (2.2 mmol/L). Initial symptoms reflect the compensatory sympathetic discharge and include feeling faint, dizzy, or "wobbly," sweating, tremulousness, and hunger. More severe symptoms reflect glucose deprivation to the central nervous system and include lethargy, bizarre behavior and—ultimately—coma or seizures. Unlike adults and older children, in young children the behavioral and neuroglycopenic symptoms predominate over autonomic symptoms.

Treatment of a hypoglycemic episode is easily achieved at an early stage by administration of a sugary drink, glucose tablet, or glucose polymer gel, which is well absorbed via the buccal mucosa. At a later stage, if consciousness is impaired or

there is lack of cooperation, IV glucose or 1 mg of IM glucagon is administered. Eating a sugary snack just before exercising reduces the risk of exercise-induced hypoglycemia.

Diabetic ketoacidosis

This can occur at presentation or complicate established diabetes (e.g., if there is poor compliance or intercurrent illness). It is considered in Chapter 26.

Late complications of diabetes

Intensive insulin control—checking the blood sugar level multiple times per day and taking 3–4 insulin injections daily—reduces the incidence of long-term vascular complications of diabetes, such as:
- Retinopathy.
- Nephropathy.
- Neuropathy.

The degree of intensive control has to be weighed against the risk of hypoglycemia in young children because intensive control is associated with greater incidence of hypoglycemic episodes. This is usually acceptable only in older children.

Hypoglycemia not associated with diabetes mellitus

As a distinct problem, hypoglycemia has many causes beyond just diabetes. It is a common problem in the newborn (see Chapter 25) but is still seen occasionally in infants and children. It is important to diagnose because it is easy to treat and has serious consequences if unrecognized.

The various causes are best understood in relation to the normal factors determining glucose homeostasis. The major causes are listed in Fig. 21.3.

Clinical features

Early symptoms reflect the compensatory sympathetic response and include dizziness, faintness, and hunger. Signs include tachycardia, sweating, and pallor. Late features are neuroglycopenia: altered behavior and consciousness, headache, and seizures.

Diagnosis

The precise definition of hypoglycemia is problematic, but a useful working definition is a blood glucose less than 2.6 mmol/L. This corresponds to changes in the EEG. Measurements

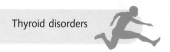

Causes of hypoglycemia beyond the neonatal period

Metabolic
Ketotic hypoglycemia
Liver disease
Inborn errors of metabolism (e.g., glycogen storage diseases)

Hormonal
Deficiency
- Adrenocortical insufficiency (e.g., Addison disease, congenital adrenal hyperplasia)
- Panhypopituitarism
- Growth hormone deficiency
Hyperinsulinism
- Islet cell adenoma
- Exogenous insulin-treated IDDM

Fig. 21.3 Causes of hypoglycemia beyond the neonatal period.

made using a glucose-sensitive strip should always be verified by a laboratory measurement. Serum and urine should be taken during the attack for further diagnostic testing (e.g., for metabolic disorders).

Management
If the child is alert, then giving a sugary drink is the first step; an unconscious child should be given 2–3 mL/kg 10% dextrose IV. Higher concentrations have been associated with rebound hypoglycemia and should be avoided. Blood glucose should be monitored closely, and a maintenance infusion of glucose can be given if the hypoglycemia persists. Glucagon can be used in cases where glycogen stores are not depleted (e.g., insulin overdose).

Ketotic hypoglycemia
The most common cause of hypoglycemia in children 1–4 years of age, this ill-defined entity is the result of diminished tolerance of normal fasting. The typical child is short and thin and becomes hypoglycemic after a short period of starvation—for example, in the early morning. Insulin levels are low, and there is ketonuria. Treatment is with frequent snacks and extra glucose drinks during intercurrent illness. Spontaneous resolution occurs by the ages of 5–8 years.

Regarding hypoglycemia, at the time of blood glucose measurement, samples should be sent for measurement of:
- Plasma insulin, growth hormone, and cortisol.
- β-hydroxybutyrate.
Urine should be tested for ketones.

Thyroid disorders

Thyroid hormone is critical for normal growth and neurologic development in infants and children. Conditions causing hypothyroidism and hyperthyroidism occur, and the gland can also be the site of benign and malignant tumors. Worldwide, the most important condition affecting the thyroid gland is iodide deficiency, estimated to affect at least 800 million people.

Hypothyroidism
This may be present at birth (congenital hypothyroidism) or develop at any time during childhood or adolescence (acquired hypothyroidism).

Congenital hypothyroidism
This has an incidence of 1 in 4000 live births. The causes include:
- Developmental defects: thyroid agenesis or failure of migration.
- Dyshormonogenesis: inborn error of thyroid hormone synthesis (accounts for 15%, a goiter usually occurs).
- Transient congenital hypothyroidism: (e.g., ingestion of maternal goitrogens).
- Congenital pituitary lesions (rare).
- Maternal iodide deficiency: the most common cause worldwide.

Clinical features
Infants may appear clinically normal at birth. The clinical features that develop include:
- Prolonged neonatal jaundice.
- Feeding problems.
- Constipation.
- Coarse facies, large fontanelle, large tongue, hypotonia, and goiter.

177

Diagnosis and treatment

As congenital hypothyroidism is common and treatable, neonatal screening is undertaken in the USA. Most laboratories test for raised levels of thyroid-stimulating hormone (TSH), although some measure both TSH and thyroxine (T_4). With neonatal screening and early treatment with oral thyroxine, neurological function and intelligence are within the normal range. Acquired hypothyroidism is treated with thyroxine. Monitoring of treatment is by regular assessment of TSH and T_4.

Hyperthyroidism

Neonatal hyperthyroidism can occur in the infants of mothers with Graves' disease from the transplacental transfer of thyroid-stimulating immunoglobulins.

Juvenile hyperthyroidism

This is most commonly caused by Graves' disease, an autoimmune condition in which one type of antibody (human thyroid stimulating immunoglobulins) mimics TSH by binding and activating the TSH receptor. It usually presents during adolescence and is much more common in girls than boys.

The clinical features are similar to those seen in adults and can also include deteriorating school performance; puberty may be delayed or accelerated.

On laboratory testing, serum levels of thyroxine (T_4) and triiodothyronine (T_3) are elevated and TSH levels are depressed. Antimicrosomal antibodies are often present.

Medical therapy with propylthiouracil (PTU) or methimazole (MMI) is the first line of treatment. β-blockers can be added for relief of severe symptoms but should be discontinued when thyroid function is controlled. Subtotal thyroidectomy or radioiodine treatments are options for relapse after medical treatment. Radioiodine has not been shown to be harmful in children.

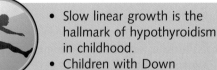

- Slow linear growth is the hallmark of hypothyroidism in childhood.
- Children with Down syndrome have an increased incidence of hypothyroidism and hyperthyroidism.

Adrenal disorders

Disorders of the adrenal cortex can result in deficiency or excess of adrenocortical hormones. The latter causes Cushing syndrome, the most common cause of which is chronic administration of corticosteroids. Disorders of the medulla (e.g., pheochromocytoma) are exceedingly rare.

Cortisol, the major glucocorticoid, is stimulated by pituitary adrenocorticotrophic hormone (ACTH) under a negative feedback loop. Aldosterone is the principal mineralocorticoid and is controlled by the renin–angiotensin system. The major sex steroids produced by the adrenal glands are androgens.

Adrenocortical insufficiency

Diminished production of adrenocortical hormones may arise from:
- Congenital adrenal hyperplasia (CAH): an inherited inborn error of metabolism in biosynthesis of adrenal corticosteroids.
- Primary adrenal cortical insufficiency: Addison's disease.
- Secondary adrenal insufficiency: ACTH deficiency due to pituitary disease or long-term corticosteroid therapy.

Congenital adrenal hyperplasia (CAH)

This is a group of disorders caused by a defect in the pathway that synthesizes cortisol from cholesterol. Approximately 90% of cases are caused by a deficiency in 21-hydroxylase, and 5–7% are due to 11-hydroxylase deficiency. Other defects are seen but are rare. Prevalence is approximately 1 in 10,000, and newborn screening is available in some centers. The condition is autosomal recessive, and the gene is found on chromosome 6.

Clinical features

Clinical features are due to androgen excess and cortisol deficiency:
- Female virilization.
- Salt-wasting crises due to mineralocorticoid deficiency (this is less common with 11-hydroxylase deficiency). This leads to volume depletion, electrolyte imbalances, and shock.
- Cortisol deficiency.

It is difficult to diagnose male infants with this disorder because they have few clinical manifestations at birth. For this reason, screening programs are currently being evaluated.

Diagnosis
Diagnosis rests on the demonstration of markedly elevated levels of 17 α-hydroxyprogesterone in the serum. In the "salt-losing" form, the characteristic electrolyte disturbance of hyponatremia, hypochloridemia, and hyperkalemia provides a clue to the diagnosis.

Management
Initial management of a "salt-wasting" crisis involves volume replacement with normal saline and systemic steroids. Parents are also taught to recognize early signs of illness and children should carry a card or wear a medical alert bracelet/necklace to alert health professionals.

Long-term treatment involves:
- Cortisol replacement with hydrocortisone: to suppress ACTH and androgen overproduction. Growth is used as a monitor of therapy.
- Mineralocorticoid replacement: Florinef if there is salt wasting.
- Surgical correction of female genital abnormalities.

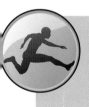
Congenital adrenal hyperplasia is a potentially lethal but treatable cause of vomiting and dehydration in young infants.

Primary adrenal insufficiency
Addison's disease is rare in children but can be caused by:
- Autoimmune disease.
- Hemorrhage and infarction (Waterhouse-Friderichsen syndrome).
- Tuberculosis (rare).

Physical findings include postural hypotension and increased pigmentation. Intercurrent illness or trauma can trigger an adrenal crisis (characterized by vomiting, dehydration, and shock).

Secondary adrenal insufficiency
This is most commonly caused by prolonged glucocorticoid use in diseases not involving the adrenal gland (e.g., severe chronic asthma). The risk is increased by increased duration of treatment, but courses less than 10 days have a low risk. Reduction of steroid doses should be slow after a prolonged course and tailored to the underlying disease. This also rarely occurs with high-dose inhaled steroids.

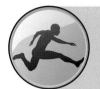
Steroid administration must not be stopped suddenly. If the child is sick, an increased dose may be needed.

Cushing syndrome
This is a cluster of symptoms and signs caused by glucocorticoid excess, due either to endogenous overproduction of cortisol or exogenous treatment with pharmacologic doses of corticosteroids. The causes are listed in Fig. 21.4.

Clinical features
The clinical features include:
- Short stature.
- Truncal obesity, "buffalo" hump.
- Rounded "moon" facies.
- Signs of virilization, striae.
- Hypertension.

Diagnosis
Elevated serum cortisol levels are found with absence of the normal diurnal rhythm (low morning levels). A prolonged dexamethasone suppression test may be required to distinguish Cushing disease (ACTH-driven bilateral adrenal hyperplasia: suppressible by dexamethasone) from Cushing syndrome (adrenal tumor: cortisol levels not suppressed by dexamethasone). CT or MRI of the adrenal and pituitary glands may identify an

Causes of Cushing syndrome	
Primary	Adrenal tumor
Secondary	ACTH secretion from: Pituitary tumor Ectopic ACTH production
Iatrogenic	Long-term glucocorticoid administration

Fig. 21.4 Causes of Cushing syndrome.

adrenal tumor or pituitary adenoma. Treatment depends on the cause and may involve surgical resection and radiotherapy.

Disorders of the pituitary gland

The pituitary gland has two distinct portions: the anterior and posterior lobes. These have different embryonic origins and separate hormonal functions. Pituitary disorders in childhood are rare.

Anterior pituitary disorders
A deficiency of the anterior pituitary hormones is more common than an excess of these and may involve individual hormones or all (panhypopituitarism). Hypopituitarism in children can be caused by:
- Cranial defects (e.g., septo-optic dysplasia and agenesis of corpus callosum).
- Tumors (e.g., craniopharyngioma).
- Idiopathic hormone abnormalities.
- Trauma/surgery and radiation.

Growth retardation is a common feature. Thyroid, adrenal, and gonadal dysfunction, depending on the pattern of deficiency, is also common. Isolated idiopathic growth hormone (GH) deficiency accounts for most cases of GH deficiency.

Posterior pituitary disorders
The posterior lobe (neurohypophysis) secretes arginine, vasopressin (also called antidiuretic hormone [ADH]), and oxytocin.

Diabetes insipidus
This results from deficiency of ADH. It may occur as an isolated idiopathic defect or in association with anterior pituitary deficiency (e.g., due to tumors, infections, or trauma).

It presents with polydipsia and polyuria. Several conditions mimic diabetes insipidus, including hypercalcemia, chronic renal disease, and psychogenic water drinking. Diagnosis is by a water deprivation test.

Syndrome of inappropriate secretion of ADH (SIADH)
Diagnosis consists of:
- Hypo-osmolality with hyponatremia.
- Normal or increased volume status.
- Normal renal, thyroid, and adrenal function.
- Elevated urine sodium and osmolality.

Symptoms occur due to effects of water intoxication: these include vomiting, behavioural changes and seizures.

SIADH is a common sequela of several underlying conditions, including:
- CNS disease: meningitis, brain tumors, or head trauma.
- Lung disease: pneumonia.

Treatment is by treating the underlying cause and fluid restriction.

Disorders of the gonads

These cause abnormalities of sexual differentiation (which usually present in the newborn) and disorders of puberty, which may be precocious or delayed.

Disorders of sexual differentiation
Abnormal sexual differentiation results in a newborn with ambiguous genitalia (intersex). Congenital adrenal hyperplasia leading to a virilized female is the most common cause. The causes can be classified as shown in Fig. 21.5.

Complete diagnostic evaluation should be undertaken as soon as possible. A definite sex cannot and should not be assigned immediately. It is worth remembering that "sex" is determined at

Causes of abnormal sexual differentiation
46XY males with testes and incomplete masculinization due to:
• Defects in testosterone synthesis
• Defects in androgen (e.g., 5α-reductase deficiency)
• Androgen resistance (testicular feminization syndrome)
46XX females with ovaries who are masculinized due to:
• Congenital adrenal hyperplasia
• Maternal androgen exposure

Fig. 21.5 Causes of abnormal sexual differentiation.

many different levels (Fig. 21.6). Naming and announcement of the child's sex should be delayed until the diagnostic work-up is complete. Investigations will include:
- Chromosomal analysis.
- Hormone levels: testosterone, luteinizing hormone, follicle stimulating hormone, 17-hydroxyprogesterone.
- Pelvic ultrasonography.

Management is multidisciplinary, involving:
- Endocrinology.
- Psychology.
- Pediatric urology and gynecology.

Disorders of puberty

During normal puberty, secondary sex characteristics are acquired and reproductive capacity is attained. Features of normal puberty in males and females are listed in Fig. 21.7. Puberty can be precocious or delayed.

Precocious puberty

This refers to the development of secondary sexual characteristics before the age of 8 years in girls or 9 years in boys. There is an associated growth spurt. It should be differentiated from:
- Premature thelarche: isolated breast development in a very young girl. A nonprogressive, benign condition.
- Premature adrenarche: isolated early appearance of pubic hair in either sex. A benign, self-limiting condition due to early maturation of adrenal androgen secretion, although an adrenal tumor may need to be excluded.

The causes of precocious puberty are shown in Fig. 21.8. In females, it is usually due to early onset of normal puberty. In boys, it is usually pathologic and must be investigated.

Treatment depends on cause. Gonadotropin-releasing hormone analogs (GnRHa) can be used to prevent puberty from progressing.

Delayed puberty

This can be defined as the absence of secondary sex characteristics at 14 years of age in girls or 15 years of age in boys. The problem is more common in boys, and the majority of adolescents affected are normal. The causes are listed in Fig. 21.9.

Assessment should include pubertal staging and examination to exclude systemic disease. If indicated, helpful investigations are:
- Chromosomal analysis.
- Measurement of gonadotropin levels.

Treatment is often not required for constitutional delay, but hormone therapy (e.g., oxandrolone or low-dose testosterone) can be used to accelerate growth and induce secondary sexual characteristics in boys. Estrogen therapy can be used in girls, but care must be taken to prevent premature closure of the epiphyses.

Sex differentiation
An individual's sex is determined at many different levels: • Chromosomal • Gonadal (testis, ovary) • Anatomic (internal and external genitalia) • Hormonal • Psychological • Sex of rearing

Fig. 21.6 Sex determination.

Fig. 21.7 Features of puberty.

Features of puberty	
Male genitalia	First sign is testicular growth Followed by penis enlargement Growth spurt reached 2 years later than females
Female genitalia	First sign is breast development (breast buds) Followed by development of pubic and axillary hair Menses occur late

Causes of precocious puberty

Gonadotropin-dependent
- Idiopathic, familial
- CNS lesions (e.g., postirradiation, surgery, tumors, hydrocephalus)

Gonadotropin-independent
- McCune–Albright syndrome (polycystic fibrous dysplasia of bone)
- Tumors of adrenals or gonads

Fig. 21.8 Causes of precocious puberty.

Causes of delayed puberty

Central causes—gonadotropins low
- Constitutional delayed puberty
- Hypothalamopituitary disorders (e.g., panhypopituitarism, intracranial tumors, isolated gonadotropin deficiency)
- Severe systemic disease (e.g., cystic fibrosis, severe asthma, starvation)

Gonadal failure—gonadotropins high
Chromosomal abnormalities (e.g., Klinefelter syndrome [47,XXY], Turner syndrome [45,XO])

Fig. 21.9 Causes of delayed puberty.

- Precocious puberty is more common in girls.
- Delayed puberty is more common in boys.

Inborn errors of metabolism

This term is used to describe any of the inherited disorders that result in a defect in normal biochemical pathways. Several hundred of these conditions have been described. Individually they are rare, although certain ethnic groups are at increased risk for specific diseases.

Inborn errors of metabolism are usually autosomal recessive, although some are X-linked. The main categories are listed in Fig. 21.10.

The clinical effects may be caused by accumulation of excess precursors, toxic metabolites or metabolic energy insufficiency.

Categories of inborn errors of metabolism	
Category	**Examples**
Amino acid metabolism	Phenylketonuria
Organic acid metabolism	Maple syrup urine disease
Urea cycle disorders	Ornithine transcarbamylase
Carbohydrate metabolism	Galactosemia Glycogen storage diseases
Mucopolysaccharidosis	Hurler syndrome

Fig. 21.10 Categories of inborn errors of metabolism

Clinical manifestations are nonspecific and often mistaken for sepsis. Metabolic stress often precipitates symptoms, e.g., weaning, intercurrent infections, and commonly during the neonatal period.

Features that should raise the suspicion of a metabolic error in the neonate include:
- Parental consanguinity.
- Previous sudden infant death.
- Previous multiple miscarriages.
- Encephalopathic episodes.
- Severe disease for which a diagnosis has not been forthcoming.

Investigations may reveal severe metabolic acidosis, hypoglycemia, or hyperammonemia. In older children, they should be considered as a cause of:
- Progressive learning difficulties.
- Developmental delay.
- Seizures.
- Failure to thrive.
- Coarse facies.
- Hepatosplenomegaly.

Investigations that should be undertaken for an initial screen include:
- Urea and electrolytes, liver function tests, lactate and ammonia levels.
- Acid–base status and anion gap.
- Cerebrospinal fluid (CSF) lactate.
- Blood levels of glucose and amino acids.
- Urine amino acids and organic acids: ketonuria is abnormal as neonates do not readily produce ketones in the urine.

Treatment is to stop feeds and administer dextrose to stop metabolic load and further catabolism. Correction of metabolic disturbances and ventilatory and renal support may be necessary.

Although in many conditions the prognosis is very poor, the diagnosis should be made so that prenatal diagnosis can be performed in future pregnancies.

Examples of individual inborn errors of metabolism are considered briefly in turn.

Phenylketonuria (PKU)

This autosomal recessive trait has an incidence of 1 in 10,000 live births with a carrier rate of 1 : 50. In most cases, the defect lies in the enzyme phenylalanine hydroxylase, which normally converts phenylalanine to tyrosine. Hyperphenylalaninemia occurs, with a build-up of toxic byproducts, such as phenylacetic acid, which are excreted in the urine (hence phenylketonuria).

As PKU is relatively common and is treatable, newborn screening is carried out by the Guthrie test. This is carried out when the child is a few days old because it is necessary for the infant to have been fed milk, which contains phenylalanine.

Infants with PKU are clinically normal at birth. Symptoms and signs appear later in infancy and even childhood if the disorder is undetected and untreated. These include:

- Neurologic manifestations: moderate to severe mental retardation, hypertonicity, tremors, behavior disorders, and seizures.
- Growth retardation.
- Hypopigmentation: fair skin, light hair (due to the block in tyrosine formation that is required for melanin production).

Treatment consists of dietary manipulation. The phenylalanine content of the diet is reduced. This should start early in infancy and is continued until at least 6 years of age. Some authorities recommend lifelong dietary restriction, but the diet is unpalatable. Females with PKU must be on dietary restriction if planning a pregnancy, because maternal hyperphenylalaninemia is associated with spontaneous abortion, microcephaly, and congenital heart disease.

Galactosemia

This causes neonatal liver disfunction, coagulopathy, and cataracts. It has an association with *E. coli* sepsis. It is diagnosed by the presence of reducing substances in the urine and galactose-1-phosphate uridyltransferase in red cells. A high suspicion of this disorder should be considered in all cases of severe neonatal jaundice. Treatment is by a lactose-free diet, and it is an absolute contraindication to breastfeeding.

Glycogen storage diseases

This group of conditions is caused by defects in the enzymes involved in glycogen synthesis or breakdown. There is an abnormal accumulation of glycogen in tissues. The pattern of organ involvement depends on the enzyme defect and may include liver, heart, brain, skeletal muscle, or other organs. There are at least six varieties, some of which have eponyms (e.g., type 1A, or von Gierke's disease; glucose-6-phosphatase deficiency). Affected children have growth failure, hypoglycemia, and hepatomegaly. Treatment is by frequent feeds throughout day and night.

Mucopolysaccharidoses (MPS)

This group of disorders is caused by defects in enzymes involved in the metabolism and storage of mucopolysaccharides. They are progressive multisystem disorders that can affect the central nervous system, eyes, heart, and skeletal system. Characteristic features are:

- Developmental delay in the first year.
- Coarse facies: develop in most cases although children are normal at birth.

There are numerous types, many of which have eponymous designations (e.g., MPS I, or Hurler syndrome, which is autosomal recessive). Affected children develop coarse facial features, corneal opacities, hepatosplenomegaly, kyphosis, and mental retardation.

Diagnosis is made by identifying the enzyme defect and identifying the excretion in the urine of the major storage substances, the glycosaminoglycans. Treatment is by bone marrow transplant if performed early.

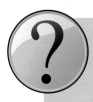

- How would you diagnose diabetes in children?
- What insulin regimen would you use in a newly diagnosed diabetic aged 5 years?
- Why is close control of blood sugar difficult in young children?
- What long-term complications of diabetes are found in adulthood?
- What are the clinical manifestations of hypoglycemia?
- Why is neonatal thyroid screening important?
- How do neonates with inborn errors of metabolism present?
- What inborn errors of metabolism are screened for? Why?

Further reading

Devendra D, Liu E, Eisenbarth GS. Type I diabetes: recent developments. *British Medical Journal* 2004; 328:750–754.

Wraith JE, Cleary MA, Chakrapani A. Detection of inborn errors of metabolism in the newborn. *Archives of Diseases in Childhood. Fetal Neonatology Edition* 2001.

22. Disorders of Emotion and Behavior

Major psychoses rarely present during childhood, although disturbed emotions and behavioral problems are very prevalent. The conditions encountered are, not surprisingly, age-related and range from the toddler who will not sleep to deliberate self-harm in an adolescent.

A child's personality, behavior patterns, and emotional responses are determined by an interplay between nature (genetic endowment) and nurture (environment, e.g., parents). The relative importance of genes and environment remains the subject of debate and current research.

An infant's first relationship is usually with the mother, and separation anxiety typically becomes evident at about 6 months to 1 year. By the second year, emotional attachments are extended to the father and other family members, and by the age of 4–5 years separation from parents can be tolerated for several hours as occurs with school attendance.

With entry into school, the importance of others—such as teachers and fellow school children—in shaping the child's psychosocial development increases.

Early, strong, emotional bonding underpins normal emotional development.

Nature

Some children have a temperament that in itself can make it difficult for the parents to maintain a positive, loving relationship. Features may include:
- Predominantly negative mood.
- Intense emotional reactions.
- Poor and slow adjustment to new situations.

Developmental delay (e.g., slow language development) can also cause problems.

Nurture

Families are the most powerful environmental influence on a child's emotional and behavioral development. Adequate parenting will endeavor to:
- Provide love and affection.
- Provide food and shelter and protect children from physical harm.
- Exert authority to establish reasonable limits on behavior.

Risk factors with an adverse influence are shown in Fig. 22.1.

Problems of early childhood

Behavioral problems can relate to sleeping or eating, and tantrums are common. The rare disorder of autism may present at this time.

Sleep-related problems
Babies
An average baby sleeps for 15 hours a day in the first 2–3 months of life, sleeping for about 4 hours and waking for 3 hours at a time. At about 4 months, night-time breastfeeds are often discontinued, and the baby may sleep through for 8 hours. Some babies are "quiet wakeners"; some are not and appear to sleep less.

Toddlers
Problems include:
- Difficulty in settling to sleep at night.
- Waking at night.
- Nightmares and night terrors.

Difficulty in getting to sleep at night
A child may not settle at night for many reasons including:
- Separation anxiety.
- Fear of darkness and silence.
- Erratic bedtime routine.
- Use of the bedroom as punishment.

Factors associated with disturbed emotional and behavioral development

Parental factors
- Maternal depression
- Marital discord
- Divorce or bereavement
- Intrusive overprotection or emotional rejection
- Inconsistent discipline

Socioeconomic factors
- Poverty, poor housing

Fig. 22.1 Factors associated with disturbed emotional and behavioral development.

Helpful strategies include creating a predictable structure around bedtime and leaving the child alone to settle for lengthening periods.

Nightmares and night terrors

Nightmares are bad dreams that can be recalled by the child. They are common and normal unless very frequent or stereotyped in content. Reassurance is usually sufficient.

Night terrors are a form of parasomnia in which there is rapid emergence from the initial period of deep, slow-wave sleep into a state of high arousal and confusion. The child usually cries out and is found sitting up with open eyes but disoriented and unresponsive. The child settles, with no subsequent recall of the episode. Waking the child briefly before the night terror is expected to occur may break the pattern. Normally, night terrors resolve without intervention—just patience.

Food refusal

Meal times can easily become a battleground. Parents often find that their toddler refuses to eat the meals provided or is a fussy eater. The child is invariably well nourished or small with a normal rate of weight gain. Advice can be given to avoid:

- Excessive food and drink between main meals.
- Irregular meal times.
- Unsuitable food or unreasonably large portions.
- Punitive methods (e.g., forcing a child to eat cold food).

Small amounts of food with gradual introduction of new foods in a relaxed, nonbargaining atmosphere is the best approach. No preschool child will voluntarily starve him- or herself, although some mothers find this difficult to believe.

Tantrums

Toddlers normally go through a period in which they are disinclined to comply with their parents' demands; this phase is sometimes referred to as "the terrible twos," although it may occur between 18 months and 4 years. Temper tantrums can occur in response to frustration. Parents may become demoralized in their attempts to assert control.

Management

Management strategies for "toddler taming" include:

- Praising compliance and rewarding good behavior.
- Avoiding threats that are not carried out.
- Setting reasonable limits.
- Giving clear commands.

A tantrum itself can be dealt with by ignoring it (this can be difficult, especially in a public place) or by giving the child a "time-out" (removing him or her from social interaction for a short period— for example, in a separate room).

Autistic spectrum disorder

This rare, pervasive condition presents in early childhood with a triad of difficulties that is usually evident before the age of 3 years. It is part of a spectrum of disorders characterized by profound impairment of social interactions.

The prevalence is 0.7–21 cases out of 10,000 children with an excess of males (M : F ratio = 4 : 1). Autism is an organic neurodevelopmental disorder, with a strong genetic component in its causation in most cases. On occasion, an identifiable cause or coexisting condition is present. No association with immunization has been found. Autistic features are found in patients with:

- Fragile X syndrome.
- Tuberous sclerosis.
- Untreated phenylketonuria.

The four main features include:

- Impaired social interaction: poor interactions with others and avoiding eye contact.
- Impaired communication: delayed speech and language development with poor comprehension.
- Restricted pattern of behavior and interests: stereotypical patterns and lack of imaginative play and behavior.
- Onset before 3 years of age.

In addition to these features, about two-thirds of affected children have a severe learning disability and a quarter of autistic individuals develop epileptic seizures during adolescence.

Autism is one end of a spectrum of disorders. Children can have autistic features and be socially and functionally impaired without fulfilling criteria for a diagnosis of autism. Children with Asperger's syndrome, for example, have near normal IQ and speech but impaired social and communication skills and obsessional interests. This syndrome tends to be recognized in later childhood.

Autism is characterized by:
- Delayed and abnormal language.
- Difficulty relating to others—poor social reciprocity.
- Restricted, stereotyped interests and activities.

Management
There are no drug treatments for autism, but medical treatment for coexisting conditions, such as seizures, may be necessary. However, specific indications do exist for symptomatic treatment of problems such as extreme anxiety or disruptive behavior. Special education programs are required to meet the complex needs of the individual child. A variety of behavioral treatment programs have been tried, and it is vital that parents receive strong professional support. Only 15% of affected individuals are independent in adult life; a further 15–20% function well with support.

Improved outcomes are seen if communicative speech is present by 5 years of age.

Problems of middle childhood

Continence disorders
Enuresis
Enuresis is the involuntary discharge of urine at an age after continence has been reached by most children. Enuresis is usefully subcategorized as shown in Fig. 22.2.

Classification of enuresis

Primary or secondary?
Children with primary enuresis have never been continent for a period of at least 3 months
Secondary enuresis is incontinence after a prolonged period of bladder control

Nocturnal or diurnal?
Nocturnal enuresis occurs only at night (85% of enuretic children)
Diurnal enuresis occurs during the day (5% of enuretic children)
10% have a mixed type

Fig. 22.2 Classification of enuresis.

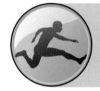
Urinary continence (dryness) is achieved by most girls by age 5 years and boys by age 6 years.

Nocturnal enuresis
Nocturnal enuresis, or "bedwetting," is the involuntary voiding of urine during sleep beyond the age at which dryness at night has been achieved in a majority of children. Children under 5 years of age who regularly wet the bed can be regarded as normal. About 1 in 6 five-year-olds regularly wets the bed; this drops to 1 in 20 at age 10 years.

Nocturnal enuresis is usefully classified into:
- Primary, in which dryness has never been achieved.
- Secondary, in which it dryness has occurred but is no longer achieved.

The etiology of primary nocturnal enuresis is multifactorial with genetic, emotional, and cultural factors contributing. Organic causes of either are uncommon but include:
- Urinary tract infection.
- Polyuria due to diabetes mellitus or chronic renal failure.
- Neuropathic bladder.
- Genital abnormalities.
- Fecal retention causing bladder neck dysfunction.

History and examination

The history should establish the frequency (50% or more wet nights over 2 weeks is severe) and time of night that wetting occurs. The presence of any daytime urgency or wetting should be established as this suggests an underlying cause. A family history may be present, and an assessment should be made of any emotional stresses either at school or at home.

Physical examination must include:
- A review of growth and measurement of blood pressure to identify unrecognized renal failure.
- Careful abdominal palpation to exclude an enlarged bladder.
- Inspection of the genitalia.

The spine and overlying skin should be inspected for any deformity, hairy patch, or sinus, and the neurology of the lower limbs should be examined thoroughly. Investigation should include:
- Urinalysis: tests for proteinuria and glycosuria.
- Microscopy and culture of a clean catch midstream urine.

Management

Important general measures include the establishment of a supportive and trusting relationship with the child and parents. A simple explanation of how the bladder works as a muscular balloon and the problem of being unaware of a full bladder during sleep should be given. Parental intolerance should be discouraged (by a reminder of how common enuresis is) and "functional payoffs" (e.g., sleeping in parents' bed) should be identified and stopped. A diary of wetting should be kept for at least 4 weeks, and frequent, regular supervision by the doctor should be arranged.

Further management is age-dependent:
- Under 5 years: the situation should improve with reassurance.
- Over 5 years: in addition to the above methods, star charts and appropriate praise may be of value.
- Over 7 years: in addition to the above methods, alarms can be used. A choice of body-worn or pad and buzzer type alarm should be offered. The alarm rings when urination begins, causing the child to wake up and "hold-on" to the

sensation of a full bladder. A high degree of compliance and motivation is required, and 60–70% of children will attain dryness after a few months.

Tricyclic antidepressants are sometimes used in the treatment of enuresis. Desmopressin (a synthetic analog of antidiuretic hormone) is available in tablet form and provides effective short-term relief. A percentage of patients who attain dryness on desmopressin remain dry when it is stopped.

Encopresis (fecal soiling)

Encopresis is involuntary fecal soiling at an age beyond which continence should have been achieved (normally about 4 years). Children with encopresis fall into two main groups:
- Retentive: those with a rectum loaded with feces. There is overflow incontinence (the majority).
- Nonretentive: children without constipation or a loaded rectum who have a neurogenic sphincter disturbance or psychiatric illness.

A number of factors predispose to chronic stool retention. These include:
- Environmental problems: lack of toilet facilities, harsh toilet training.
- Idiopathic: some children's rectums only empty occasionally, perhaps due to poor coordination with anal sphincter relaxation.
- Transient constipation: an episode of constipation due to dehydration or an anal fissure may lead to chronic retention.
- Organic constipation: associated with Hirschsprung's disease, drugs, or hypothyroidism.

Once established, a large bolus of feces in the rectum may be impossible for the child to expel. The loaded rectum becomes dilated and may habituate to distention, so the child is unaware of the need to empty it. Psychological factors can be both a cause and a result of encopresis. Soiling disturbs the child and can have a profound impact in school, socially, and in the family.

Onset of soiling in middle childhood, without a previous history of constipation, suggests a primary psychiatric cause. It may occur in the setting of a chaotic family with high levels of emotional deprivation, neglect, and disturbed behavior.

Diagnosis
Assessment must include a full bowel history, assessment of the family's psychological functioning, and careful examination of the neurologic system and abdomen. Rectal examination and abdominal palpation will determine whether there is fecal retention.

Management
The key objective in management of encopresis due to fecal retention is to empty the rectum as soon as possible. This may require an enema but can often be achieved by a combination of stool softener (e.g., lactulose) and laxative (e.g., senna). Regular defecation should then be encouraged by:
- Star charts.
- Sitting on the toilet after meals.
- Dietary changes: increased fiber.

The distended rectum will take several weeks to shrink to normal size. It is unusual for the problem to persist into adolescence.

Attention-deficit hyperactivity disorder (ADHD)
The three hallmarks of ADHD are:
- Inattention beyond the child's norm for age.
- Hyperactivity.
- Impulsiveness.

Incidence and etiology
In the USA, this diagnosis is applied if either inattention or hyperactivity and impulsiveness persist in two or more situations.

Twin studies suggest a genetic contribution to etiology. Perinatal problems and delays in early development appear to be common.

Clinical features
Features of ADHD:
- Inattention: manifests as an easily distracted child who changes activity frequently and does not persist with tasks.
- Hyperactivity: an excess of movement with persistent fidgeting and restlessness that can be distinguished from normal high-spirited,

energetic behavior by the interference with normal social functioning.
- Impulsiveness: acting without reflection; affected children act impetuously and erratically.

Although these features may be present in the preschool years, they often come to clinical attention with the increased demands of the classroom. Physical examination should include a search for:
- Developmental delay, clumsiness.
- Deficits in hearing or vision and specific learning difficulties.
- Dysmorphic features.

Most children do not have a sudden onset or an identifiable brain disorder and do not need special investigations such as electroencephalography or brain imaging. Between 18 and 35% will have an additional psychiatric disorder.

Management
A behavior-modifying and educational approach is the mainstay of treatment, but drug treatment should be considered if these strategies fail. It is important to explain the nature of the disorder to the parents and school staff. Parent support groups may provide reassurance and help.

Behavioral therapy
About 50% of children respond to behavioral therapy comprising:
- A structured environment.
- Positive reinforcement.
- Cognitive approaches emphasizing relaxation and self-control.

Extra help in the classroom and modification of the curriculum may be required.

Drug therapy
Studies have shown that the addition of drugs to behavioral therapy is effective. These are central stimulant drugs such as methylphenidate (Ritalin). Side effects include slowing of growth, hypertension, and arrhythmias; an ECG should be done.

Alternative therapies
Numerous alternative therapies have been advocated. Diets can have a role in a minority of

children, and the parents' observations that a particular food aggravates hyperactivity should be heeded. A trial of an exclusion diet may be warranted. (Few children react to additives alone, and a diet just excluding foods with synthetic dyes or preservatives is unlikely to be helpful.)

Hyperactivity itself does not usually persist as a predominant feature into adulthood. However, affected children tend to do poorly at school, and low self-esteem together with antisocial traits lead to disadvantaged adults.

Symptoms diminish over time, but approximately half will continue to have symptoms in adolescence and adulthood.

Recurrent pain syndromes

Recurrent pain without an organic cause is not uncommon in children. The usual sites are the abdomen, head, or limbs.

A strict dichotomy between organic and psychological causation for recurrent pain is

- Apley's law: the further the pain is from the umbilicus, the more likely it is to be organic.
- The more localized limb pain is, the less likely it is to be "growing pains."
- Measure the blood pressure and examine the fundi in a child with recurrent headaches.

unhelpful and explains only a minority of cases. In most cases the pain is best explained as dysfunctional, a result of mild individual differences in physiology that render the child vulnerable to pain in response to stress.

Clinical features and diagnosis

The history should establish:
- Onset, frequency, and duration of the pain and associated symptoms.
- Family functioning.
- Stressors (e.g., bullying at school).

Physical examination is directed towards excluding an organic cause (Fig. 22.3). Investigations have a low yield if physical examination is normal and should be kept to a minimum. Full blood count, erythrocyte sedimentation rate, and urinalysis may be indicated.

Management

For dysfunctional pain, normal activity should be encouraged. Symptomatic relief should be offered (e.g., mild analgesics) and the patient should be encouraged to keep a symptom diary.

School refusal

Repeated absence from school may be due to illness or truancy but in a few cases it is due to school refusal, i.e., an unwillingness to attend because of anxiety. School refusal may be associated with:
- Separation anxiety (under 11 years).
- Adverse life events (bereavement, moving).
- Stressors (bullying).

Organic causes of recurrent pain	
Site	**Cause**
Abdominal pain	Genitourinary problems: UTI, obstructive uropathy Gastrointestinal disorders: inflammatory bowel disease, peptic ulcer
Headache	Refractive disorders Migraine Hypertension Raised intracranial pressure
Limb pain	Neoplastic disease (e.g., leukemia, bone tumor) Orthopedic: Osgood–Schlatter disease

Fig. 22.3 Organic causes of recurrent pain.

School refusers tend to be good academically but oppositional at home.

True school phobia is seen in older, anxious children, who typically have problems beginning school in the autumn and returning to school after weekends and holidays. Unlike school refusal, they are poor academically.

Management

Management requires an early, graded return to school with support for the parents and treatment of any underlying emotional disorder. Two-thirds of school refusers will return to school regularly.

Adolescent problems

Adolescence is a period during which a number of important disorders may present, including emotional disorders such as anxiety and depression, conduct disorders, and eating disorders.

Eating disorders
Anorexia nervosa

This eating disorder is characterized by:

- Refusal to maintain an expected bodyweight for height with weight less than 85% of expected bodyweight.
- Intense fear of gaining weight or being fat.
- Disturbed body image: feeling fat when actually emaciated.
- Denial of the danger of serious weight loss of low bodyweight.
- Amenorrhea for at least three cycles (in postmenarchal girls).

The prevalence rate is 1% with a peak age of onset of 14 years (and girls outnumbering boys by 20 to 1). The etiology is unknown. The patient often displays obsessive, overachieving, perfectionist, and controlling personality traits.

Clinical features and diagnosis

Physical examination may reveal:

- Emaciation and muscle wasting.
- Fine lanugo hair over trunk and limbs.
- Bradycardia and poor peripheral perfusion.
- Slowly relaxing tendon reflexes.

Laboratory investigations may reveal:

- Reduced plasma proteins, vitamin B12 and ferritin.

- Endocrine abnormalities: elevated cortisol, reduced T_4, luteinizing hormone, and follicle stimulating hormone.

In boys, cranial computed tomography should be undertaken to exclude a brain tumor.

Management and prognosis

The immediate goal is to make a therapeutic alliance with the patient to restore normal bodyweight by refeeding. This can be attempted initially as an outpatient, aiming at a gain of 500 g per week. Failure to meet this target necessitates hospital admission for refeeding under nursing supervision. This can be difficult because affected young people may hide food and lie about their weight. Tube feeding may be required if there is continued weight loss in hospital.

Once weight gain is achieved, psychotherapeutic approaches are adopted. This aims to provide counseling on handling conflict, relationships, and personal autonomy.

Prognosis is variable with an eventual 5% mortality rate from malnutrition, infection, or suicide. Fifty percent make a good recovery, 30% show partial improvement, and 20% have a chronic relapsing course. Good prognostic factors are:

- Young age at onset.
- Supportive family.
- Less denial and improved self-esteem.

Emotional disorders
Depression

Depression as a clinical syndrome is more than just a transitory low mood or misery in response to adverse life circumstances. It is characterized by:

- Persistent feelings of sadness or unhappiness.
- Ideas of guilt, despair, and lack of self-worth.
- Social withdrawal.
- Lack of motivation and energy.
- Disturbances of sleep, appetite, and weight.

It is increasingly recognized in prepubertal children but is predominantly a problem of adolescence. Etiology is multifactorial, but there is a clear genetic contribution. Dysfunctional families or adverse life events may contribute.

Management

Treatment includes selective serotonin re-uptake inhibitor (SSRI) antidepressants and family therapy.

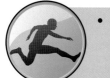

- Suicide is the third most common cause of death in adolescents and young adults.
- Most intentional overdoses are not taken with suicidal intent but an important minority are, so psychiatric evaluation is important in all cases.

Conduct disorder

This is a syndrome characterized by the persistent (6–12 months) failure to control behavior within socially defined rules. This involves three overlapping domains of behavior:

- Defiance of authority.
- Aggressiveness.
- Antisocial behavior: violating other people's property, rights, or person.

This affects approximately 4% of all children and is more prevalent in boys. The etiology is multifactorial, with genetic and environmental contributions. In many children, it is preceded by oppositional defiant disorder, i.e., children who demonstrate a persistent pattern of angry, negative, vindictive, and defiant behavior.

Management and prognosis

Family behavioral therapy with social support is helpful. A significant number (40%) of children with conduct disorder become delinquent young adults with ongoing behavior problems and disrupted relationships. Those with onset before adolescence are most at risk.

Psychosis

Chronic disorders such as schizophrenia and bipolar affective disorder may present in adolescence. The prevalence of drug abuse in this age group renders drug-induced psychosis an important problem.

- How would you manage nocturnal enuresis?
- Describe the clinical features of ADHD.
- Formulate a management plan for a child with eating difficulties.

Further reading

Evans JHC. Evidence based management of nocturnal enuresis. *British Medical Journal* 2001; 323:1167–1169.
Volkmar FR, Pauls D. Autism. *Lancet* 2003; 362:133–141.

23. Social and Preventive Pediatrics

This includes all aspects of promoting health and preventing illness such as well child visits, immunization, health education, and accident prevention. In addition, community pediatric services are closely involved with the problems of child abuse, adoption and foster care, and children with special needs. Important legislation concerns child abuse, foster care, adoption, informed consent and confidentiality, and children with disabilities.

Prevention in child health

There remains a high level of morbidity from preventable conditions, including:
- Infectious diseases.
- Congenital disorders.
- Accidents.
- Malnutrition.
- Smoking in teenagers.

Strategies for prevention include:
- Immunization.
- Screening.
- Well child visits.
- Health promotion and education.

Immunization

Immunization has probably conferred more benefit on the world's children than any other medical advance or intervention. It has allowed the prevention of many major diseases, such as diphtheria and polio, which killed or crippled millions of children, and the complete eradication of smallpox. In recent times, the highly successful introduction of immunization against *Haemophilus influenzae* type B (Hib) has dramatically reduced the incidence of invasive infections such as Hib meningitis and epiglottitis.

Immunization is effective against major bacterial diseases, such as diphtheria and tuberculosis (TB), and viral diseases, such as measles, mumps, rubella, and hepatitis. Bacille Calmette–Guérin (BCG) vaccination against TB is effective in some parts of the world but is not routinely used in the USA. However, a vaccine has yet to be developed against the important parasitic disease, malaria.

Immunity: active and passive

Immunity can be induced either actively (long term) or provided by passive transfer (short term) against a variety of bacterial and viral agents.

Active immunity is induced by using:
- A live, attenuated form of the pathogen (e.g., oral poliomyelitis vaccine [OPV], measles, mumps, rubella vaccine [MMR], BCG vaccine for TB).
- An inactivated organism (e.g., inactivated poliomyelitis vaccine [IPV], pertussis).
- A component of the organism (e.g., Hib, pneumococcal vaccine, hepatitis B, meningitis C).
- An inactivated toxin (toxoid) (e.g., tetanus vaccine, diphtheria vaccine).

In many individuals, live, attenuated viral vaccines promote a full, long-lasting antibody response after one dose. Several doses of an inactivated version or toxoid are usually required.

Passive immunity is conferred by the injection of human immunoglobulin. There are two main types:
- Human normal immunoglobulin (HNIG).
- Specific immunoglobulins for tetanus, hepatitis B, rabies, and varicella zoster (VZIG).

Routes of administration are:
- By mouth: oral polio vaccine.
- Intradermal: BCG.
- Subcutaneous or intramuscular injection: all other vaccines.

In infants, the upper outer quadrant of the buttock or the anterolateral aspect of the thigh are the recommended sites for the injection of vaccines.

US immunization schedule	
Vaccine	**When to give in routine cases**
Hepatitis B	Birth, 1–2 months, 6–18 months (3 doses)
DTaP (diphtheria, tetanus, acellular pertussis)	2, 4, 6, 15–18 months and 4–6 years (5 doses) plus tetanus booster (Td) every 10 years
Haemophilus influenzae type b	2, 4, 6, 12–15 months (4 doses)
Inactivated polio virus (IPV)	2, 4, 6–18 months, and 4–6 years (4doses)
Measles, mumps, rubella (MMR)	12–15 months and 4–6 years (2 doses)
Pneumococcus spp. (heptavalent)	2, 4, 6, 12–15 months (4 doses)
Varicella	12–18 months (1 dose)

Fig. 23.1 US immunization schedule.

Immunization schedule

In the USA, the schedule for primary immunization with DTaP (diphtheria, tetanus, acellular pertussis), Hib, and polio starts at 2 months with an interval of at least 1 month between the first three doses (4 doses for Hib and IPV). This accelerated schedule was adopted to provide earlier and more effective protection against haemophilus and pertussis infections, which are more dangerous to the very young. Added benefits have included fewer side effects and better completion of the full course.

The schedule is shown in Fig. 23.1.

> The timing of childhood immunization is critical: too early and the immune response may be inadequate, too late and the child could acquire the disease before being protected.

Indications for immunization

Every child should be protected against infectious diseases, and a denial of immunization should not be allowed without serious consideration of the consequences.

Special risk groups can be identified for whom the risk of complications from infectious disease is high and who should be immunized as a priority.

These include children with:
• Chronic lung and congenital heart disease.
• Down syndrome.
• HIV infection.
• Low birth weight.
• No spleen or hyposplenism.

In addition to the routine schedule, these children should have vaccines against pneumococcus and meningococcus.

Contraindications for immunization

General contraindications include:
• Acute illness with fever >38°C: postpone until recovery has occurred.
• A definite history of a severe local or general reaction to a preceding dose.

Live vaccines pose a risk for certain individuals whose immunity is impaired. These include children:
• Being treated with chemotherapy or radiotherapy for malignant disease.
• On immunosuppressive treatment after organ or bone marrow transplant.
• On high-dose systemic steroids.
• With impaired cell-mediated immunity (e.g., severe combined immunodeficiency syndrome or DiGeorge syndrome).

Children positive for antibodies to HIV, with or without symptoms, should be given all vaccines except BCG (there have been reports of dissemination of BCG in HIV-positive individuals), yellow fever, and oral typhoid.

- Immunization should be postponed if the child has an acute febrile illness.
- Premature babies can be immunized following the recommended schedule according to chronologic age, i.e., immunization should not be postponed.
- Live vaccines are contraindicated in immunocompromised children.

Particular vaccines are contraindicated in certain circumstances:

- Measles vaccination is contraindicated if there is allergy to neomycin. MMR is safe for those with egg allergies. If there is concern, immunization should be given under hospital supervision.
- Pertussis: it has never been conclusively demonstrated that this vaccine ever causes permanent brain damage. There are no specific contraindications (in particular, a family or personal history of epilepsy is not a contraindication). Immunization is best delayed in patients with progressive neurological disease until the condition is stabilized.

The following factors are *not* contraindications to immunization:

- Family history of adverse reaction to immunization.
- Prematurity.
- Stable neurologic conditions (e.g., cerebral palsy).
- Asthma, eczema, hay fever.

- Under a certain weight.
- Over the age recommended in standard schedule.
- Minor afebrile illness.
- Child's mother being pregnant.

Adverse reactions associated with specific vaccines are shown in Fig. 23.2.

Screening

An effective and worthwhile screening program should satisfy certain criteria:

- The condition screened for should be an important health problem.
- There should be a sensitive and specific test.
- Treatment should improve the condition.
- It should be cost-effective.
- The screening method should be acceptable to child and parents.

Screening can be targeted at a "high-risk" population or carried out opportunistically when a patient presents for some other reason at the relevant age.

Child health promotion: the well-child visit

A program of health surveillance is undertaken to identify important conditions that have a better outcome if diagnosed and treated early (e.g., congenital dislocation of the hip and deafness). This program includes:

- Newborn examination.
- 0- to 2-week examination.
- 2-month examination.
- 4-month examination
- 6-month examination.

Adverse reactions associated with specific vaccines		
Vaccine	Minor reaction	Major reaction
Diphtheria/tetanus	Local	Neurologic (very rare)
Pertussis	Fever, crying	Seizures (1 : 300,000) Encephalopathy (very rare)
Polio	—	Vaccine-associated polio (1 in 2 million)
MMR	Fever, rash, arthropathy	Encephalopathy (very rare) Thrombocytopenia
BCG	Local abscess	Adenitis

Fig. 23.2 Adverse reactions associated with specific vaccines.

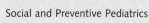

- 9-month examination.
- 12-month examination.
- 15-month examination.
- 18-month examination.
- 24-month examination.
- 3-year examination.
- Annual examination thereafter.

Newborn examination

Full physical examination looking for congenital anomalies such as congenital dislocation of the hips, undescended testes, and absence of the red reflex. A test of hearing (otoacoustic emission test) is scheduled if not done in hospital before discharge.

Newborn screening before hospital discharge includes sending of blood samples to the laboratory to screen for congenital diseases. The specific diseases tested vary from state to state. Examples include:

- Guthrie test: a heel prick blood sample is taken to screen for phenylketonuria and hypothyroidism.
- Screening for cystic fibrosis and muscular dystrophy is done in certain centers.

Every well-child visit

Physical examination with emphasis on:
- Surveillance for congenital anomalies (e.g., cardiac, undescended testes, and dislocated hips).
- Growth: vital signs, weight, length, and head circumference (up to 2 years).
- Development: domains of gross motor, fine motor, language, and social. The Denver Development Assessment (Denver 11) Chart is commonly used.
- Vision and hearing (explore parental concerns).
- Anticipatory guidance (e.g., feeding, sleeping, safety and injury prevention, elimination and toilet training).
- Behavior and emotional assessment of patient and family. Assessment should be made of the family's adjustment to the new infant, quality of parent–child interactions, and signs of maternal depression.

Child abuse

Although children have been abused throughout history, it is only in the past few decades that the extent to which children can be abused by their

Types of abuse
Physical (nonaccidental injury)
Sexual
Emotional
Neglect
Munchausen by proxy (fictitious illness)

Fig. 23.3 Types of abuse.

parents or caregivers has been recognized. Several types of abuse are recognized, and these often occur together (Fig. 23.3).

Diagnosis

Certain families and children are at particular risk. Adults who abuse are often young, immature, isolated, poor, and subject to social or marital stress. Alcoholism, drug abuse, and personality or psychiatric disorders (e.g., postnatal depression) may be contributory. Young children under the age of 3 years, babies born prematurely, and children with physical handicaps are at particular risk.

Child abuse may present directly to the pediatrician or emergency department doctor, or a health visitor, social services, police, school, relative, or even neighbor may raise a suspicion of abuse. Diagnosis is difficult and, of course, false accusations cause great anguish. Each type of abuse is considered in turn.

Types of abuse
Physical abuse or nonaccidental injury (NAI)

Certain features in the history of a physical injury should raise the suspicion that it may be nonaccidental (Fig. 23.4). Actual injuries can include bruises (Fig. 23.5), bite marks, burns or scalds, and fractures or head injuries. Accidental fractures of long bones are rare in babies but common in mobile children aged 3–4 years. Metaphyseal fractures and posterior rib fractures should raise the suspicion of NAI. Direct blows to the mouth or forcing a bottle into the mouth can tear the frenulum. Violent shaking of a baby may tear the vessels that cross the subdural space, leading to subdural hemorrhage (Fig. 23.6). This is known as shaken baby syndrome and is associated with irritability or lethargy, poor feeding, and signs of raised intracranial pressure (increasing head circumference, tense fontanelle, and retinal hemorrhages).

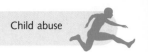

Features of nonaccidental injury

History
- Delay in seeking medical help
- Injury inconsistent with history or changing story
- Cause of trauma inappropriate for age and activity
- Previous unexplained injury
- Parents unconcerned or concerned about minor unrelated problem

Examination
- Signs of neglect
- Withdrawn personality
- Frenulum lacerations
- Genital injury
- Old injuries

Fig. 23.4 Features of nonaccidental injury.

Features of nonaccidental bruises

Any bruise in a (nonmobile) baby
Bruises on face, back, buttocks as opposed to forehead and shins in toddler
Bruises in pattern of fingertips, hand print, belt (follow shape and size of object used)
Bruises of different ages

Fig. 23.5 Features of nonaccidental bruises.

Neglect and emotional abuse

Neglect can manifest as failure to thrive, developmental delay, and poor hygiene. Emotional abuse includes rejection and withdrawal of love and persistent malicious criticism or threats. The child typically improves when taken to a different environment (e.g., hospital).

Fabricated or induced illness

This was previously called "Munchausen syndrome by proxy." The caregiver, usually the mother, fabricates illness in the child by inducing or faking symptoms and signs (e.g., by putting blood or sugar in the urine or contaminating microbiologic specimens). This can result in a wide range of clinical symptoms, and significant harm may also come from investigating such symptoms. Harm to the child can also result from treatments used. As diagnosis can be difficult, consultation with other members of the child health team and other specialists may be useful.

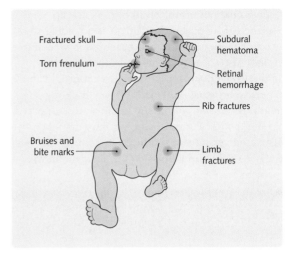

Fig. 23.6 Battered or shaken baby syndrome.

Sexual abuse

Child sexual abuse (CSA) can involve either sex and at any age, but is more common in girls. It has been defined as the involvement of dependent, immature children or adolescents in sexual activities that they do not fully understand and to which they are unable to give informed consent. It should be remembered that medical examination is rarely diagnostic. Physical findings such as tears or abrasions around genitalia, bruising around the genitalia, or genital infection are present in less than 30% of abused children. Vulval soreness is very common in young girls and is rarely due to abuse; 80% of sexual abuse is perpetrated by someone the child knows.

Management

Extra care should be taken to record the history and physical findings in detail and with great accuracy. Physical findings should be measured, drawn, and—if appropriate—photographed (with parental consent). As always, all notes should be dated, timed, and signed, as this is particularly important in relation to any subsequent legal proceedings. If child abuse is suspected, the state welfare department must be informed.

Treatment of physical injury may be required and, if abuse is suspected, a decision made as to whether the child needs immediate protection. This may mean admission to hospital or placement in a foster home; if parental consent is not given, legal enforcement may be necessary. Senior staff should be involved from the beginning because experience is required in handling what is always a very difficult situation.

Investigations are often indicated. In the presence of suspicious bruising it is advisable to do a complete blood count and coagulation screen to exclude thrombocytopenia and other bleeding diatheses, which often present with multiple and excessive bruising. A skeletal survey by x-ray should be carried out in any infant with suspected physical abuse. Forensic samples must be taken in suspected sexual abuse. Emergency protection is available to secure admission for abused children.

Sudden infant death syndrome (SIDS)

This is defined as the sudden death of an infant under 1 year of age, which remains unexplained after the performance of a complete post-mortem examination and examination of the scene of death. In the USA, SIDS occurs in 1.4 of 1000 live births; specific etiology is unknown.

Risk factors are numerous but include:
- Sleeping prone.
- Maternal smoking.
- Overheating at home.
- Bed sharing.
- Preterm birth.

All pediatric units should have a protocol on dealing with SIDS, and a senior pediatrician must fully examine the child, take appropriate laboratory specimens, and inform the coroner.

The family needs support and counseling, and there are numerous agencies that provide ongoing help and support.

Children and the law

Foster care
The purpose of foster care is to provide a safe, temporary placement for a child who is at physical, emotional, or social risk. Common reasons for foster placement include:
- Child abuse.
- Death or absence of parents.
- Babies awaiting adoption.

Foster care does not provide legal rights, which remain with the natural parents, local authority, or courts.

Adoption
Most children available for adoption are in local authority care, either with foster parents or in a group home. Unfortunately, the children available for adoption—many of whom are older or disabled or have suffered abuse or neglect—are not always the kind that adopting couples are looking for.

Adoption is a legal procedure encompassing several important features:
- It is arranged by registered agencies.
- Adopters must be over 21 years old.
- An adoption cannot be reversed except in exceptional circumstances.
- An adopted child loses all legal ties with his or her birth parents (i.e., has no claim to maintenance or inheritance) and becomes a full member of the new family, taking on the nationality of the adoptive parents.
- The original parents have no right of access, although contact for older children is sometimes maintained.
- The natural parents must give informed consent, unless they cannot be found or are judged unlikely to ever be able to look after the child adequately.
- The child usually lives with the adoptive parents before the order is finalized.

Consent to medical care
A person older than 18 years can legally give his or her own consent. Below the age of 18, the consent of a parent or guardian (person with parental responsibility for the child) is required unless:
- Emergency treatment is required.
- If the parent(s) of a child younger than 18 years refuse a life-saving treatment, a court can give consent.

 If a child is deemed competent, the parents cannot override consent.

Confidentiality
A person aged 18 years and over has full rights to confidentiality. However, the duty of confidentiality owed to a patient under 18 years old is as great as that owed to any other person. Information can be disclosed to parents if it is in the interests of the child.

The child with a disability

Many children have complex and long-lasting neurodevelopmental disabilities that require early identification and support in the community. It is useful to define some of the terms used:

- Impairment: any loss or abnormality of physiological or anatomical structure.
- Disability: any restriction or loss of ability in performing an activity (considered normal for a particular age) that is caused by an impairment.
- Handicap: a disadvantage for an individual arising from a disability that prevents the achievement of desired goals.

For example, an intraventricular hemorrhage with periventricular leukomalacia (impairment of motor tracts) may cause a hemiparesis (the disability), resulting in difficulty playing the piano (handicap). The use of the term "handicap" with its connotation of dependency has fallen out of favor.

Disabilities can give rise to "special needs," which are educational needs not usually met by the normal provisions for a child of that age and protected by law.

Presentation of children with disabilities

The kinds of conditions under consideration include:
- Speech and language problems.
- Behavioral problems.
- Down syndrome.
- Cerebral palsy.
- Spina bifida.
- Hearing or visual impairment.
- Learning disability.

Examples of how different problems tend to present at different ages are shown in Fig. 23.7.

Telling parents about a disability

Diagnosis of a disability may be sudden and unexpected or the culmination of protracted concern and investigation. In any event, the news is likely to provoke reactions of grief accompanied by anger, guilt, despair, or denial. The initial interview requires sensitive handling.

Breaking news to parents about a disability:
- They should be told as soon as possible.
- They should be told together, not separately.
- Tell them in a quiet place with a colleague (e.g., a nurse).
- Adopt an honest and direct approach.
- Arrange a period of privacy for the parents after the initial interview.
- Arrange a second meeting to allow questions after the news has been assimilated.

Presentation of disabilities by age	
Age	**Disability**
Neonatal period	Chromosomal abnormality or syndrome (e.g., Down syndrome) Hypoxic–ischemic syndrome
Infancy	Cerebral palsy Severe visual or hearing impairment
Preschool	Speech and language delay Abnormal gait Global delay Loss of skills from neurodegenerative disorder
School age	Learning difficulties—specific or general Clumsiness

Fig. 23.7 Presentation of disabilities by age.

Assessment

It is necessary to assess what a child is able to do and what the main difficulties are in several areas:

- Hearing, language, and communication.
- Vision and coordination.
- Physical health and mobility.
- Behavior and emotions.
- Social interactions and self-care, including continence.
- Learning disabilities.

Medical problems commonly encountered in children with disabilities are shown in Fig. 23.8.

Management: the multidisciplinary team

Management of a severe or complex disability requires a multidisciplinary clinical team, working in concert with the social services, local education authorities, and voluntary agencies. The balance changes with age:

- Preschool children: community-led child development team, voluntary agencies.
- School-age children: education authorities, community health services.
- College-age/young adults: social services, community disability teams.

Members of the child development team will usually include:

- Pediatricians.
- Physical therapists.
- Occupational therapists.
- Speech and language therapists.

Medical problems in children with neurodisdability	
System	**Problem**
Nervous system	Vision and hearing impairment Seizures Behavioral disorders
Skeletal	Postural deformities (e.g., scoliosis)
Gastrointestinal	Feeding difficulties Gastroesophageal reflux Constipation or fecal incontinence
Respiratory	Recurrent aspiration pneumonia
Genitourinary	Renal failure Urinary incontinence

Fig. 23.8 Medical problems in children with neurodisability.

- Psychologists.
- Social workers.
- Nurses and health visitors.

"Statementing"

Education authorities have a duty to identify children with special needs and provide appropriate resources. A detailed assessment is undertaken with reports from the educational psychologist, members of the multidisciplinary team and the parents. The resulting "statement" sets out the child's educational and noneducational needs and the provision of services required to meet those needs. Regular reviews of the statement are also undertaken.

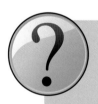

- Describe the immunization schedule in infants.
- What are the contraindications for immunization?
- What are not contraindications for immunization?
- Describe some complications of immunization.
- How does child abuse manifest?
- What is the immediate management of an abused child?
- What are the features of nonaccidental injury?
- Can a child give consent to treatment?
- When can a parent override consent?

24. Genetic Disorders

The human genome comprises 46 chromosomes, which include 22 pairs of autosomes and 1 pair of sex chromosomes. With the recent mapping of the human genome, our understanding of genetics will increase greatly over the next few years. Many genetic disorders are common during childhood and infancy; those that are associated with a poor prognosis and a short lifespan are not seen during adulthood. As our understanding of genetics has advanced, many new diagnostic technologies have become clinically relevant, and therapies for genetic diseases are emerging.

Clinical manifestations are highly variable, but it is worth remembering that many dysmorphic syndromes have a genetic basis.

Dysmorphism and syndromes:
- Dysmorphism is an abnormality in form or structural development, often manifested in the facial appearance and often due to an underlying genetic disorder.
- A syndrome is a recognizable pattern of structural and functional abnormalities or malformations known or presumed to be the result of a single cause. Dysmorphism is often a feature.
- Syndromes may be of unknown cause, due to teratogens (e.g., fetal alcohol syndrome), chromosomal anomalies (e.g., Turner syndrome), or single gene disorders (e.g., Marfan syndrome).

Basic genetics

Some useful definitions are shown in Fig. 24.1. The key symbols used in drawing a family tree are shown in Fig. 24.2.

Single gene disorders

Disorders of single nuclear genes are recognizable because of their Mendelian pattern of inheritance, which can be:
- Autosomal dominant.
- Autosomal recessive.
- X-linked.

Examples of important single gene disorders are shown in Fig. 24.3.

Autosomal dominant disorders

An affected person has just one copy of the abnormal gene. The disease is manifested in the heterozygote. Each offspring has a 50% chance of inheriting the abnormal gene. Thus, each child of an affected individual has a 50% chance of being affected. A typical pedigree of an autosomal dominant (AD) disorder is shown in Fig. 24.4. The features of an AD pedigree are:
- Each generation with affected individuals.
- Equal numbers of males and females are affected.
- Male-to-male transmission occurs.

Several complicating factors can occur. These include:
- Variable expression: the pattern and severity of disease varies in affected individuals within the same family.
- Nonpenetrance: some individuals with the disease allele have no clinical signs or symptoms.
- Sporadic cases: a new mutation in the ovum or spermatocyte of a parent will give rise to a "sporadic" case with no family history of the disease. The recurrence risk for new offspring from those parents is then very low.

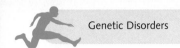

Basic genetics—some definitions	
Term	Definition
Karyotype	A display of the set of chromosomes extracted from a eukaryotic somatic cell arrested at metaphase
Genome	The totality of the DNA contained within the diploid chromosome set of a eukaryotic species and within extranuclear structures such as the mitochondrial genome
Gene	A sequence of DNA occupying its own place (locus) on a chromosome and containing the information necessary for biosynthesis of a gene product such as a protein or ribosomal RNA molecule
Allele	Any one of the variations of a gene or polymorphic DNA marker found in the members of a species. Numerous alleles may exist, but any individual usually possesses at most two alleles of the gene or polymorphic marker
Genotype	The pair of alleles of a variable gene possessed by an individual, or the pairs of alleles of any number of variable genes possessed by an individual
Phenotype	The entire physical, biochemical, and physiologic make-up of an individual as determined by genotype and environment

Fig. 24.1 Basic genetics: some definitions.

New mutations are common in some AD disorders. For example, over 80% of individuals with achondroplasia have unaffected parents.

Achondroplasia

This autosomal dominant disorder is characterized by short limbs, large head, and abnormalities in neurology. The gene is found on the short arm of chromosome 4 and is a fibroblast growth receptor gene (FGFR3 gene). It affects 1 in 2500 births; typical clinical features are shown in Fig. 24.5.

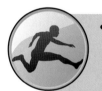

- Autosomal dominant disorders are often caused by mutations in a gene encoding a structural protein.
- Autosomal recessive disorders are often caused by mutations in a gene encoding a functional protein, such as an enzyme.

Autosomal recessive disorders

An affected individual has two copies of the abnormal gene. The affected person has inherited an abnormal allele from each parent and is said to be homozygous for the disease alleles. The parents are heterozygous carriers. Many recessive disorders are caused by mutations in the genes coding for enzymes. As half of the normal enzyme activity is usually sufficient, a person with only one mutant allele will not normally be affected.

A typical pedigree of an autosomal recessive disorder is shown in Fig. 24.6.

The risk of each child being affected when both parents are carriers is 25%. Males and females are equally likely to be affected. There is often no positive family history other than affected individuals within the sibship.

Parental consanguinity increases the risk of a recessive disease occurring in the offspring. Everyone probably carries at least one recessive disease gene allele. A couple who are first cousins, for example, are more likely to have inherited the same abnormal recessive disease gene allele from their common ancestor.

Certain recessive disorders show a founder effect. Affected individuals have inherited a

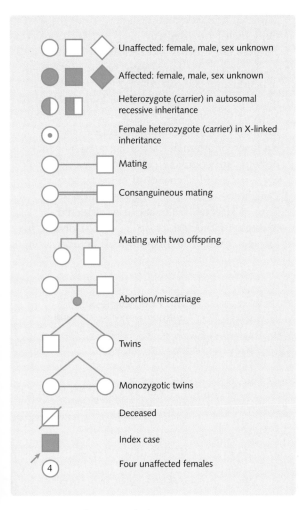

Unaffected: female, male, sex unknown

Affected: female, male, sex unknown

Heterozygote (carrier) in autosomal recessive inheritance

Female heterozygote (carrier) in X-linked inheritance

Mating

Consanguineous mating

Mating with two offspring

Abortion/miscarriage

Twins

Monozygotic twins

Deceased

Index case

Four unaffected females

Fig. 24.2 Pedigree symbols.

Single gene disorders: examples

Autosomal dominant (total number approximately 3000)
Myotonic dystrophy
Marfan syndrome
Neurofibromatosis type 1
Tuberous sclerosis
Achondroplasia

Autosomal recessive (total number approximately 1500)
Cystic fibrosis
Thalassemia
Sickle-cell disease
Congenital adrenal hyperplasia
Inborn errors of metabolism (majority; e.g., phenylketonuria)

X-linked recessive (total number approximately 300)
Hemophilia A and B
Duchenne muscular dystrophy
Fragile X syndrome
Glucose-6-phosphate dehydrogenase (G6PD) deficiency
Color blindness (red-green)

Fig. 24.3 Single gene disorders: examples.

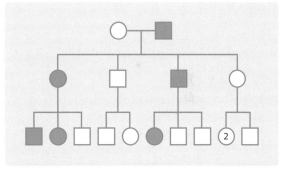

Fig. 24.4 Typical pedigree with autosomal dominant inheritance.

founder mutation that occurred on an ancestral chromosome many generations ago. Carrier rates may be high within inbred populations (e.g., Tay–Sachs disease in Ashkenazi Jews).

Important autosomal recessive diseases are described elsewhere, including cystic fibrosis (Chapter 14), thalassemia, sickle-cell disease (Chapter 19), congenital adrenal hyperplasia (Chapter 21), and inborn errors of metabolism (Chapter 21).

X-linked disorders

Several hundred disease genes are found on the X chromosome and give rise to the characteristic pattern of X-linked inheritance. Most X-linked

disorders are recessive. In the carrier female there is a disease allele on one X chromosome, but the normal allele on her other X chromosome provides protection from the disease. The male is hemizygous for the gene because he has only a single X chromosome. The abnormal allele is not balanced by a normal allele and he manifests the disease.

A typical pedigree for X-linked recessive inheritance is shown in Fig. 24.7.

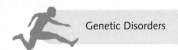

Major clinical features of achondroplasia	
Limbs	Shortened limbs: proximal > distal Bow legs
Neurologic	Hydrocephalus Motor development delay Normal intelligence
Spine	Short stature Thoracolumbar kyphosis Lumbar lordosis
Ear	Recurrent otitis media

Fig. 24.5 Major clinical features of achondroplasia.

The characteristic features are:
• Only males are affected.
• Females are carriers and are usually healthy.
• Females may show mild signs of the disease depending on the pattern of X-chromosome inactivation (note that the Lyon hypothesis suggests that only one of the two X chromosomes in any cell is transcriptionally active).
• Each son of a female carrier has a 50% chance of being affected, and each daughter of a female carrier has a 50% chance of being a carrier.
• Daughters of affected males are all carriers.
• Sons of affected males are never affected because a father passes his Y chromosome to his son (i.e., there is no male-to-male transmission).

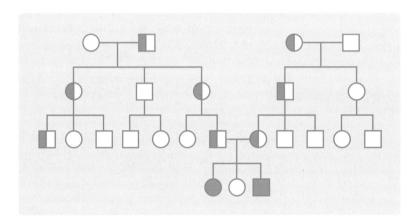

Fig. 24.6 Pedigree of an autosomal recessive disorder.

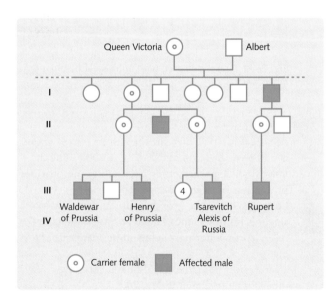

Fig. 24.7 Typical pedigree for X-linked recessive inheritance. Hemophilia in a royal family.

New mutations are common, so there may be no family history. Several important X-linked recessive diseases, including hemophilia (Chapter 19) and Duchenne muscular dystrophy (Chapter 17), are discussed elsewhere. Additional examples are fragile X syndrome and ornithine transcarbamylase deficiency.

Fragile X syndrome

This is an example of a trinucleotide repeat disorder. After Down syndrome, this is the most common cause of severe learning impairment (mental retardation) with an incidence of 1 in 1000 males and 1 in 2000 females. The disorder is due to expansion of a triplet repeat (CGG) in the FRAXA gene FMR1.

The clinical features of fragile X syndrome are listed in Fig. 24.8.

A number of unusual features are accounted for in part by the triplet repeat amplification:

- The number of repeats determines status: normal individuals have fewer than 50 triplet repeats, carriers with a "pre-mutation" have 50–200 triplet repeats, and affected men or women have over 200 triplet repeats.
- The number of repeats becomes amplified when the gene is inherited from a mother but not usually when inherited from a father.
- One-third of obligate female carriers have mild learning difficulties.
- "Normal transmitting males" occur, who pass the disorder on to their grandchildren through their daughters.
- Cytogenetic analysis or direct DNA analysis confirms the diagnosis.

Ornithine transcarbamylase deficiency

This is an X-linked recessive disorder caused by mutations in the gene for the urea-cycle enzyme that causes hyperammonemia. Males are most severely affected and usually present with an overwhelming and sometimes fatal illness a few days after birth when protein-containing feeds are given.

Up to 30% of female carriers manifest symptoms, depending on the pattern of lyonization in hepatic cells (the enzyme is expressed in the liver). They may present with learning difficulties or headache and vomiting after high-protein meals.

Multifactorial disorders

These conditions are believed to be caused by a combination of genetic susceptibility, due to the interaction of several genes (polygenic), and environmental (nongenetic) factors. Multifactorial inheritance accounts for several common birth defects as well as a number of other important diseases with onset in childhood or adult life (Fig. 24.9).

A feature of the familial clustering of multifactorial diseases is that the recurrence risk is low, often in the range 3–5% (most significant for first-degree relatives and decreases rapidly with more distant relatedness). Factors that increase the risk to relatives include:

Clinical features of fragile X syndrome

More common in males
Learning difficulty (IQ 20–80, mean 50)
Autistic features and hyperactivity
Physical features
- Dysmorphic facial appearance (i.e., large forehead, long face, large prominent ears)
- Macrocephaly
- Macro-orchidism—more common after puberty

Fig. 24.8 Clinical features of fragile X syndrome.

Conditions with multifactorial inheritance

Congenital malformations
Neural tube defects
Orofacial clefts (lip and palate)
Pyloric stenosis
Talipes

Common diseases
Asthma
Insulin-dependent diabetes mellitus (IDDM)
Epilepsy
Hypertension
Atherosclerosis
Psychiatric disorders (e.g., autism)

Fig. 24.9 Conditions with multifactorial inheritance.

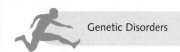

Chromosomal disorders			
Type	Class	Name	Defect
Numerical	Autosomal	Down syndrome Edwards syndrome Patau syndrome	Trisomy 21 Trisomy 18 Trisomy 13
	Sex chromosome	Klinefelter syndrome Turner syndrome	47, XXY 45, XO
Structural	Deletions	Prader–Willi syndrome Cri-du-chat syndrome Wilms' tumor with aniridia	15q deletion 5p deletion 11p deletion

Fig. 24.10 Chromosomal disorders.

- Severely affected proband (e.g., greater in bilateral cleft lip and palate than unilateral cleft lip).
- Multiple affected family members.
- The affected proband is of the more often affected sex (if there is a difference in the M : F ratio of affected individuals).

In many multifactorial disorders, the environmental factors remain obscure.

Chromosomal disorders

Humans normally have 22 pairs of autosomes and 1 pair of sex chromosomes. An alteration in the amount or nature of the chromosomal material is seen in 5 in 1000 live births and is usually associated with multiple congenital anomalies and learning difficulties. A high proportion (40%) of all spontaneous abortions are caused by chromosome abnormalities.

Most chromosome defects arise de novo. They are classified as abnormalities of number or structure, and may involve either the autosomes or the sex chromosomes. Examples of important chromosomal disorders are shown in Fig. 24.10.

The indications for chromosome analysis are shown in Fig. 24.11. Chromosome studies are carried out on dividing cells. Most commonly, T cells from peripheral blood are used after stimulation of mitosis with phytohemagglutinin.

Chromosomal abnormalities

Three autosomal trisomies are found in live born infants; others are not compatible with life and are

Indications for chromosome analysis
- Phenotype consistent with known chromosomal disorder - Multiple congenital abnormalities - Dysmorphic features - Recurrent pregnancy losses - Spontaneously aborted or stillborn fetuses - Bone marrow in leukemia, solid tumors

Fig. 24.11 Indications for chromosome analysis.

found only in spontaneously aborted fetuses. The three are:
- Down syndrome: trisomy 21 (1 : 700 live births).
- Edward syndrome: trisomy 18 (1 : 8000 live births).
- Patau syndrome: trisomy 13 (1 : 15,000 live births).

Trisomy refers to the fact that three, rather than the normal two copies of a specific chromosome are present in the cells of an individual. Trisomies occur because of a meiotic error called nondysjunction in the gamete of the mother or father.

Down syndrome
Trisomy 21 is the most common autosomal trisomy compatible with life. The extra chromosomal material can result from nondysjunction, translocation, or mosaicism.

Nondysjunction
Ninety-five percent of children with Down syndrome have trisomy 21 due to nondysjunction.

The pair of chromosomes 21 fails to separate at meiosis, so one gamete has two copies of chromosome 21. Fertilization of this gamete gives rise to a zygote with trisomy 21.

Ninety percent of nondysjunctions are maternally derived, and the risk rises with maternal age, increasing steeply in mothers over 35 years (Fig. 24.12). However, because a higher proportion of pregnancies occur in younger women, most children with trisomy 21 are born to women under 35 years of age. The recurrence risk for parents of children with trisomy 21 increases to 1–2% (unless the age-related risk is higher).

Translocation

Four percent of Down syndrome children have 46 chromosomes with a translocation of the third number 21 chromosome to another chromosome (most commonly 14). Three-quarters of cases are de novo and, in one-quarter, one of the parents has a balanced translocation involving one chromosome 21. If the mother is the translocation carrier, the recurrence risk may be as high as 15%; if the father is the carrier, the risk is 2.5%.

Mosaicism

In 1% of cases the nondysjunction occurs during mitosis after formation of the zygote so that some cells are normal and some show trisomy 21. The phenotype may be milder in mosaicism.

Clinical features

Down syndrome is often suspected at birth because of the characteristic facial appearance but the diagnosis can be difficult on clinical features alone. Chromosome analysis takes several days. The phenotypic features are listed in Fig. 24.13.

Risk of Down syndrome (for live births) by maternal age at delivery	
Maternal age (years)	**Risk**
All ages	1 : 700
30	1 : 900
35	1 : 380
40	1 : 110
44	1 : 37

Fig. 24.12 Risk of Down syndrome (for live births) by maternal age at delivery.

Clinical features of Down syndrome	
Dysmorphic facial features	Round face Epicanthic folds, flat nasal bridge Protruding tongue Small ears Brushfield spots on iris
Other dysmorphic features	Single palmar crease Flat occiput Incurved little fingers Flap between first and second toes (sandal toe gap) Small stature
Structural defects	Cardiac defects in 50% Duodenal atresia
Neurologic features	Hypotonia Developmental delay Mean IQ = 50
Late medical complications	Increased risk of leukemia Respiratory infections Hypothyroidism Alzheimer's disease Atlantoaxial instability

Fig. 24.13 Clinical features of Down syndrome.

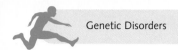

Management and prognosis

Parents need information about the implications of the diagnosis and the assistance available from professionals and self-help groups. Feelings of disappointment, anger, and guilt are common. Genetic counseling for recurrence risks will be required. Life expectancy in Down syndrome has increased, and issues relating to employment and living situations in adulthood will need to be addressed.

Sex chromosome disorders

Turner syndrome

In this condition, there is only one normal X chromosome. It affects 1 in 2500 live born females. Various underlying chromosomal defects are seen:

- In 55% of girls, the karyotype is 45, XO.
- In 25%, there is a deletion of the short arm of one X chromosome, or a so-called isochromosome with duplication of one arm and loss of the other.
- In 15%, there is mosaicism due to postzygotic mitotic nondysjunction. (45, XO/46, XY).

The incidence does not increase with maternal age, and the recurrence risk is the same as the general population risk.

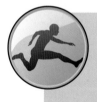

The hallmarks of Turner syndrome are short stature and primary amenorrhea. Intelligence is normal, but there may be specific learning difficulties.

Clinical features and diagnosis

The clinical features are shown in Fig. 24.14. Diagnosis may be made:

- Prenatally by ultrasound scan.
- At birth by presence of puffy hands and feet (lymphedema).
- During childhood because of short stature.
- In adolescence because of primary amenorrhea and lack of pubertal development.

Diagnosis is confirmed by a peripheral blood karyotype.

Clinical features of Turner syndrome

Dysmorphic features
Lymphedema of hands and feet (at birth)
Neck webbing
Widely spaced nipples
Wide carrying angle (cubitus valgus)
Short stature
Structural and functional abnormalities
Gonadal dysgenesis
Congenital heart disease, particularly coarctation of the aorta
Renal anomalies

Fig. 24.14 Clinical features of Turner syndrome.

Management

Therapy with growth hormone improves final height. Ovarian hormones are not produced due to the gonadal dysgenesis (streak ovaries). Estrogen therapy is given at the appropriate age (11 years) to produce maturation of secondary sexual characteristics including breast development. Toward the end of puberty, progesterone is added to maintain uterine health and allow monthly withdrawal bleeds (menses). Although pregnancy can occur naturally, most patients are infertile. Pregnancy can be achieved with in vitro fertilization.

Structural chromosomal abnormalities

These arise from chromosome breakage and include deletions, duplications, inversions, and unbalanced translocations. Deletions are the most common. Most arise de novo, but they can also arise from inheritance of an unbalanced translocation. Examples of conditions associated with chromosomal deletions include:

- Cri-du-chat syndrome: caused by deletion of the short arm of chromosome 5 (5p–). Affected children have profound mental retardation and a cat-like cry.
- Prader–Willi syndrome: caused by deletions of the paternal copy of 15q11–13.
- Angelman syndrome: caused by deletions of the maternal copy of 15q11–13.

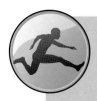

Imprinting:
- Some genes are "imprinted." The copy derived from one parent (either male or female) is active, and the other is not.
- Deletions of chromosomal regions that are "imprinted" have different effects according to the parent of origin of the deleted chromosome.
- The best-known example is deletion of 15q11–13. Paternal chromosome deletion causes Prader–Willi syndrome (obesity, learning difficulties). Maternal chromosome deletion causes Angelman syndrome (happy puppet syndrome: ataxia, learning difficulties, "happy" disposition).

Mitochondrial inheritance

Mitochondrial disorders are inherited maternally. Examples include:
- Mitochondrial encephalopathy, lactic acidosis, stroke-like episodes (MELAS).
- Mitochondrially inherited diabetes mellitus.

The mitochondria contain genetic material as a 16.5 kilobase circular chromosome. They have no introns and a mixture of normal and abnormal mitochondria (heteroplasmy) can exist within tissues. It is worth noting the similarities between mitochondrial and prokaryotic genetics.

Polymerase chain reaction

This is a technique of obtaining a large amount of DNA copied from a small initial sample. It has applications in detection of specific DNA sequences or differences in genes. Its main clinical use is in detection of mutations and rapid diagnosis of bacterial or viral infection. It has a very high sensitivity and is being increasingly used in clinical practice.

Genetic counseling

Genetic counseling is usually carried out as a specialist service by trained medical staff and specialist nurses. The main aim is to provide information about hereditary disorders so that parents will have greater autonomy and choice in reproductive decisions.

The basic elements of counseling include:
- Establishing a diagnosis: this may involve physical examination of proband and family members and special investigations including DNA, cytogenetic, and biochemical analysis.
- Estimation of risk: the risk for future offspring is determined by the mode of inheritance of the disease.
- Communication: information must be conveyed in an unbiased and nondirective way, and all the possible options should be discussed.

Information base in genetic counseling:
- Magnitude of risk.
- Severity of disorder.
- Availability of treatment.
- Parental cultural and ethical values.

Options in antenatal genetic counseling:
- Not to have offspring.
- To ignore the risk.
- Antenatal diagnosis and termination of pregnancy.
- Pre-implantation diagnosis.
- Artificial insemination by donor or ovum donation.

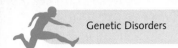

- List the differences between autosomal dominant, recessive, and X-linked disorders.
- Why are females not affected by X-linked disorders?
- What are the clinical features of Turner's syndrome?
- What is genomic imprinting?
- How are mitochondrial disorders inherited?
- Describe a clinical use of the polymerase chain reaction.

25. The Newborn

Fetal life and neonatal life are best regarded as a continuum, and the term "perinatal" medicine is sometimes used to encompass the care of the pregnant mother and fetus as well as the newborn infant. Many factors from before conception to delivery influence the health of the newborn infant.

Introduction: perinatal statistics and definitions

Terms used in perinatal statistics are defined in Fig. 25.1.

Nearly half of all neonatal deaths occur in the first 24 hours. The perinatal mortality rate in developed countries has fallen steadily over the past 20 years and seems to be approaching a lower limit set by deaths from lethal malformations. However, disadvantaged people continue to have the highest rates of perinatal deaths and congenital malformations.

Maternal and fetal health

Mother and fetus are a single physiologic unit, and any serious maternal disease or condition can affect the fetus. Action to optimize the chances of a healthy baby can begin even before conception. The chance of a good outcome can be enhanced by:
- Avoiding smoking, excess alcohol and medication.
- Avoiding infections: rubella immunization before pregnancy, avoiding exposure to toxoplasmosis (via cat's litter) and avoiding exposure to listeriosis (unpasteurized dairy products).
- Folic acid supplements reduce the risk of neural tube defects.
- Optimizing treatment of maternal conditions such as hypertension and diabetes mellitus.
- Genetic counseling for couples at risk of inherited diseases.

Fetal assessment and antenatal diagnosis

Methods for assessing the growth, maturation, and well-being of the fetus include:
- Ultrasound: for assessing age and growth.
- Doppler blood flow studies.

Antenatal diagnosis is now available for many disorders using the methods shown in Fig. 25.2.

Antenatal diagnosis can allow the option of termination to be offered in certain disorders, therapy to be given or neonatal management to be planned in advance. Medical treatment can be given to the fetus via the mother or directly (e.g., fetal blood transfusion for anemia in severe rhesus isoimmunization).

Maternal conditions affecting the fetus

The fetus can be affected by:
- Maternal diseases: diabetes mellitus, thyrotoxicosis, and autoimmune disorders (e.g., systemic lupus erythematosus, myasthenia gravis, and thrombocytopenia).
- Maternal drugs (e.g., medications, alcohol, and narcotics).
- Maternal infections: congenital infections.

Thus, many conditions affecting the first and second trimesters lead to organ dysfunction or structural abnormality.

Maternal diseases
Diabetes mellitus
The outlook for the infant of a mother with insulin-dependent diabetes mellitus has improved greatly and is enhanced by good diabetic control during the pregnancy. Potential fetal problems include:
- Congenital malformations: there is a three-fold increase (there is a particular increased incidence of cardiac malformations).
- Macrosomia: the fetal insulin response to hyperglycemia promotes excessive growth, which predisposes to difficulties during delivery.

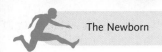

Definitions for perinatal statistics	
Term	**Definition**
Still birth	A fetus born after 24 weeks of gestation who shows no signs of life after delivery
Low birth weight	A baby weighing 2500 g or less at birth
Preterm	A baby born at any time before 37 weeks' gestation
Term	A baby between 37 and 42 completed weeks' gestation
Post-term	A baby born after 42 weeks' gestation
Neonatal period	First month of life
Perinatal mortality rate	Still births and deaths within the first 6 days per 1000 live and still births (i.e., total births)
Neonatal mortality rate	Deaths of liveborn infants during the first 28 days of age per 100 live births

Fig. 25.1 Definitions for perinatal statistics.

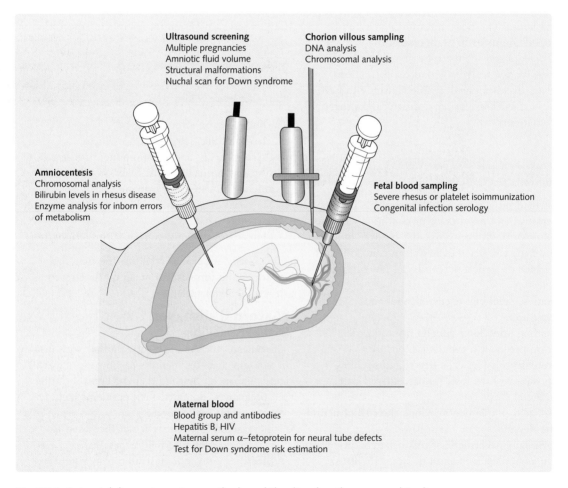

Ultrasound screening
Multiple pregnancies
Amniotic fluid volume
Structural malformations
Nuchal scan for Down syndrome

Chorion villous sampling
DNA analysis
Chromosomal analysis

Amniocentesis
Chromosomal analysis
Bilirubin levels in rhesus disease
Enzyme analysis for inborn errors
of metabolism

Fetal blood sampling
Severe rhesus or platelet isoimmunization
Congenital infection serology

Maternal blood
Blood group and antibodies
Hepatitis B, HIV
Maternal serum α–fetoprotein for neural tube defects
Test for Down syndrome risk estimation

Fig. 25.2 Antenatal diagnosis: various methods and the disorders they are used to diagnose.

Potential neonatal problems include:
- Hypoglycemia: transient early hypoglycemia occurs due to fetal hyperinsulinism; early feeding can usually prevent this.
- Respiratory distress syndrome (RDS).
- Polycythemia (hematocrit >65%).

Maternal drugs affecting the fetus

Drugs taken by the mother may cause congenital malformations (Fig. 25.3), adverse effects by their pharmacologic action on the fetus or placenta, or transient problems at birth.

Maternal drugs and the fetus:
- Teratogenic drugs taken during organogenesis can cause spontaneous abortions or congenital malformations.
- Drugs given during labor can have adverse effects, (e.g., analgesics and anesthesia can suppress spontaneous breathing at birth, sedatives can cause sedation, hypotension).
- IV fluids: excess hypotonic fluids can cause hyponatremia.

Maternal infections and the fetus

A number of infections acquired by the mother could affect the fetus or newborn (Fig. 25.4). Transmission can occur in utero, during labor, or postpartum (Fig. 25.5).

Rubella

For rubella, see Chapter 10.

Varicella zoster

More than 85% of women of childbearing age have evidence of past infection with chickenpox, so a minority of pregnant women are at risk. Infection in the first trimester does not usually cause fetal damage but about 5% develop the so-called "congenital varicella syndrome" characterized by:
- Cicatricial skin lesions (scars).
- Malformed digits.
- Cataracts.
- CNS damage, chorioretinitis.

The principal problem is infection acquired late in pregnancy, particularly within 5 days before and 2 days after delivery. The fetus receives a high viral load but little in the way of maternal antibodies. Severe infection can ensue with a mortality rate of up to 5%.

Maternal medications that may harm the fetus	
Drug	**Adverse effects**
Cytotoxic agents	Congenital malformations
Phenytoin	Fetal hydantoin syndrome (growth retardation, microcephaly, hypoplastic nails)
Sodium valproate	Neural tube defects
Carbamazepine	Growth retardation, craniofacial abnormalities
Warfarin	Interferes with cartilage formation, risk of cerebral hemorrhage, and microcephaly
Progestens (androgenic)	Masculinization of fetus
Diethylstilbestrol	Adenocarcinoma of vagina
Thalidomide	Limbs shortening (phocomelia)
Drug abuse	
Alcohol	Fetal alcohol syndrome (characteristic facies, septal defects, mental retardation)
Opiates (heroin/methadone)	Growth retardation, prematurity, drug withdrawal in neonate (tremors, hyperirritability, seizures)
Cocaine	Spontaneous abortion, prematurity, cerebral infarction

Fig. 25.3 Maternal medication that can harm the fetus.

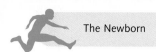

Maternal infections transmitted to the fetus in utero
Toxoplasmosis
Rubella
Cytomegalovirus
Varicella zoster
HIV
Treponema pallidum (syphilis)
Listeria monocytogenes

Fig. 25.4 Maternal infections transmitted to the fetus in utero.

Infections acquired during delivery
Group B hemolytic streptococci
E. coli
HIV
Hepatitis B
Herpes simplex
Gonococci
Chlamydia trachomatis
Echoviruses

Fig. 25.5 Infections acquired during delivery.

Exposed susceptible women can be treated with varicella zoster immune globulin (VZIG) and acyclovir. Infants exposed in the high-risk period should also be treated with VZIG. Intravenous acyclovir should be used if lesions develop in the newborn infant.

Cytomegalovirus

For cytomegalovirus, see Chapter 10.

Human immunodeficiency virus (HIV)

Vertical transmission from mother to infant can occur in utero, during birth, or postnatally by breastfeeding. The exact risk of infection by each of these routes is uncertain, but overall vertical transmission rates are now less than 1% (see Chapter 10).

Administration of zidovudine to the mother during pregnancy and delivery and to the neonate for the first 6 weeks of life reduces the transmission risk.

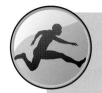

- Diagnosis of HIV during infancy is rendered difficult by the passage of maternal antibody, which can persist for up to 18 months.
- Breastfeeding can increase the risk of vertical transmission by 15%.

Toxoplasmosis

Infection with the protozoan parasite *Toxoplasma gondis* occurs from the ingestion of raw or undercooked meat, or from oocytes excreted in the feces of infected cats. Most infections are asymptomatic. Serologic epidemiologic studies show that in some countries (e.g., France and Austria), 80% of women of childbearing age are immune, whereas in the USA only 10–20% have antibodies.

About 40% of women who acquire an acute infection during pregnancy transmit the infection to the fetus. The risk of severe damage is highest following infection in the first trimester. About 10% of infected infants have clinical manifestations at birth, which can include:

- Hydrocephalus.
- Intracranial calcification.
- Chorioretinitis.
- Neurologic damage.

Infants with asymptomatic infection may still develop chorioretinitis in later life.

In some countries, serologic screening for infection is carried out during pregnancy. If positive (and fetal infection is confirmed by cordocentesis), termination can be offered. An infected newborn infant is treated with alternating courses of pyrimethamine with sulphadiazine or spiramycin until the age of 1 year.

Normal neonatal anatomy and physiology

There are characteristic features of newborn anatomy and physiology that are important and these are considered in turn.

Size and growth

The average term infant in the USA weighs about 3500 g. Boys weigh approximately 250 g more than girls. Infants of 2500 g or less are classified as "low birth weight." This important category is considered separately.

During the first 3–5 days, up to 10% of birth weight is lost. This is regained by 7–10 days. In the first month, average weight gain per week is 200 g.

Skin

The newborn skin is immature, with a thin epithelial layer and incompletely developed sweat and sebaceous glands. Combined with the high surface area to body mass ratio, this renders the baby prone to heat and water losses.

Numerous benign skin lesions occur (see Chapter 12). The skin is covered with a greasy protective layer, the vernix caseosa.

Head

The average occipitofrontal head circumference is 35 cm. Significant molding of the head may occur during birth. Two soft spots or fontanelles are present. The anterior fontanelle closes between 9 and 18 months of age and the posterior closes by 6–8 weeks.

Respiratory system

Changes occur at birth that allow the newborn to convert from dependence on the placenta to breathing air for the exchange of respiratory gases:

- In utero, the airways and lungs are filled with fluid that contains surfactant.
- The lung fluid is removed by the squeezing of the thorax during vaginal delivery and by reduced secretion and increased absorption mediated by fetal catecholamines during labor and after birth.
- Surfactant lines the air–fluid interface of the alveoli and reduces the surface tension thereby facilitating lung expansion. This is associated with a fall in pulmonary vascular resistance.

Newborn infants breathe mainly with the diaphragm. The rate is variable and normally ranges between 30–50 breaths/minute. Brief (up to several seconds) self-limiting apneic spells may occur during sleep. Babies are obligate nose-breathers.

Cardiovascular system

Major changes in the lungs and circulation allow adaptation to extrauterine life.

In the fetal circulation, the right-sided (pulmonary) pressure exceeds the left-sided (systemic) pressure. Blood flows from right to left through the foramen ovale and ductus arteriosus (Fig. 25.6). At birth, these relationships reverse:
- Left-sided (systemic) pressure rises with clamping of umbilical vessels.
- Right-sided (pulmonary) pressure falls as the lungs expand and the rising PO_2 triggers a prostaglandin-mediated vasodilatation.
- The foramen ovale and ductus arteriosus close functionally shortly after birth. The ductus closes due to muscular contraction in response to rising oxygen tension.

Gastrointestinal system

Most infants over 35 weeks' gestation have developed the coordination necessary to "latch on" and feed from breast or bottle. At term, the secretory and absorbing surfaces are well developed, as are digestive enzymes, with the exception of pancreatic amylase.

Meconium is usually passed within 6 hours and delay beyond 24 hours is considered abnormal.

With normal feeding, "changing stools" replace meconium on day 3 or 4, and thereafter the yellowish stools of the milk-fed infant develop.

Immaturity of the liver enzymes responsible for conjugation of bilirubin is responsible for the "physiological jaundice," which can occur from the second day of life.

Genitourinary system

Urine production is occurring during the second half of gestation and accounts for much of the amniotic fluid. The infant may micturate during delivery (unnoticed) and should void within the first 24 hours of life. Renal concentrating ability is diminished in neonates.

Hematopoietic and immune system

The newborn's red cells contain fetal hemoglobin (HbF) which has a higher affinity for oxygen than adult hemoglobin. The hemoglobin concentration of cord blood ranges from 15–20 g/dL (mean 17 g/dL). A large volume of blood is present in the placenta and late cutting causes this blood to enter

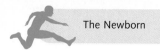

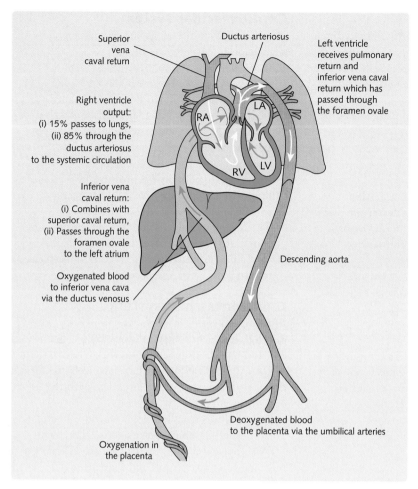

Fig. 25.6 Fetal circulation.

Superior vena caval return

Ductus arteriosus

Left ventricle receives pulmonary return and inferior vena caval return which has passed through the foramen ovale

Right ventricle output:
(i) 15% passes to lungs,
(ii) 85% through the ductus arteriosus to the systemic circulation

Inferior vena caval return:
(i) Combines with superior caval return,
(ii) Passes through the foramen ovale to the left atrium

Oxygenated blood to inferior vena cava via the ductus venosus

Descending aorta

Deoxygenated blood to the placenta via the umbilical arteries

Oxygenation in the placenta

RA LA RV LV

the baby. This can lead to polycythemia, which in the preterm baby is advantageous.

The neonatal immune system also is incomplete compared to older children and adults:
- Impaired neutrophil reserves.
- Diminished phagocytosis and intracellular killing capacity.
- Decreased complement components.
- Low IgG_2, leading to infections with encapsulated organisms.

The presence of maternal antibody in babies born greater than 30 weeks gestational age provides some protection against infection.

Central nervous system

The central nervous system (CNS) is relatively immature at birth. Myelination is incomplete and continues during the first 2 years of life.

A limited behavioral response repertoire is sufficient for survival, comprising a sleep and wake cycle, sucking and swallowing, and crying:
- Newborn infants sleep for a total of 16–20 hours each day.
- The touch of a nipple on the baby's face initiates the sequence of rooting, latching on and the complex coordination of lip, tongue, palate, and pharynx required for sucking and swallowing.
- Crying (without tears) is the main means of communication. Usually this is in response to hunger, thirst, or pain, but some newborns cry without obvious reason and are difficult to pacify.

Birth

The short journey down the birth canal from the intrauterine environment to the external world is

Apgar score evaluation of the newborn			
	Score		
Criteria	0	1	2
Heart rate	Absent	<100 beats/min	>100 beats/min
Respiratory effort	Absent/weak	Irregular/gasping	Regular
Muscle tone	Limp	Some flexion	Active movements
Reflex response to stimulation	None	Weak	Cries
Color	Blue or pale	Extremities blue	Pink

Fig. 25.7 Apgar score evaluation of the newborn.

potentially hazardous. Various risk factors can be identified during labor; the most important of which is prematurity. The problems of the preterm infant are dealt with separately. Here we consider the:

- Normal care and resuscitation of the term newborn.
- Problems of birth asphyxia and birth injuries.

Assessment and care at a normal birth

The infant is usually delivered after a short period of oxygen deprivation and begins to breathe within a few seconds. The Apgar score is a useful quantitative assessment of the infant's condition (Fig. 25.7) and is commonly determined at 1 and 5 minutes after birth. The Apgar score is influenced by several factors including intrapartum asphyxia, maternal sedation or analgesia, the gestational age, and any cardiac, pulmonary, or neurological disease in the infant. Most babies will establish respirations spontaneously after delivery or, if apneic, will respond to airway opening maneuvers. However, a few will need more extensive resuscitation (see Fig. 25.9).

Birth asphyxia

This refers to a condition in which the fetus is acutely deprived of oxygen and is commonly due to uteroplacental insufficiency. The incidence has fallen to 1.5–6 per 1000 live births. In 75% of newborns neurological damage is antenatal, 20% is antenatal and intrapartum, and only 5% is intrapartum alone.

Asphyxia (which literally means "absent pulse" and was a term for "suffocation") is manifested

Complications of perinatal asphyxia (severe)	
Organ	Complication
Brain	Hypoxic–ischemic encephalopathy
Heart	Hypoxic cardiomyopathy, hypotension
Lungs	Persistent pulmonary hypotension
Intestines	Ileus and necrotizing enterocolitis
Kidneys	Acute tubular necrosis
Blood	Disseminated intravascular coagulation

Fig. 25.8 Complications of perinatal asphyxia (severe).

during labor by various fetal responses (previously termed "fetal distress"). These responses are fetal hypoxia, hypercapnia, and acidosis, which may be detected by:

- Abnormalities in fetal heart rate: there may be fetal bradycardia (rate under 120 beats/minute), fetal tachycardia (rate over 160 beats/minute) or an abnormal pattern of deceleration during or after uterine contractions.
- Acidosis: sampling of fetal blood from scalp or cord will demonstrate significant acidosis (pH < 7.20).
- Meconium staining: the asphyxiated infant passes meconium.

These signs are an indication for prompt delivery of the fetus. The effects of asphyxia are seen in Fig. 25.8. Resuscitation is described in Fig. 25.9.

The postnatal symptoms and signs of asphyxia vary with the degree of asphyxia, which can be classified as mild, moderate or severe. "Neonatal

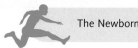

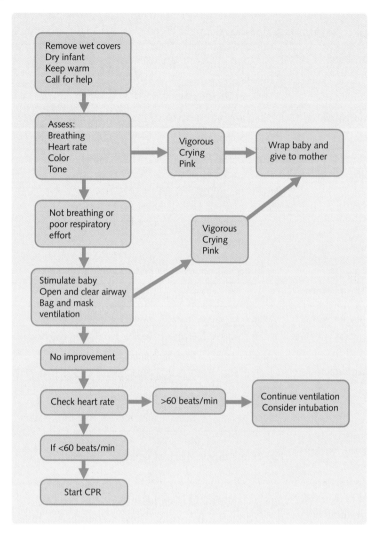

Fig. 25.9 Neonatal resuscitation.

encephalopathy" is the term used to describe the neurologic manifestations.

Neonatal encephalopathy (hypoxic–ischemic encephalopathy)

The manifestations of the effects of asphyxia on the brain vary with its severity:

- Mild: initial lethargy followed by a period of hyperalertness with irritability, staring of the eyes and impaired feeding for 1–2 days. There are no focal signs. Prognosis is good.
- Moderate: as above with generalized seizures occurring 12–24 hours after the episode of asphyxia and resolving within a few days. Depressed level of consciousness. Variable prognosis.

- Severe: coma and intractable seizures worsening over 1–3 days as delayed or "secondary" injury develops. Multiorgan failure is often present. Death is common and survival is associated with poor long-term outcome.

As neuronal injury continues after resuscitation, good supportive care is required. Management involves:

- Respiratory support.
- Anticonvulsants for seizures.
- Fluid restriction.
- Circulatory support with inotropes if necessary.

MRI and EEG can assist in predicting the outcome. Cystic lesions or cerebral atrophy may appear in the ensuing weeks.

Birth injury

Physical injury during labor and delivery is now relatively uncommon, partly because the availability of cesarean section obviates the need for heroic attempts at vaginal delivery. Predisposing factors include:
- Breech presentation.
- Cephalopelvic disproportion.
- Assisted delivery: manual or instrumental (forceps or vacuum extraction). Injuries can occur to soft tissues, nerves or bones.

Diseases of the newborn

Much neonatal care is directed toward the problems of low birth weight infants, especially those born prematurely, many of whom require intensive care. It is therefore useful to consider the disorders of low birth weight and term infants separately, although there is, of course, significant overlap.

Size and gestational age
Newborn infants may be small because they have been born preterm or because they are small in relation to their gestational age (small for dates). Some useful definitions are shown in Fig. 25.10.

Small for gestational age infants
These infants have intrauterine growth retardation (IUGR), which can be caused by:

- An intrinsic fetal problem: poor growth is symmetrical, with head circumference proportionally reduced (e.g., chromosomal disorders, small normal fetus, and congenital infections).
- Placental insufficiency: poor growth is asymmetrical, with brain growth relatively spared (an adaptive response, e.g., maternal pre-eclampsia, hypertension, renal disease, sickle-cell disease, and multiple pregnancy).

The fetus with IUGR is at risk from hypoxia and death and is closely monitored using cardiotocography and Doppler ultrasound to profile blood flow velocity in the uterine and umbilical arteries.

Postnatal problems encountered by the fetus with IUGR include:
- Hypothermia.
- Hypoglycemia from low fat and glycogen stores.
- Hypocalcemia.
- Polycythemia (hematocrit >65%).

Large for gestational age infants
The most common cause of macrosomia is maternal diabetes mellitus. Potential associated problems include birth asphyxia from a difficult delivery and birth trauma, especially from shoulder dystocia.

The preterm infant
About 3 in every 100 babies are born prematurely (before 37 weeks' gestation) and are classified as "preterm." Most weigh less than 2500 g and are therefore "low birth weight" babies. These infants

Definitions for size and gestational age	
Term	**Definition**
Preterm	Gestation <37 completed weeks
Post-term	Gestation >42 completed weeks
Low birth weight	<2500 g
Very low birth weight	<1500 g
Extremely low birth weight	<1000 g
Small for gestational age	Birth weight <10th percentile for gestational age
Large for gestational age	Birth weight >90th percentile for gestational age

Fig. 25.10 Definitions for size and gestational age.

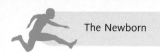
Major problems in preterm infants	
Temperature	Hypothermia
Respiratory	Respiratory distress syndrome Pneumothorax Chronic lung disease Pneumonia Pulmonary hypertension
Cardiac	Patent ductus arteriosus Hypotension
Gastrointestinal	Feed intolerance Vomiting and gastroesophageal reflux Jaundice Necrotizing enterocolitis
Infection	Group B streptococci *Staphylococcus epidermidis* Gram-negative cocci Fungi (e.g., *Candida* species)
Nervous	Intraventricular hemorrhage Retinopathy of prematurity Developmental delay
Bone	Osteopenia of prematurity
Fluids and electrolytes	High transepidermal water loss Hypoglycemia
Hematology	Anemia

Fig. 25.11 Major problems in preterm infants.

provide much of the work in neonatal units and account for 60% of neonatal deaths.

The major problems encountered by preterm infants are determined by the immaturity of their organ systems, particularly the lungs (Fig. 25.11). The limits of viability are currently in the region of 23–24 weeks' gestation.

Characteristics of the preterm infant
A typical infant of 28 weeks' gestation would have the following features:
- Large head in relation to the chest, which is small and narrow.
- Shiny, smooth skin.
- Skull soft, ears floppy and lacking cartilage.
- Eyes closed.
- Extended posture, jerky, frog-like movements.
- Weak cry.

The physiology of the major organ systems and bodily functions are immature as shown by:

- Temperature control: heat production is low (no brown fat, limited muscle activity). Heat loss is high (high surface area to volume, lack of fat insulation).
- Blood and circulation: hypotension, easy bruising and bleeding.
- Respiratory system: narrow nasal airways, soft thoracic cage, poor cough reflex, unstable respiratory drive with irregular breathing and apnea. Alveolar collapse due to surfactant deficiency.
- Gastrointestinal tract: uncoordinated suck or swallow (before 32–34 weeks). Regurgitation common. Increased severity and incidence of "physiologic" jaundice.
- Renal function: tendency to lose sodium but unable to excrete fluid load. Edema and hyponatremia may occur.
- Immune system: active and passive immunity are both limited.

General care of the preterm infant
Some basic principles apply to the care of all preterm infants. These are considered separately from the specific problems that arise in different systems. Attention must be paid to:
- Prevention and predelivery care.
- Resuscitation at birth.
- Maintaining body temperature.
- Avoiding infection.
- Nutrition and fluids.
- Physiologic monitoring.

Prevention and predelivery care
Preterm labor can be avoided in the presence of risk factors by bed rest and β-mimetic drugs. Once labor has started, it can be delayed by using the same group of drugs. This may give time for the administration of a corticosteroid to reduce the risk of respiratory distress syndrome (hyaline membrane disease).

Resuscitation at birth
Delivery should ideally take place in a location with full pediatric back-up, including a neonatal special care unit. At birth the baby should be handled gently, dried and placed under a source of radiant heat.

Many preterm infants of 32 weeks' gestation or less will not achieve adequate spontaneous ventilation and intermittent positive pressure ventilation or nasal continuous positive airways pressure is advisable. Surfactant administration in <29 weeks should be considered at this stage.

Body temperature

Preterm infants rapidly lose heat through evaporation, radiation, and convection and have limited heat-production mechanisms. Strategies for maintaining body temperature have to take into account the need for observation and access. They include:

- Ambient temperature: incubators provide a controlled microenvironment.
- Insulation with clothing: monitoring equipment can be attached to a clothed infant so most do not need to be kept naked. A bonnet prevents excessive loss from the relatively large head.
- Radiant heat: this is useful in the resuscitation area as access is optimized, but it causes excessive fluid loss over prolonged periods.

Body temperature in the preterm infant:
- Heat loss is excessive due to high surface area to volume ratio, poor insulation and transepidermal water loss.
- Heat generation is limited by reduced muscular activity, lack of brown fat, and inability to shiver.

Avoiding infection

Meticulous attention to hand-washing before and after handling is the most important safeguard against transmitting infection. Obviously, staff with skin or bowel infections should not be at work until clear. Good skin care will reduce the incidence of *Staphylococcus epidermidis* infection.

Nutrition and fluids

Infants of 35 weeks' gestation or more are usually able to take oral feeds of milk from breast or bottle without difficulty. Although preterm infants can digest and absorb enteral feeds, their sucking and swallowing reflexes may be ineffective and some or all of the feeds must be delivered through a small-bore polyethylene tube passed via the nose or mouth into the stomach. The approach to giving nutrition and fluids therefore depends on the size and maturity of the individual baby.

Enteral feeding in very low birth weight babies should be slow to allow the gut to adapt to feeds.

The majority of small preterm infants (under 1500 g) require their fluid and calorie requirements to be given intravenously during the first few days. Feeds should be slowly introduced and in the <1000 g babies parenteral nutrition commenced early as full enteral feeding will take longer to establish.

If enteral feeds by mouth or nasogastric tube are not tolerated, more prolonged maintenance of nutrition is achieved by total parenteral nutrition. A mixture of amino acids, dextrose, lipids, and electrolytes is given intravenously via a long line, the lumen of which is placed centrally in the vena cava or right atrium.

Which milk for preterm infants? Although breast milk alone does not provide enough calories or minerals, it is better tolerated than artificial feeds and its use is encouraged in the early setting for this reason, and to protect against necrotizing enterocolitis (NEC). Once feeding is established, a preterm formula to increase calories and electrolytes can be added.

Supplements. Breastfed preterm infants need supplements of phosphate and vitamin D to ensure adequate bone mineralization. A multivitamin preparation is usually given from the third week and an iron supplement from 4–6 weeks of age onwards. This is continued until 1 year of life but vitamins can be for up to 5 years.

Disorders of the preterm infant

Respiratory disorders
Surfactant deficiency (hyaline membrane disease, respiratory distress syndrome [RDS])
This syndrome is caused by a deficiency of surfactant associated with immaturity of the type II alveolar cells. Surfactant is a lipoprotein that lowers surface tension in the alveoli and prevents collapse of the alveoli during expiration. At postmortem, an exudate of proteinaceous hyaline material is seen in the alveoli and terminal

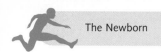

bronchioles (hence, the alternative term "hyaline membrane disease" for this disorder).

Surfactant deficiency is uncommon in term infants but will occur in the majority born before 30 weeks' gestation. It tends to be worse in boys and hypoxia, acidosis, or hypothermia exacerbates surfactant deficiency.

Clinical features

Respiratory distress is the major feature. This may be present from birth or could develop within the first 4 hours. The signs include:

- Tachypnea.
- Cyanosis.
- Subcostal and intercostal retractions.
- Expiratory grunting.

The disease displays a spectrum of severity from mild to severe and life-threatening. A chest x-ray (CXR) will show a diffuse granular or "ground glass" appearance of the lungs and air bronchograms outlining the larger airways.

Management

Glucocorticoids given antenatally for 48 hours stimulate fetal surfactant production but, of course, many preterm births occur without this period of warning. Effective resuscitation at birth of infants at risk reduces the severity of the disease.

The mainstays of management include:

- Surfactant therapy.
- Oxygen.
- Assisted ventilation.

Exogenous surfactant therapy Given after birth reduces mortality and morbidity and many babies can be rapidly weaned off ventilatory support after treatment.

An increased concentration of inspired oxygen is required and in more severe disease this needs to be supplemented with continuous positive airways pressure via the nasal airways or intermittent positive pressure ventilation via an endotracheal tube. Ventilation is guided by monitoring of the arterial blood gas tensions (PaO_2 and $PaCO_2$). High frequency oscillatory ventilation can be used as the sole mode of ventilation but often reserved for severe lung disease. Complications of RDS are shown in Fig. 25.12.

RDS resolves spontaneously in 3–7 days as endogenous surfactant is produced. Extremely preterm, very low birthweight infants, have lungs

Complications of respiratory distress syndrome	
Pulmonary	Pneumothorax
	Interstitial emphysema
	Secondary infection
	Chronic lung disease
Nonpulmonary	Intraventricular hemorrhage
	Patent ductus arteriosus

Fig. 25.12 Complications of respiratory distress syndrome.

that are both anatomically immature as well as surfactant deficient. Also, ventilation itself can cause lung injury so ventilatory support may be required for weeks or months and chronic lung disease may ensue.

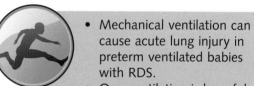

- Mechanical ventilation can cause acute lung injury in preterm ventilated babies with RDS.
- Overventilation is harmful and contributes to chronic lung disease.
- A lower oxygen saturation limit should be used to minimize ROP and to reduce mechanical ventilator requirements.

Apneic attacks

Many small, preterm infants display "periodic respiration" with some spells of very shallow breathing or complete cessation of breathing for up to 20 seconds. This reflects immaturity of the respiratory center.

Apneic is defined as cessation of respirations for at least 20 seconds and may be associated with bradycardia and desaturations. Predisposing factors include:

- Respiratory distress syndrome.
- Hypoxia.
- Infection.
- Cranial pathology, especially hemorrhage.

The differential diagnosis includes seizures, which can mimic apneic attacks.

Apnea alarms set to respond at an appropriate interval are useful for alerting staff to the need for action. Breathing will usually start again with physical stimulation. If frequent, and in the absence of an underlying cause, they can be prevented by oral caffeine. Ventilatory support may be needed if severe.

Cardiovascular problems
Patent ductus arteriosus
A patent ductus arteriosus (PDA) is a common problem in preterm infants and is often associated with RDS. Failure of closure occurs because of gestational immaturity and hypoxia. Presentation occurs after 2–3 days.

As the pulmonary vascular resistance falls, blood is shunted across the ductus from left to right. The clinical features are a widened pulse pressure with prominent peripheral pulses, tachycardia, and a continuous murmur. This shunt often causes difficulty in weaning ventilated infants. Diagnosis is by echocardiography.

Treatment
Spontaneous closure is the rule but treatment is used if the baby is ventilated or cardiac failure occurs. Fluid restriction and diuretics may be sufficient initially but a prostaglandin inhibitor, such as indomethacin or ibuprofen, could be used to facilitate closure. (The local action of prostaglandin maintains an open ductus.) Surgical closure may occasionally be required.

Intracranial lesions
Preterm infants are at risk of:
- Intracranial hemorrhage: into the germinal matrix or ventricles.
- Ischemia: of the periventricular white matter.

Risk factors for both include pneumothorax, asphyxia, hypovolemia, hypotension, and hypoxia in association with RDS.

Gastrointestinal problems
Necrotizing enterocolitis (NEC)
This is a necrosis of the intestine involving usually the distal ileum or proximal colon. The etiology is uncertain, but established predisposing factors include:
- Preterm birth.
- Polycythemia.
- PDA.
- Asphyxia.
- Early rapid oral feeding with formula milk: early feeding with breast milk is protective.

Clinical features include abdominal distention, vomiting, and bloody stools. Abdominal x-rays may show intramural gas, a pathognomonic finding. Bowel perforation may occur in 20–30%.

Treatment
This comprises:
- Gastric aspiration and parenteral nutrition.
- Antibiotics: penicillin, gentamicin, and metronidazole.
- In severe cases, surgical resection of the necrosed segment may be required.

Prognosis and long-term sequelae
Although the majority of preterm infants survive intact without sequelae, a number of significant problems can persist, especially in the very low birth weight group. These include:
- Retinopathy of prematurity (retrolental fibroplasia).
- Chronic lung disease of prematurity (bronchopulmonary dysplasia).
- Neurodevelopmental problems.

Retinopathy of prematurity
This comprises a spectrum of vascular abnormalities of the retina that occur in preterm infants in response to various injurious factors especially hyperoxia ($PaO_2 > 12$ kPa). There is abnormal vascular proliferation, which may progress to fibrosis, retinal detachment, and blindness.

All infants weighing less than 1500 g or <32 weeks gestational age should have their eyes screened 6–8 weeks after birth by indirect ophthalmoscopy until 36 weeks corrected gestational age. Most cases resolve spontaneously but laser therapy may be indicated for severe disease.

Chronic lung disease of prematurity
Chronic lung disease of prematurity or bronchopulmonary dysplasia occurs in newborns who for any reason require prolonged assisted ventilation with high pressures and high concentrations of oxygen. It is particularly common

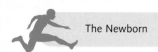

in very low birth weight infants and positive pressure ventilation is believed to be the main causative factor. The CXR shows widespread opacities with patchy translucent areas.

Treatment
- Initially, there may be a continued requirement for assisted ventilation or continuous positive airways pressure and supplemental O_2.
- Dexamethasone is effective in weaning from ventilatory support but increases the risk of neurodevelopmental impairment, so is used only in severe cases.
- Strict attention to nutrition.

Complete recovery of lung function occurs over several months but severely affected babies are at high risk of respiratory infections, which carry a high mortality rate.

Neurodevelopmental problems
The prospects for normal survival in preterm infants are good, especially for those weighing more than 1500 g at birth. However, very low birth weight infants and those with a gestation period of under 28 weeks are at risk of a range of neurodevelopmental problems, including:
- Cerebral palsy.
- Cognitive delay.
- Visual impairment.
- Hearing loss.
- Seizures.
- Behavioral problems.
- Educational difficulties.

Of infants born at ≤25 weeks gestational age, 23% have severe neurologic disability. This improves with babies born later but all should have regular monitoring of developmental progression. Low birth weight infants also show educational disadvantages into adulthood.

Disorders of the term infant

Respiratory disorders
Respiratory distress in term infants is characterized by:
- Tachypnea.
- Cyanosis.

Respiratory distress in term infants
Pulmonary Transient tachypnea of the newborn Pneumonia Pneumothorax Meconium aspiration Persistent fetal circulation Milk aspiration Diaphragmatic hernia
Nonpulmonary Congenital heart disease Severe anemia Metabolic acidosis

Fig. 25.13 Respiratory distress in term infants.

- Nasal flaring and retraction.
- Expiratory grunting.

The causes are considered in Chapter 9 and are listed again in Fig. 25.13.

The pulmonary causes are considered in turn.

Transient tachypnea of the newborn
This is caused by delay in reabsorption of fetal lung fluid and is more common after birth by cesarean section. There is early onset of mild to moderate respiratory distress and the CXR shows prominent pulmonary vasculature and fluid in the horizontal fissure. Treatment with increased ambient oxygen may be required. The condition usually settles spontaneously but antibiotics may be given because infection cannot be ruled out in the early stages.

Pneumonia
Early-onset, congenital pneumonia is acquired prenatally, especially when the membranes have been ruptured for more than 24 hours before the onset of labor. It is most commonly caused by the group B hemolytic streptococci. Respiratory distress is the chief sign, and the condition can mimic surfactant deficiency in preterm infants. Preterm infants with respiratory distress are therefore given antibiotics.

Chlamydia should be suspected if there is concurrent purulent conjunctivitis.

Treatment
This comprises:
- Physiotherapy to prevent local accumulation of secretions.

- Respiratory support with oxygen and ventilation if severe.
- Careful fluid balance and nutrition.
- Intravenous antibiotics.

Pneumothorax

A pneumothorax can occur spontaneously but is most commonly seen as a complication of positive pressure ventilation. Tension pneumothorax results in partial collapse of the lung with a sudden deterioration in the infant's condition manifested by cyanosis and hypotension. Diagnosis is confirmed by transillumination with a fiberoptic cold light source, or CXR. Urgent treatment by insertion of a chest tube is indicated for tension pneumothorax.

Meconium aspiration

Passage of meconium into the amniotic fluid is triggered by fetal distress in term or post-term infants. The infant is at risk of inhaling meconium and developing meconium aspiration syndrome. This severe condition causes respiratory distress and cyanosis and has a high mortality rate. It can be ameliorated by suctioning thick meconium from the upper airway as soon as the head is delivered and by suctioning any meconium from the trachea under direct vision after delivery. However, most severe cases are probably due to antenatal aspiration in utero and cannot be prevented by suction at delivery.

Persistent fetal circulation

This condition is characterized by high pulmonary vascular resistance and is usually found in term or post-term infants. There is right-to-left shunting of blood at atrial and ductal levels with severe cyanosis. Persistent fetal circulation may be primary or secondary to birth asphyxia, meconium aspiration, or respiratory distress syndrome.

A CXR shows a normal cardiac shadow and decreased pulmonary vascular markings, and an echocardiogram may be necessary to exclude cyanotic congenital heart disease.

Treatment

This includes:
- Assisted ventilation.
- Inhaled nitric oxide for pulmonary vasodilatation.
- Extracorporeal membrane oxygenation for severe cases.

Milk aspiration

Aspiration of milk or stomach contents into the lungs may occur especially in:
- Preterm infants with RDS or neurologic problems.
- Infants with chronic lung disease of prematurity.
- Infants with cleft palate.
- Infants with tracheoesophageal fistula.

Diaphragmatic hernia

See Chapter 9. This congenital malformation:
- Occurs in 1 in 4000 live births.
- Is usually left-sided.
- Can be diagnosed on antenatal ultrasound.
- Is repaired surgically.
- Has a high mortality due to coexisting pulmonary hypoplasia.

Gastrointestinal and hepatic disorders

Congenital anomalies of the gastrointestinal tract including cleft lip and palate, tracheoesophageal fistula, duodenal stenosis or atresia, and exomphalos or gastroschisis are considered in Chapter 9.

Small bowel obstruction

This presents with:
- Persistent, bile-stained vomiting.
- Delayed or absent passage of meconium.
- Abdominal distention.

Important causes are listed in Fig. 25.14.

Diagnosis is made on clinical features and abdominal x-ray. Treatment depends on the cause and is often surgical. Administering gastrograffin contrast medium may relieve meconium ileus.

Causes of small bowel obstruction
Duodenal atresia
Midgut volvulus and malrotation
Gastroschisis and exomphalos
Meconium ileus

Fig. 25.14 Causes of small bowel obstruction.

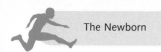
Large bowel obstruction

Hirschsprung's disease or rectal atresia can cause this.

Hirschsprung's disease

Congenital aganglionic megacolon, or Hirschsprung's disease, is a genetic disorder in which there is absence of ganglion cells from the myenteric and submyenteric plexuses of a segment of the large bowel (see Chapter 15).

Clinical features. Presentation is usually in the neonatal period with failure to pass meconium in the first 24 hours followed by abdominal distension and bile-stained vomiting. Diarrhea may occur and alternate with periods of constipation. A major complication is enterocolitis.

Diagnosis. A unprepped barium enema can suggest the diagnosis, but definitive diagnosis requires demonstration of the absence of ganglion cells on a suction rectal biopsy.

Management. Treatment is surgical. A preliminary colostomy is usually performed in the neonatal period followed later by an operation to anastomose normally innervated bowel to anus.

Jaundice

Clinical jaundice appears in newborns when the serum bilirubin exceeds 80–120 μmol/L. The causes are considered in Chapter 9.

Jaundice is important because it may be indicative of underlying problems such as infection and because unconjugated bilirubin can be deposited in the brain and cause bilirubin encephalopathy (previously called "kernicterus"). Causative conditions are most usefully considered by age of onset of the jaundice.

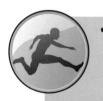

- Physiologic jaundice is the most common cause of jaundice in the newborn. It is associated with unconjugated hyperbilirubinemia.
- Conjugated hyperbilirubinemia, in excess of 15% of total serum bilirubin, suggests cholestasis due to hepatobiliary disease.

Jaundice in the first 24 hours

This is always pathologic. The most common cause is hemolysis, which can be due to:
- Hemolytic disease of the newborn: Rhesus or ABO incompatibility.
- Intrinsic red cell defects: spherocytosis, G6PD deficiency, or pyruvate kinase deficiency.

Congenital infections can also cause early-onset jaundice.

Hemolytic disorders. Isoimmune hemolysis is caused by the destruction of fetal and neonatal red blood cells by maternal IgG antibodies that cross the placenta during pregnancy. Maternal sensitization is caused by fetal–maternal transfusion during current or previous pregnancies or from mismatched blood transfusions.

The incidence of Rhesus (Rh) hemolytic disease has fallen since the introduction of anti-D immune globulin, which is given to the Rh-negative mother immediately after birth of a Rh-positive infant. Affected infants are usually diagnosed antenatally and given fetal therapy as necessary. Severe hemolysis causes anemia and hydrops fetalis, which is treated by intrauterine blood transfusion.

ABO incompatibility is more common than Rh hemolytic disease. The usual combination is a group O mother with a group A, or less commonly group B infant. The anti-A or anti-B hemolysins are comparatively weak. There is mild anemia, no organomegaly, a weakly positive Coombs' test, and mild jaundice peaking in the first few days.

G6PD deficiency and congenital spherocytosis can cause neonatal jaundice.

Jaundice at 2 days to 2 weeks of age

The most common cause is physiological jaundice, due to the combination of liver enzyme immaturity and an increased load of bilirubin from red cell breakdown. Prematurity, bruising, or polycythemia (hematocrit >65%) can exacerbate it. Physiologic jaundice usually peaks on the third day of life.

Infection, particularly of the urinary tract, also causes unconjugated hyperbilirubinemia at this time.

Jaundice at more than 2 weeks of age

Persistent (prolonged, protracted) jaundice is usually an unconjugated hyperbilirubinemia, which can be due to:
- "Breast milk" jaundice: affects 15% of healthy breastfed infants. The cause is unknown. It usually resolves by 3–4 weeks of age.

- Infection: particularly of urinary tract.
- Congenital hypothyroidism: this should have been detected on neonatal screening.

Prolonged conjugated hyperbilirubinemia is usually associated with dark urine and pale stools. Causes include neonatal hepatitis syndrome and biliary atresia. Early diagnosis of biliary atresia is important because delay in surgical treatment beyond 6 weeks of age compromises outcome.

Management of neonatal jaundice

Investigations are directed towards establishing the cause (see Chapter 9). Clinical estimation of the severity is unreliable and a plasma bilirubin must be measured in any significantly jaundiced infant. The main concern is to prevent bilirubin encephalopathy.

Bilirubin encephalopathy occurs when unconjugated bilirubin is deposited in the brain, especially in the basal ganglia and cerebellum. This presents initially with lethargy, rigidity, eye-rolling, and seizures. The long-term sequelae include choreoathetoid cerebral palsy, sensorineural deafness and learning difficulties.

Many factors in addition to the bilirubin level influence this risk. These include:

- The infant's gestational age: risk increases for preterm infants.
- The postnatal age: risk decreases with increasing postnatal age.
- The serum albumin level: risk increases with hypoalbuminemia.
- Coexistent asphyxia, acidosis, or hypoglycemia.

Charts exist indicating levels at which treatment should be initiated, bearing those factors in mind.
Treatment options are:
- Phototherapy.
- Exchange transfusion.

Phototherapy. Blue light (not ultraviolet) of wavelength 450 nm converts the bilirubin in the skin and superficial capillaries into harmless water-soluble metabolites, which are excreted in urine and through the bowel. The eyes are covered to prevent discomfort and additional fluids are given to counteract increased losses from skin.

Exchange transfusion. This is required if the bilirubin rises to levels considered dangerous despite phototherapy. It rapidly reduces the level of circulating bilirubin, and in isoimmune hemolytic disease also removes circulating antibodies and corrects anemia. Techniques vary, but conventionally the exchange is done via umbilical artery and vein catheters. Aliquots of baby's blood (10–20 mL) are withdrawn, alternating with infusions of donor blood of the same volumes. Twice the infant's blood volume (i.e., 2×80 mL/kg) is exchanged over about 2 hours.

Hematologic disorders

Hemolytic diseases of the newborn are considered with jaundice.

Hemorrhagic disease of the newborn

This is caused by a relative deficiency of the vitamin K-dependent coagulation factors II, VII, IX, and X. It characteristically affects the fully breastfed infant between the third and sixth day of life, because breast milk does not contain adequate amounts of vitamin K. Mothers taking anticonvulsant drugs that interfere with vitamin K metabolism, such as phenytoin, are at increased risk.

Bleeding usually occurs from the gastrointestinal tract but can rarely be intracranial or from the umbilical stump.

A single intramuscular dose of vitamin K prevents this disease but three doses of oral vitamin K can also be given. It is important that all three doses are administered.

Infections

The newborn infant is vulnerable to infection by bacteria, viruses, and fungi. In utero, infection can take place across the placenta or by ascending the birth canal.

After birth, the skin and umbilicus are colonized by staphylococci, the gut by *Escherichia coli*, and the upper respiratory tract by streptococci. Important bacterial pathogens in the neonate include:

- Group B β-hemolytic streptococci.
- *Escherichia coli*.
- *Staphylococcus epidermidis*: found in preterm babies on intensive care.

The range of acquired infections in the newborn is shown in Fig. 25.15. Signs suggestive of neonatal infections are summarized in Fig. 25.16.

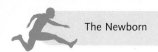

Acquired infections in the newborn
Minor infections
Skin pustules
Paronychia
Acute mastitis
Conjunctivitis
Thrush
Major infections
Septicemia
Meningitis
Pneumonia
Urinary tract infection
Ophthalmia neonatorum

Fig. 25.15 Acquired infections in the newborn.

Signs suggestive of neonatal infection
Irritability or lethargy
Persistent tachycardia
Tachypnea or grunting
Frequent apneas or bradycardias and desaturation
Poor response to handling
Acute onset of pallor
Temperature instability
Feeding intolerance

Fig. 25.16 Signs suggestive of neonatal infection.

Minor infections

Skin pustules and paronychia

These are caused by staphylococcal infection and typically occur in moist areas such as the groin and axillae. Inflammation of the skin in the area of a nail fold may evolve into a pustular lesion. Treatment with oral cephalexin is indicated in severe cases, but most resolve spontaneously.

Acute mastitis

This is an inflamed swelling under the nipple in a febrile infant. It is usually caused by *Staphylococcus aureus* infection in an engorged neonatal breast. Cephalexin is the antibiotic of choice.

Conjunctivitis

A "sticky eye" in the first day or two of life is often due to chemical irritation and clears spontaneously. Conjunctivitis with a purulent discharge may be due to:

- Staphylococci, streptococci, *Escherichia coli*.
- Gonococci: ophthalmia neonatorum (see below)—usually between days 2 and 5 of life.
- *Chlamydia trachomatis*: usually between days 7 and 10 of life.

Gonococcal and chlamydial infections need systemic antibiotic treatment because the risk of scarring and blindness is high. Erythromycin or a cephalosporin is used and ophthalmologic evaluation is mandatory. It is also important to treat the parents.

Thrush (moniliasis)

Infection with *Candida albicans* can affect the mouth or diaper area. Oral thrush appears as white plaques on the tongue and inside of the mouth. Nystatin suspension, 1 mL (100,000 units) after feeds for 7–10 days, is usually effective. Perineal thrush responds to topical nystatin.

Major infections

Septicemia

Neonatal sepsis carries a high mortality and morbidity and can be rapid and fulminant. As signs are nonspecific, a low threshold for investigation and empirical treatment with antibiotics is needed. As this results in a high number of treated infants, to reduce unnecessary antibiotic usage antibiotics should be stopped if cultures are negative in 48 hours. Unlike adults, the incidence of false-negative blood cultures is less in neonates.

The incidence of serious acute infections in the newborn period is about 3 per 1000 live births in the USA.

Initial presentation is often nonspecific with:
- Lethargy and drowsiness or excessive irritability.
- Poor feeding, vomiting.
- Temperature and cardiovascular instability.
- Pallor.
- Acidosis or glucose instability.

Specific signs relating to a site of infection may then emerge. These include:
- Tense fontanelle, seizures: meningitis.
- Respiratory distress: pneumonia.

Group B streptococcal infection

Genital tract colonization with this organism is found in 20–30% of all women and infection carries a high mortality and morbidity. It presents in two ways: early (within the first week) or late (after the first week). Early disease is associated with a worse outcome but can be reduced with preventive measures.

Diagnosis. If systemic infection is suspected, prompt investigation is essential. The following investigations are performed to confirm the diagnosis and identify a causative organism.

- "Septic" screen: blood culture, urine culture, lumbar puncture, and cerebrospinal fluid culture. Swabs from the throat, nose, and ear.
- Rapid antigen testing on blood and cerebrospinal fluid (CSF).
- Gram stain of CSF.

Treatment. Group B streptococcal (GBS) infection is usually sensitive to penicillin and aminoglycosides are added for additional synergistic effects. Cephalosporins can be also used for their high CSF penetration but they are associated with secondary coliform infections.

Meningitis

Neonatal meningitis is usually due to a different range of pathogens from that in the older infant or child. In infants, the infective organisms include:

- *Escherichia coli.*
- Group B streptococci.
- *Listeria monocytogenes.*

Meningeal infection usually follows a septicemic stage. Clinical features include poor feeding, pallor, and temperature instability. Fullness of the anterior fontanelle and seizures are late signs.

Diagnosis. Lumbar puncture is required to confirm the diagnosis.

Treatment and outcome. High-dose intravenous antibiotics for 14–21 days are required. Penetration of drugs occur through the inflamed meninges. Mortality is 30–60% and a high incidence of neurological impairment occurs in survivors.

Pneumonia

This is most commonly due to the group B streptococci. Respiratory distress is the chief presenting sign together with features of septicemia.

Urinary tract infection

The most common pathogen is *Escherichia coli*, although other Gram-negative organisms are occasionally responsible. There is a relatively high incidence of underlying congenital anomalies or vesicoureteral reflux.

Symptoms and signs are usually nonspecific. Urine must be cultured in all infants with poor feeding, lethargy, vomiting, failure to thrive, and jaundice.

The optimal way of obtaining a specimen is catheterization of a suprapubic aspirate. Any growth is diagnostic of a UTI.

IV antibiotics are used for treatment and imaging of the renal tract to look for structural abnormalities once the infant has recovered.

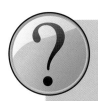

- Describe effects of maternal drugs on neonates.
- What are the clinical features of respiratory distress syndrome (RDS)?
- Describe the natural history of RDS.
- What are the complications of neonatal intensive care?
- What nonrespiratory complications are found on preterm neonates?
- How is group B streptococcal infection manifest?
- What are the consequences of birth asphyxia?
- How is jaundice assessed and treated?

Further reading

Gomella TG. Neonatology: management, procedures, on-call problems. In *Diseases and Drugs*, 4th edn. Philadelphia, PA: Appleton Lange, 1999.

Hack M et al. Outcomes in young adulthood for low birthweight infants. *New England Journal of Medicine* 2002; 346:149–157.

MacLennan A. A template for defining a causal relation between acute intrapartum events and cerebral palsy: international consensus statement. *British Medical Journal* 1999; 319:1054–1059.

Wood NS et al. for the EPICure study group. Neurological and developmental disability after extremely preterm birth. *New England Journal of Medicine* 2000; 343:378–384.

26. Accidents and Emergencies

Accidents

Accidents in children are extremely common and are the leading cause of death between the ages of 1 and 14 years. The pattern of accidents varies with age (Fig. 26.1). Road traffic accidents account for the majority of fatal accidents (Fig. 26.2). Child abuse needs to be considered in any child presenting with injury.

Trauma

Physical trauma causing multiple serious injuries is an important cause of death; early, appropriate management of the multiply injured child is vital to reduce mortality and long-term morbidity. Injuries to the head are the most important class of local injury.

Major trauma

Initial assessment and management is described in Fig. 26.3. Events during the first "golden hour" determine the outcome. Once the initial steps of immediate resuscitation have been carried out, a careful secondary survey of the complete child must be undertaken to detect and treat all injuries (Fig. 26.4).

Head injury

Minor head injuries in children are very common and most children recover without ill effect. A small minority, about 1 in 800 of those admitted, develops serious complications such as intracranial hemorrhage. Causes of head injury include:

- Motor vehicle accidents (MVAs): the most common cause of severe and fatal head injuries.
- Falls from trees, walls, bicycles, etc.
- Child abuse: especially "shaking" injuries in infants.

Damage to the brain may be primary or secondary (Fig. 26.5).

The history should establish:
- The mechanism of injury.
- Was consciousness lost?
- Subsequent symptoms: vomiting, drowsiness, seizures, bleeding from nose or ears.
- Anterograde amnesia >30 minutes.

Clinical features

Clinical examination should look for the following signs:
- Head: external injury, including hematoma, laceration, depressed fracture. In babies, the anterior fontanelle tension provides a useful indicator of intracranial pressure, as does the head circumference. Look for blood or cerebrospinal fluid leak from the ears or nose.
- Central nervous system: assess Glasgow coma scale/AVPU scale, fundi and pupillary reflexes. Examine for focal neurologic signs.
- General: full examination to exclude other injuries.

Diagnosis

Investigations include:
- Skull x-ray: now not routinely indicated, useful only if nonaccidental injury is suspected.
- Cranial computed tomography (CT): if fracture seen on x-ray, decreased conscious level, seizures, amnesia, or focal neurologic signs.

Management

Minor and moderate injuries. These are the majority. Admit to hospital for observation if:
- History of seizure or loss of consciousness.
- Declining level of consciousness.
- Severe headache or persistent vomiting.
- Skull fracture.
- Suspected nonaccidental injury.
- Child has a bleeding tendency.
- Supervision at home is inadequate.

If the child is not admitted, the parents should be given written instructions to bring the child back if there is severe headache, recurrent vomiting, or a declining level of consciousness.

If admitted, neurologic observations should be made at intervals dictated by the child's clinical state.

Accidents in Childhood

Toddlers are prone to:
Falls
Scalds
Drowning
Accidental ingestion
Choking

School-age children are prone to:
Falls while climbing
Road traffic accidents

Fig. 26.1 Accidents in childhood.

Causes of fatal accidents

Age range	Leading cause of death (highest at top)
4–52 weeks	Congenital abnormalities SIDS Infection
1–4 years	Trauma Congenital abnormalities Cancer Infection
5–14 years	Trauma Cancer Congenital abnormality Infection

Fig. 26.2 Causes of fatal accidents.

Severe injuries. These usually occur in the context of major trauma requiring intensive care.

Additional measures in severe head injury are directed toward the management of complications such as raised intracranial pressure, intracranial bleeding, seizures, and risk of infection.

Urgent referral to a neurosurgeon is indicated if there is any evidence of an expanding hematoma, such as:
- Declining level of consciousness.
- Focal neurologic signs.
- Depressed skull fracture.
- Signs of rising intracranial pressure: bradycardia, rise in systolic blood pressure, and irregular respirations.

Burns and scalds

Scalds from contact with hot liquids are the most common form of thermal trauma in childhood (most of the fatalities are from house fires but those are due to gas and smoke inhalation rather than burns). Burns and scalds can be nonaccidental. Toddlers are most at risk of accidental scalds.

- Electrical burns are usually full thickness.
- Most scalds are deep, partial thickness.

Assessment

The extent, depth, and distribution of the injury should be estimated (Figs. 26.6 and 26.7).

Diagnosis

Investigations should include:
- Complete blood count: packed cell volume is increased with significant hypovolemia.
- Urea and electrolytes.
- Type and cross (if burns are greater than 15–20%).
- Serum albumin.

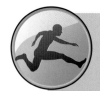

Location of the burn is important as well as extent:
- Face—potential airway involvement, scarring
- Hands—contractures and functional loss
- Genitalia—difficult to nurse, risk of infection

Management

Recommended first aid is:
- Run cold water over the affected part for 5 minutes.
- Cover the burn with a clean dressing.

Admit to burns center if:
- The extent is over 5% full thickness or over 10% partial thickness.
- A difficult area is involved (e.g., face, hands and feet, perineum, or genitalia).
- There is any inhalational injury (e.g., smoke inhalation).

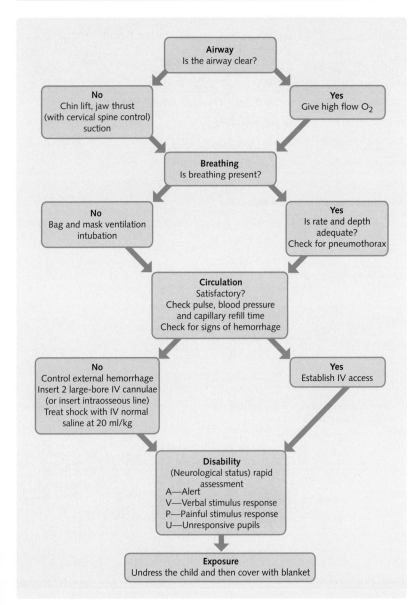

Fig. 26.3 Major trauma. Initial assessment and management (ABCDE).

Airway
Is the airway clear?

No
Chin lift, jaw thrust
(with cervical spine control)
suction

Yes
Give high flow O_2

Breathing
Is breathing present?

No
Bag and mask ventilation
intubation

Yes
Is rate and depth
adequate?
Check for pneumothorax

Circulation
Satisfactory?
Check pulse, blood pressure
and capillary refill time
Check for signs of hemorrhage

No
Control external hemorrhage
Insert 2 large-bore IV cannulae
(or insert intraosseous line)
Treat shock with IV normal
saline at 20 ml/kg

Yes
Establish IV access

Disability
(Neurological status) rapid
assessment
A—Alert
V—Verbal stimulus response
P—Painful stimulus response
U—Unresponsive pupils

Exposure
Undress the child and then cover with blanket

The important aspects of management are shown in Fig. 26.8.

Near drowning

Drowning is more common in boys than girls. It is the third most common cause of childhood accidental death in the USA. Drowning incidents are more common in freshwater canals and lakes, swimming pools, and domestic baths than in the sea.

The two principal problems in near drowning are:
- Hypoxia: laryngospasm results in asphyxia. Only a small amount of water initially enters the lungs.
- Hypothermia: this leads to bradycardia and asystole (extreme hypothermia can be protective).

Hemolysis or electrolyte problems caused by the ingestion or inhalation of large amounts of water are unusual.

Management

Skilled resuscitation and warming is vital. Cervical injury should be assumed. All children should be hospitalized for at least 24 hours. Patients admitted

233

Secondary survey and treatment—multiple trauma	
Head	Examine for bruising, lacerations, CSF leak from ears or nose. Mini-neurologic exam
Face	Look for bruising, factures, and loose teeth
Neck	Cervical spine stabilization. Examine for bony tenderness, bruising, or wounds
Chest	Look for wounds, bruising. Feel trachea and auscultate
Abdomen	Observe movement and bruising, palpate for tenderness
Pelvis	Inspect perineum and for bone deformity. Look for blood at urethral meatus
Spine	Done by log-rolling: look for swelling, palpate vertebrae, and assess motor and sensory function
Extremities	Assess movement deformity, bruising, and tenderness Test sensation and peripheral circulation
Radiologic investigations as needed and a full history	

Fig. 26.4 Secondary survey and treatment—multiple trauma.

Brain damage in head injury	
Primary damage	Cerebral laceration and contusion Diffuse axonal injury Dural sac tears
Secondary damage	Ischemia from shock, hypoxia, or raised intracranial pressure Hypoglycemia CNS infection Seizures Hyperthermia

Fig. 26.5 Brain damage in head injury.

Assessment of the depth of burn		
Superficial	**Partial thickness**	**Full thickness**
Red	Pink or mottled	White or charred
No blisters	Blisters	Painless
Affects only epithelial layer	Some dermal damage	Full dermal and nerve damage

Fig. 26.6 Assessment of the depth of burn.

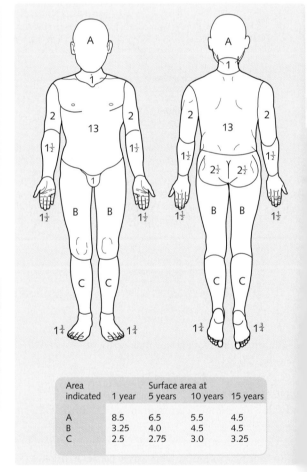

Area indicated	Surface area at			
	1 year	5 years	10 years	15 years
A	8.5	6.5	5.5	4.5
B	3.25	4.0	4.5	4.5
C	2.5	2.75	3.0	3.25

Fig. 26.7 Assessment of the extent of a burn. The percentage body surface area affected is calculated from this standard body diagram. Note that the area corresponding to head and lower limbs (A, B, C) changes with age. The small child has a relatively big head and short legs.

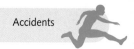

in asystole or respiratory arrest should undergo cardiopulmonary resuscitation in the normal way. Resuscitation must be continued until the core temperature has been raised to above 32°C because many arrythmias are refractory at temperatures below 30°C.

Prognostic indicators of near drowning

The prognostic indicators are shown in Fig. 26.9.

Late respiratory sequelae can occur in the 72-hour period after near drowning. These include pneumonia and pulmonary edema.

Poisoning

Most cases of poisoning in young children follow accidental ingestion by an inquisitive, fearless toddler; in adolescents most poisoning is deliberate self-harm. Children can also be poisoned deliberately by their parents (or inadvertently by their doctors). Although many thousands of children are admiited each year, very few die as a result of accidental ingestion.

The history should establish:

- What was ingested: identify from carton or bottle.
- Amount ingested: usually an approximation.
- Time ingested: important in relation to management.

The toxicity of the ingested substance can then be assessed (Fig. 26.10) or the Regional Poison Information Center contacted if there is any doubt concerning the agent's identity or toxicity.

Management of burns	
Analgesia	IV morphine for major burns
IV fluids	Treat shock with 20 mL/kg If >10% burn, IV fluids are needed: Normal fluid requirements with additional fluids at: % burn × weight (kg) × 4 per day (Half of this given within 8 h) Keep urine output >1 mL/kg/h
Wound care	Sterile towels and avoid excessive re-examination.

Fig. 26.8 Management of burns.

Prognostic indicators for near drowning	
Prognostic indicators	Poor if:
Immersion time	Submerged for >8 minutes
Time to first gasp	No gasp after 40 minutes resuscitation
Rectal temperature	<33°C on arrival
Consciousness level	Persisting coma
Arterial blood pH	<7.0 despite treatment
Arterial blood O_2	<8.0 kPa despite treatment
Type of water	No difference in terms of prognosis

Fig. 26.9 Prognostic indicators for near drowning.

Poison-specific adverse effects and treatments		
Poison	Adverse effects	Specific treatment
Iron	Shock, gut hemorrhage	IV deferoxamine
Acetaminophen	Liver failure	IV N-acetylcysteine
Salicylates	Metabolic acidosis	Alkalinization of urine with bicarbonate
Ethylene glycol	Widespread cellular damage	Ethanol, dialysis if severe
Tricyclic antidepressants	Cardiac dysrhythmias	Alkalinization of urine with bicarbonate
Ecstasy	Hyperpyrexia and rhabdomyolysis Dysrhythmias Hyponatremia (secondary to excessive H_2O ingestion)	Active cooling

Fig. 26.10 Poison-specific adverse effects and treatments.

Clinical features

Examination should include the following:
- Inspect oropharynx for any vomitus.
- Assess level of consciousness.
- Look for features specific to various poisons. For example: small pupils (opiates or barbiturates), tachypnea (salicylate poisoning), or cardiac arrhythmias (tricyclic antidepressants or digoxin).

Diagnosis

Relevant investigations include:
- Blood levels (at optimum time after ingestion) can be measured for salicylates, acetaminophen, digoxin, iron, lithium, and tricyclic antidepressants.
- Keep specimens of vomitus and urine for analysis.

Management

If the agent ingested was relatively innocuous, the patient can be allowed to go home or observed briefly in hospital. Efforts should be made to remove the poison if there has been a large ingestion of a highly toxic substance. These include:
- Activated charcoal: give 1 g/kg, if necessary by nasogastric tube. It binds a wide range of toxic drugs, with the exception of iron and lithium. It is most efficacious if used within 1 hr of ingestion.

Specific treatment is indicated for certain drugs and toxins (see Fig. 26.10).

Deliberate self-poisoning in older children

This is a serious occurrence that can reflect a significant underlying psychiatric disorder such as depression. In most cases, there is no serious suicidal intent. Drug or alcohol intoxication is often a predisposing element. All children who deliberately poison themselves should be admitted to hospital and assessed by a child and adolescent psychiatrist.

Emergencies

Children differ from adults in important ways that are relevant to emergency care (Fig. 26.11).

Anatomic and physiologic characteristics of young children	
Anatomy	Airway (see Chapter 2) Large surface area to volume ratio Small airways and elastic ribs Obligate nasal breathers until 5 months old
Physiology	Increased oxygen consumption and metabolic rate Compliant chest wall: leading to airways collapse Inefficient respiratory muscles Low stroke volume: cardiac output dependent on heart rate

Fig. 26.11 Anatomic and physiologic characteristics of young children.

The seriously ill child

A seriously ill child is on one of the pathways leading to cardiopulmonary arrest (Fig. 26.12). Such arrests in children are rarely unheralded but preceded by a period of progressive circulatory, respiratory, or central neurological failure. It is vital to recognize such a critically ill child and intervene to prevent the progression to cardiac arrest.

Rapid assessment

An initial ABCD assessment should be carried out to identify features of:
- Airway and breathing: airway obstruction and hypoxia.
- Circulation: shock.
- Disability: central neurologic failure.

Airway and breathing

A critical state is indicated either by:
- An increase in the work of breathing (respiratory distress).
- Absent or decreased respiratory effort (exhaustion or respiratory depression).

Key signs include (Fig. 26.13):
- Efficacy of breathing.
- Effort of breathing.
- Signs of inadequate respiration.

Circulation

Signs of potential circulatory failure (shock) include:
- Tachycardia.
- Pulse volume reduction: absent peripheral pulses and weak central pulses are serious signs of advanced shock.

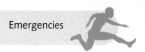

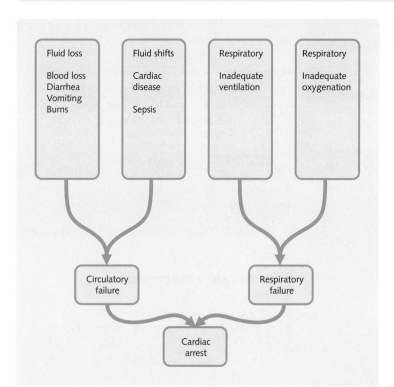

Fig. 26.12 The critically ill child: pathways to cardiopulmonary arrest.

Respiratory assessment	
Effort of breathing	Respiratory rate Inspiratory or expiratory noises Grunting Use of accessory muscles Nasal flaring
Efficacy of air entry	Presence of breath sounds Pulse oximetry
Adequacy of oxygenation	Heart rate Skin color Mental status

Fig. 26.13 Respiratory assessment.

- Capillary refill time of over 2 seconds.
- Blood pressure: hypotension is a late and preterminal sign of circulatory failure.

The effects of circulatory failure encompass:
- Metabolic acidosis with increased respiratory rate.
- Skin: mottled, cold, pale skin peripherally.
- Mental state: agitation followed by drowsiness due to reduced cerebral perfusion.
- Urine output: oliguria due to renal hypoperfusion.

 Always go back to assessing airway, breathing, and circulation (ABCs) if the child's condition changes.

Disability
Signs of potential central neurologic failure are:
- Level of consciousness: reduced.
- Posture: most are hypotonic; seizures reflect brain dysfunction.
- Pupils: most sinister signs are dilatation, unreactivity, and inequality.

Central neurologic failure has important effects on both respiration and circulation:
- Respiratory depression.
- Abnormal respiratory patterns.
- Systemic hypertension with sinus bradycardia (Cushing's response) indicates herniation of the cerebellar tonsils through the foramen magnum.

Central neurologic failure has respiratory and circulatory consequences.

Cardiorespiratory arrest

A standard procedure exists for applying basic life support in the event of a cardiorespiratory arrest (Figs. 26.14 to 26.19).

Hypoxia is the cause of the majority of arrests; a primary cardiac cause is rare.

After basic life support procedures, it may be necessary to proceed to:
• Intubation and ventilation.
• Circulatory access: venous or intraosseous.
• ECG monitoring: to identify the rhythm (asystole is most common). The protocol for drug use in asystole is shown in Fig. 26.16.

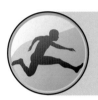

Asystole is the most common arrest rhythm in children.

Neurologic emergencies
Coma

There are many causes of a reduced consciousness level. Evaluation is done by the Glasgow coma scale or AVPU (see Chapter 5). Some are self-evident, but others may be identified only after careful clinical evaluation and special investigations.

Assessment

A rapid history should include information about:
• Chronic medical conditions such as epilepsy and diabetes mellitus.
• Any recent injury.
• Access to poisons including drugs.
• Normal neurologic state.

Clinical examination should pay attention to:
• Airway, breathing, and circulation.
• Fever or rash: especially a purpuric rash.
• Signs of injury.
• CNS: Glasgow coma score (see Fig. 5.5) or AVPU, signs of meningism (neck stiffness), focal neurologic signs and posture, pupil size and reaction to light, fundi-papilledema, or hemorrhages.

Diagnosis

Investigations are determined by the clinical evaluation and may include:
• Blood analysis for glucose, electrolytes.
• Urine for toxins.
• Lumbar puncture for suspected meningitis.
• Brain imaging: cranial CT or magnetic resonance imaging.
• EEG for seizures, metabolic encephalopathy.

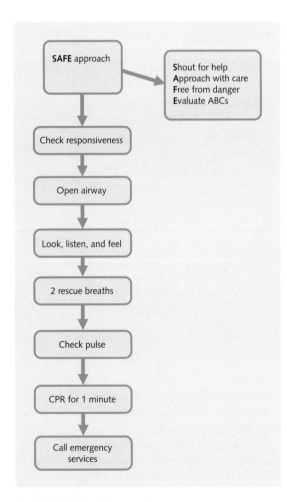

SAFE approach

Shout for help
Approach with care
Free from danger
Evaluate ABCs

Check responsiveness

Open airway

Look, listen, and feel

2 rescue breaths

Check pulse

CPR for 1 minute

Call emergency services

Fig. 26.14 Basic life support.

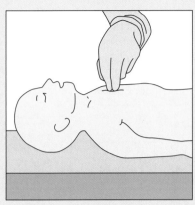

A Infant chest compression: Two finger technique

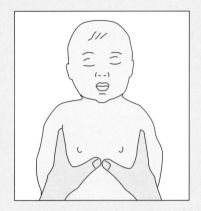

B Infant chest compression: Hand-encircling technique

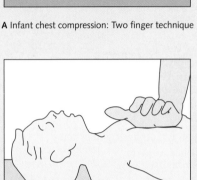

C Chest compression in small children

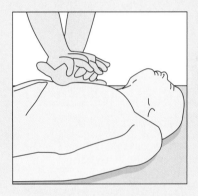

D Chest compression in older children

Fig. 26.15 Cardiac compression techniques.

Check blood sugar in a comatose or seizing child to identify treatable hypoglycemia.

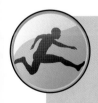

Hypoglycemia is an important cause of both coma and seizures in children. Recognition and treatment are simple. If missed, brain damage can result.

Management

Initial management should be directed towards maintaining airway, breathing, and circulation. Further specific treatment depends on etiology. All children with a GCS < 8 or P on the AVPU scale need airway protection with endotracheal intubation.

Secondary brain damage is minimized by maintaining oxygenation and perfusion.

Seizures

The causes of a seizure vary with age (Fig. 26.20). The most common cause in young children is a "febrile seizure" (see Chapter 17).

A continuous seizure lasting more than 30 minutes, or repeated seizures without recovery

239

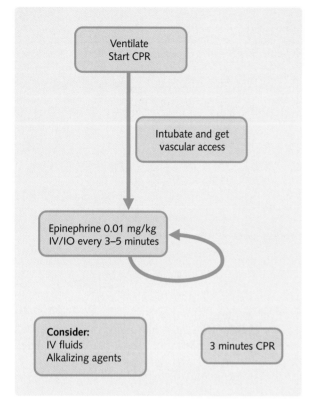

Fig. 26.16 Protocol for drug use in asystole.

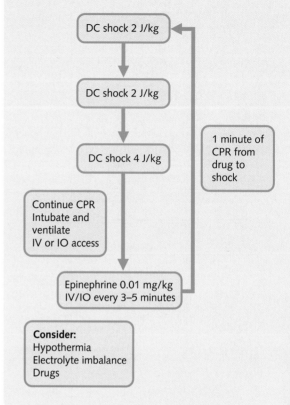

Fig. 26.17 Protocol for ventricular fibrillation.

of consciousness between attacks, is called status epilepticus (SE).

Prolonged convulsions can result in brain damage or death from hypoxia. Cerebral blood flow and oxygen consumption increase five-fold to meet the extra metabolic demand. Oxygen delivery to the brain will be impaired if there is inadequate ventilation or hypotension.

Management

An algorithm for management of the seizing child is shown in Fig. 26.21.

While initiating emergency management, establish the history and examine the child:

History

- Duration of seizure.
- History of recent trauma.
- Known epileptic? If so, medication regimen.
- Known diabetic?
- Preceding illness.

Examination

- Cardiorespiratory status.
- Signs of head trauma.
- Fever, petechial rash, meningismus.
- Nature of seizure: generalized or focal.

If lorazepam fails to stop the seizure, further options include, in order:

1. IV phenytoin: give as an infusion under ECG and blood pressure monitoring.
2. Call anesthesia.
3. If no IV access, such as in the field, rectal valium is a useful and effective choice.

Status epilepticus

Protracted seizures (of over 30 minutes) can occur in:

- Epilepsy.
- Febrile seizures.
- Head injury.

240

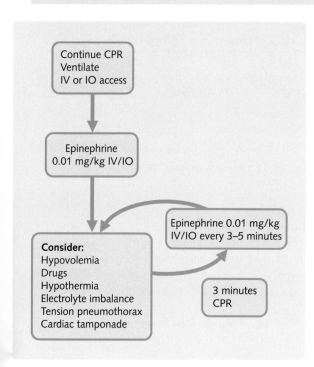

Fig. 26.18 Protocol for pulseless electrical activity.

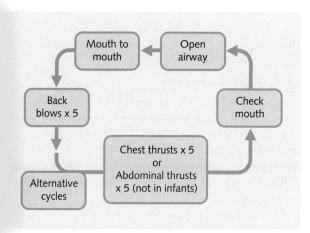

Fig. 26.19 Protocol for the choking child.

Causes of seizures	
Age	**Causes**
All ages	Hypoglycemia Head injury Poisoning Meningitis Epilepsy
Birth to 6 months	Hypoglycemia Hypocalcemia Inborn errors of metabolism Meningitis
6 months to 5 years	Febrile seizures Meningitis
>5 years	Epilepsy (most common cause)

Fig. 26.20 Causes for seizures.

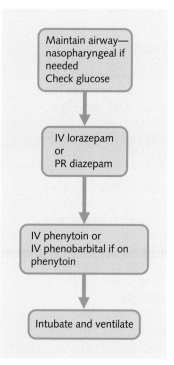

Fig. 26.21 The seizing child.

- Intracranial infection: meningitis or encephalitis.
- Metabolic seizures: hypoglycemia or poisoning.

Lorazepam, diazepam, and phenytoin are used in order, as in Fig.26.21. If seizures persist, the child should be paralyzed, ventilated, and managed on an intensive care unit where a thiopental or benzodiazepine infusion can be safely instituted.

241

Cardiac emergencies

Serious illness arising from a primary cardiac problem is uncommon outside the newborn period. The causes and management of heart failure are considered elsewhere (see Chapter 2), as is the management of circulatory failure (shock) and cardiac arrest. Cardiac arrhythmias, uncommon but treatable conditions in childhood, are considered in Chapter 13.

Respiratory emergencies

The pattern of severe respiratory illness in children is determined by features of the anatomy and physiology of their respiratory system, including:

- Small airways: easily obstructed with rapid increase in airways resistance.
- Compliant thoracic cage: reduced breathing efficiency.
- Inefficient respiratory muscles: rapid development of fatigue.
- Susceptibility to infection.

Not all respiratory distress has a respiratory cause:
- Metabolic acidosis causes deep, rapid breathing.
- Heart failure is associated with tachypnea.

The illnesses most commonly presenting as emergencies are:

- Upper airway obstruction: croup, acute epiglottitis.
- Lower airway obstruction: asthma, bronchiolitis.
- Pneumonia.

Upper airway obstruction

The cardinal sign of upper airway obstruction is stridor. This is a noise associated with breathing and due to obstruction of the extrathoracic airway. It tends to be worse on inspiration.

The important common causes of acute stridor are:

- Croup: acute laryngotracheobronchitis.
- Inhaled foreign body.
- Epiglottitis.

Features suggesting severe upper airway obstruction are shown in Fig. 26.22. Epiglottitis has become uncommon since the introduction of Hib vaccination.

Clinical features of severe upper airway obstruction
Exhaustion
Decreased consciousness level
Poor air entry on auscultation
Tachycardia
Cyanosis
Chest wall recession

Fig. 26.22 Clinical features of severe upper airway obstruction.

Croup

This is a clinical diagnosis. Investigations are not usually required. Management depends on the severity of upper airway obstruction. Children requiring hospital admission are given supportive care:

- Gentle, confident handling.
- Monitoring of transcutaneous O_2 saturation, heart rate.
- O_2 therapy.
- Nebulized budesonide or oral dexamethasone: reduces severity.
- Nebulized racemic epinephrine: gives transient relief of severe obstruction.

The differential diagnosis of severe croup includes bacterial tracheitis.

Acute epiglottitis

This now rare diagnosis is clinical. Any disturbance of the child, such as lying down, examining the throat, or venipuncture, must be avoided because total airway obstruction and death can be precipitated. The procedure is:

- Call for help: pediatric team, senior anesthetist, ENT surgeon.
- Arrange examination under anesthesia.
- If the diagnosis is confirmed, secure an airway by endotracheal intubation. Take blood cultures and start IV antibiotics (e.g., cefuroxime).

Most children can be extubated within a day or two and will have recovered fully within a week.

Lower airway obstruction
Acute asthma

An algorithm for the management of acute severe asthma is shown in Fig. 26.23. Features of life-threatening asthma are shown in Fig. 26.24.

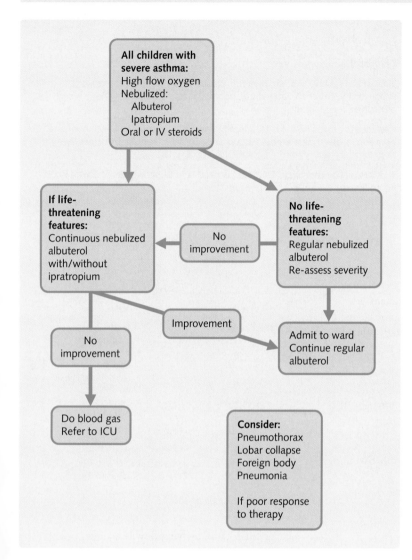

Fig. 26.23 Management of acute severe asthma.

Clinical features of life-threatening asthma
Decreased consciousness level
Exhaustion or agitation
Poor respiratory effort
Silent chest
Oxygen saturation <85% in room air

Fig. 26.24 Clinical features of life-threatening asthma.

β_2-bronchodilators, steroids, and oxygen are the mainstays of treatment of acute asthma:

- Inhaled bronchodilator therapy can be given as a spacer in nonsevere cases. Nebulizers are given in severe and life-threatening attacks.

- Steroids take 1–6 hours to exert their effect so should be given early.
- Intravenous aminophylline has a role in children who do not respond adequately to nebulizers.
- Nebulized therapy can be given continuously, but it is important to monitor for sinus tachycardia and hypokalemia. IV fluids should be two-thirds the normal requirement as there is often inappropriate antidiuretic hormone (ADH) secretion.

Antibiotics are unnecessary unless there are clear signs of infection. Mechanical ventilation is rarely required (see Chapter 14).

Three phases of shock	
Phase	**Clinicopathologic features**
Compensated shock	Vital organ function (brain, heart) is preserved by sympathetic response. Pallor, tachycardia, cold periphery, poor capillary return, but systolic blood pressure is maintained
Decompensated shock	Inadequate perfusion leads to anerobic metabolism, metabolic acidosis, and, on occasion, a bleeding diathesis. Blood pressure falls, acidotic breathing, very slow capillary return, altered consciousness, anuria
Irreversible shock	A retrospective diagnosis. Damage to heart and brain irreversible, with no improvement even if circulation is restored

Fig. 26.25 Three phases of shock.

Bronchiolitis

This is the most common, serious respiratory infection of childhood. It is predominantly a disease of infants aged 1–9 months and occurs as an annual winter epidemic. Respiratory syncytial virus is the pathogen in 75% of cases.

Clinical features. Features of severe disease include:
- Irregular breathing or recurrent apnea.
- Tachypnea: respiratory rate >60/min.
- Hypoxia: O_2 requirement >60%.

Management. Management is supportive and includes:
- Monitoring O_2 saturation by pulse oximetry: apnea alarm.
- Humidified O_2 by hood or nasal cannulas to maintain O_2 saturation above 94%.
- Fluids: nasogastric feeds or IV fluids.

Antibiotics, bronchodilators, and steroids have not been shown to be of value; the mainstay of treatment is supportive.

Shock (circulatory failure)

Shock is a clinical syndrome resulting from acute failure of circulatory function, leading to tissue hypoperfusion, and is commonly present in the critically ill child. It tends to progress through three phases (Fig. 26.25):
- Compensated.
- Uncompensated.
- Irreversible.

Causes of shock are shown in Fig. 26.26. The two most common mechanisms are hypovolemia or septicemia.

Causes of shock	
Mechanism	**Causes**
Hypovolemia	Fluid loss • Hemorrhage • Burns • Diarrhea and vomiting • Diabetic ketoacidosis Fluid shifts • Septicemia • Anaphylaxis • Peritonitis
Cardiogenic	Arrhythmias Heart failure

Fig. 26.26 Causes of shock.

Clinical features

A brief history may identify the cause. The early physical signs of shock include:
- Pallor: due to vasoconstriction.
- Tachycardia with reduced pulse volume.
- Poor skin perfusion: capillary refill time >3 seconds, core/toe temperature difference >2°C.
- Hypotension.

The late physical signs of shock include:
- Rapid, deep breathing: response to metabolic acidosis.
- Agitation, confusion: due to brain hypoperfusion.
- Oliguria: urine flow less than 2 mL/kg/hr in children.

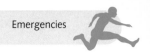

Management of shock: general

An algorithm for the general management of circulatory failure is shown in Fig. 26.27. If there is not rapid improvement or if there is evidence of organ failure, transfer to an intensive care unit will be required for assisted ventilation, intensive monitoring, and inotropic support.

> Poor capillary refill should not be used in isolation to diagnose shock. The clinician must look at heart rate, blood pressure, base excess, and clinical signs of organ perfusion (e.g., consciousness level and urine output).

Specific shock syndromes

The three important specific syndromes in which shock occurs are:

- Anaphylactic shock.
- Septicemic shock.
- Diabetic ketoacidosis.

Anaphylactic shock

See Chapter 11 for the features of anaphylaxis. The major problems are airway obstruction, bronchospasm and shock.

A protocol for management is shown in Fig. 26.28.

Septicemic shock

Septicemia is an important cause of shock in children. The main pathogens include:

- *Neisseria meningitidis.*
- *Haemophilus influenzae* (rare if Hib immunized).
- Staphylococci, pneumococci, streptococci.
- Gram-negative bacteria.

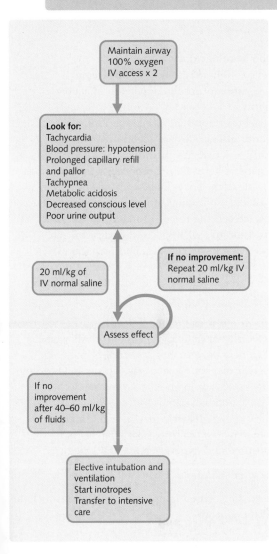

Fig. 26.27 Management of shock (ABCs).

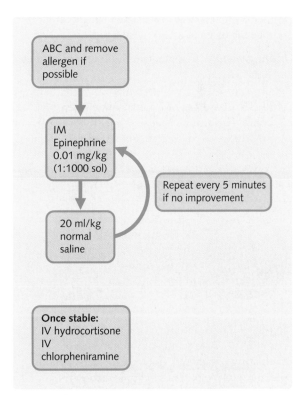

Fig. 26.28 Management of anaphylactic shock.

245

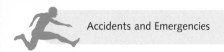

Meningococcal septicemia is the most fulminant variety. Death can occur within 12 hours of the first symptom; early diagnosis is vital.

Bacterial toxins trigger the release of various mediators and activators, which can:
- Cause vasodilatation or vasoconstriction.
- Depress cardiac function.
- Disturb cellular oxygen consumption.
- Cause "capillary leak" with hypovolemia.
- Promote disseminated intravascular coagulation.

Clinical features. The clinical features progress from early (compensated) to late (decompensated) shock:
- Early shock: increased cardiac output, decreased systemic resistance, warm extremities, high fever and mental confusion.
- Late shock: reduced cardiac output, hypotension, cool peripheries and metabolic acidosis.

The cardinal sign of meningococcal septicemia is a petechial or purpuric rash. This may be subtle in the early stages and a careful search for petechiae is required (in 10% of cases a blanching erythematous rash may occur first). An injection of ceftriaxone or penicillin G should be given immediately if a diagnosis of meningococcal septicemia or meningitis is suspected.

Management. Key points in initial management include:
- Oxygen: 100% O_2 by face mask.
- Fluids: 20 mL/kg of normal saline given as a bolus. This can be repeated but if more than 40 mL/kg is required then assisted ventilation is indicated.
- Antibiotics: IV ceftriaxone.
- Investigations (Fig. 26.29).

Outcome in septic shock is improved with aggressive fluid resuscitation and early referral to intensive care.

In severe illness, intensive care facilities are required to allow continuous monitoring of circulatory parameters (including central venous pressure), urine output, and pulse oximetry. Assisted ventilation, inotropic agents, and renal replacement therapy may be required.

Investigations in septic shock
To define the severity of disease
CBC
Electrolytes and liver function
Glucose
Blood gas
Lactate
Coagulation screen
To look for the focus of infection
Blood culture
Urine culture
Throat swabs
Rapid antigen testing and PCR
Chest x-ray
Abdominal ultrasound (if indicated)

Fig. 26.29 Investigations in septic shock.

Diabetic ketoacidosis

This is an important and life-threatening complication of insulin-dependent diabetes mellitus. It is relatively uncommon for new cases of diabetes to present in a ketoacidotic state. The majority of episodes are seen in patients known to have type 1 diabetes mellitus.

Diabetic ketoacidosis represents the end stage of insulin deficiency. Deficiency of insulin blocks use of glucose leading to hyperglycemia. As glucose levels exceed the renal threshold, an osmotic diuresis ensues with severe dehydration and electrolytes losses (sodium and potassium). Without insulin, fat is used as a source of energy leading to the generation of ketones and metabolic acidosis.

Clinical features. The clinical features evolve as the severity of dehydration and acidosis worsens.
- The new diabetic has a history of polyuria, polydipsia, and weight loss. This is followed by the rapid development of vomiting, lethargy, and abdominal pain.
- The known diabetic may have an intercurrent illness with vomiting, poor control, and documented hyperglycemia and ketonuria.

Characteristic physical signs are listed in Fig. 26.30.

Diagnosis. Essential initial investigations include:
- Blood glucose.
- Urea and electrolytes.
- Arterial blood gas analysis.
- Urine glucose and ketones.

Physical signs in diabetic ketoacidosis	
Dehydration	Dry mucous membranes Loss of skin turgor Tachycardia, hypotension if severe
Acidosis	Ketones on breath Kussmaul breathing; rapid, deep, sighing respiration
Cerebral edema	Headache Slowing of pulse rate and hypertension Decreased consciousness level Seizures and focal neurologic signs

Fig. 26.30 Physical signs in diabetic ketoacidosis.

Management of diabetic ketoacidosis	
Fluids	Treat shock Maintenance fluids: rehydrate over 48 h 0.9% saline with potassium initially Change to 0.45% saline once glucose has fallen to <15 mmol/L
Insulin	Start IV at 0.05 units/kg/hr Adjust depending on glucose; avoid drops >5 mmol/L/h
Additional	Monitor electrolytes regularly Monitor consciousness level

Fig. 26.31 Management of diabetic ketoacidosis.

The typical metabolic abnormalities in diabetic ketoacidosis, which will be revealed by these investigations, include:

- Hyperglycemia: blood glucose over 15 mmol/L and glycosuria.
- Ketoacidosis: ketonuria, metabolic acidosis on arterial blood gas analysis (ABG) (pH is low, [HCO_3] is reduced, $PaCO_2$ is low, there is respiratory compensation with hypocapnia).
- Dehydration: raised urea.
- Sodium and potassium depletion: serum sodium concentration is often slightly reduced; serum potassium concentration may be low, normal, or high, depending on renal function and the degree of acidosis.

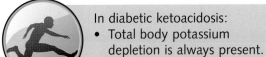

In diabetic ketoacidosis:
- Total body potassium depletion is always present.
- Cerebral edema is rare but associated with a high mortality. Its prevention is by slow metabolic correction and rehydration.
- Serum potassium concentration falls with treatment as potassium is driven into cells (with insulin action and correction of acidosis) and renal function improves.
- IV fluids need to include potassium to avoid hypokalemia as treatment proceeds.

Management. The mainstays of management are the slow and careful restoration of fluid and electrolyte status, and insulin (Fig. 26.31).

The acidosis will usually correct with correction of fluid balance and insulin therapy. Administration of bicarbonate is rarely used. A nasogastric tube should be passed if there is vomiting or evidence of gastric dilatation.

Careful monitoring is required of:
- Fluid status: weight, input and output.
- Electrolytes: check urea and electrolytes every 2–4-hours initially.
- Acid–base status: check ABG every 2–4-hours initially.
- Blood glucose: monitor hourly.
- ECG monitoring allows early identification of dysrhythmias secondary to electrolyte imbalances.
- Vital signs and neurologic observations.

Complications. Major complications include:
- Cerebral edema: manifested by reduced consciousness level, headache, irritability and fits. Attempt to prevent this by avoiding *rapid* falls in blood glucose or serum sodium concentrations.
- Cardiac dysrhythmias: usually secondary to electrolyte (potassium) disturbances. Acute renal failure is uncommon.

After the initial 24–48 hours, it is usually possible to switch to oral fluids and every 4-hours subcutaneous soluble insulin on a sliding scale determined by the blood glucose concentration.

247

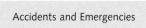

- How are the causes of death distributed in childhood?
- Describe the fluid management in burns.
- What types of burns need specialist advice?
- What are the most important assessments of any sick child?
- What are the differences between primary and secondary survey in trauma?
- How are children different from adults in critical illness?
- How is the respiratory system assessed in an ill child?
- Describe the features of severe airway obstruction.
- What is the first-line drug used for stopping convulsions?
- What are the indications for intensive care in a shocked child?
- What is the complication associated with the highest mortality in diabetic ketoacidosis?

Infants and children are more vulnerable than adults to inadequate nutrition or the derangement of fluid and electrolyte balance. Their high surface area to volume ratio is associated with a high metabolic rate, large caloric requirements, and corresponding rapid fluid turnover.

Globally, malnutrition is probably directly or indirectly responsible for half of all deaths of children under 5 years of age. In the developed world, nutrition is a vital consideration in the management of many diseases (such as cystic fibrosis) and special diets are indicated for some disorders (such as celiac disease, phenylketonuria, and food allergy).

> Breastfeeding in early infancy saves lives in developing countries. Its benefits are seen in babies who are exclusively breastfed; the addition of formula in early feeding can negate many of its benefits.

Dehydration associated with diarrheal diseases is a major killer worldwide and its treatment with oral rehydration solution represented a major advance. However, attention to fluid and electrolyte status is an important aspect of a wide spectrum of disorders, including diabetes mellitus, pyloric stenosis, and postoperative care.

Prescribing for infants and children involves many considerations unique to this age group. The route and frequency of administration must be adapted to the age, and dosage must take into account bodyweight, surface area, and age-dependent changes in drug metabolism and excretion.

Nutrition

Normal nutritional requirements

A satisfactory dietary intake should meet the normal requirements for energy and protein, together with providing an adequate supply of vitamins and trace elements. Reference values for energy and protein requirements are shown in Fig. 27.1.

Infants and children are vulnerable to undernutrition because of:

- Low nutritional stores of fat and protein.
- Growth creating high nutritional demands (at 4 months of age, 30% of an infant's energy intake is used for growth; by 3 years of age this has fallen to 2%).

Brain growth: the brain is proportionally larger in infants and is growing rapidly during the last trimester and first 2 years of life. It is vulnerable to energy deprivation during this period.

Infant feeding

An infant's primary source of nutrition is milk, either human breast milk or so-called "formula" milk based on modified cow's milk. Weaning, the introduction of solid foods, is usually initiated between the ages of 3 and 6 months.

Breastfeeding

This is the preferred method for most infants. Galactosemia is the only contraindication, but it is advised that HIV-positive mothers should not breastfeed in the Western world. The many advantages, and few disadvantages, of breastfeeding are listed in Fig. 27.2.

Reference values for energy and protein requirements

Age	Energy (kcal/kg/day)	Protein (g/kg/day)
0–6 months	115	2.2
6–12 months	95	2.0
1–3 years	95	1.8
4–6 years	90	1.5
7–10 years	75	1.2
11–14 years	60	1.0
16–18 years	50	0.8

Fig. 27.1 Reference values for energy and protein requirements.

Establishing breastfeeding:
- The baby should be put to the breast as soon as possible after birth.
- Thereafter the baby should be fed on demand (indicated by crying).
- Frequent suckling promotes lactation.
- The baby's mouth needs to be well applied around the areola, with the nipple drawn into the back of the baby's mouth.
- Colostrum (high content of protein and immunoglobulin) rather than milk is produced in first few days.
- The interval between feeds gradually lengthens from every 2–3 hours to approximately every 4 hours.

Bottlefeeding

The composition of breast milk, cow's milk, and infant formula differs significantly (Fig. 27.3). Unmodified, whole, pasteurized cow's milk is unsuitable as a main diet for infants under the age of 1 year because it:
- Contains too much protein and sodium.
- Is deficient in iron and vitamins.

Modified cow's milk formulas have a modified casein to whey ratio and reduced mineral content and are fortified with iron and vitamins.

Advantages and disadvantages of breastfeeding

Advantages
Quality:
- Breast milk has anti-infective properties, including secretory IgA, lysozyme, phagocytic cells, lactoferrin (iron-binding agent), a factor that promotes growth of nonpathogenic flora
- Breast milk has better nutritional qualities, including easily digested protein, low renal solute load, and a favorable calcium to phosphate ratio

Emotional—if successful, promotes mother–infant bonding
Reduction in risk of maternal breast cancer

Disadvantages
Volume of intake uncertain
Transmission of drugs (e.g., laxatives, anticoagulants, antineoplastics)
Nutrient deficiencies:
- Insufficient vitamin K to prevent hemorrhagic disease of the newborn
- Vitamin D deficiency (rickets) may occur if there is prolonged breastfeeding and delayed weaning

Emotional—failure to establish breastfeeding may be a cause of emotional upset

Fig. 27.2 Advantages and disadvantages of breastfeeding.

Breastfeeding mothers may be concerned about whether their baby has had an adequate milk intake. This is best measured by the baby's weight gain. Poor weight gain or weight loss may mean inadequate lactation.

Important features of bottlefeeding:
- Less restrictive for mothers as others can do the feeding.
- Available as a dry powder requiring reconstitution or as ready made liquid feeds.
- Changing "brands" in response to feeding difficulties is usually a futile gesture, but changing formula may be helpful (e.g., from cow milk based to soy based).

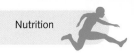

Composition of different milks (per 100 mL)			
	Breast milk	Cow's milk	Infant formula
Protein (g)	1.3	3.3	1.5
Casein : whey	40 : 60	60 : 40	Variable
Carbohydrate (g)	7.0	4.5	7.0–8.0
Fat (g)	4.2	3.6	2.6–3.8
Energy (kcal)	70	65	65
Sodium (mmol)	0.65	2.3	0.65–1.1
Calcium (mmol)	0.87	3.0	1.4
Iron (mmol)	1.36	0.9	10
Vitamin D (μg)	0.6	0.03	1.0

Fig. 27.3 Composition of different milks (per 100 mL).

Specialized milks

A variety of specialized milks exist that are used in infants who are intolerant of specific constituents. Examples include:

- Low phenylalanine milk: phenylketonuria.
- Low lactose milk: lactose intolerance.
- Soy milk: cow's milk protein intolerance. Soy-based milks have been used to prevent atopic conditions in infants and in the treatment of colic, although evidence of this effect is lacking. Infants with cow's milk intolerance often develop intolerance to soy milk.

Weaning

The introduction of solid foods (weaning) is usually undertaken after 4 months of age. At this age the infant can coordinate swallowing and has reasonable head control. After 6 months of age, breast milk alone becomes nutritionally inadequate and continued breastfeeding without introduction of solids will lead to energy, vitamin, and iron deficiency. Evidence is conflicting on late feeding and prevention of atopy.

A typical scheme for the introduction of solids is shown in Fig. 27.4.

Malnutrition

Worldwide, malnutrition due to inadequate intake (starvation) is responsible for millions of childhood deaths. However, malnutrition can also complicate many childhood diseases (Fig. 27.5) and specific nutritional deficiencies such as iron deficiency are not uncommon in the developed world.

Introduction of solids	
Age	Feeding
3–4 months	Cereals (e.g., baby rice)
4–5 months	Pureed fruit and vegetables, meat (e.g., chicken)
6–7 months	Able to chew (e.g., rusks) Introduce lumpy foods and variety of tastes and textures
8–9 months	Bread and butter, fruit
12 months	"Real" food in small bits

Fig. 27.4 Introduction of solids.

Severe malnutrition affects many body systems (Fig. 27.6).

Assessment of nutritional status

Evaluation involves:

- Dietary history.
- Anthropometry and clinical examination.
- Laboratory investigations.

Dietary history

The food intake, as recalled by the parents or recorded in a diary, is determined over a period of several days.

Anthropometry

This involves measurement of:

Malnutrition in childhood—causes

Inadequate intake
Starvation due to famine
Poverty
Restrictive diets—parental, iatrogenic, self-inflicted
Anorexia nervosa
Anorexia due to chronic illness

Malabsorption
Pancreatic disease (e.g., cystic fibrosis)
Celiac disease
Short gut (postoperative)

Increased energy requirements
Cystic fibrosis
Malignant disease
Burns
Trauma

Fig. 27.5 Malnutrition in childhood—causes.

Consequences of severe malnutrition

Impaired immunity
Delayed wound healing
Apathy and inactivity
Impaired intellectual development

Fig. 27.6 Consequences of severe malnutrition.

- Height: height for age is reduced (stunted growth) in chronic malnutrition.
- Weight: reduced weight with normal height (wasting) is an index of acute malnutrition.
- Midarm circumference: an indication of skeletal muscle mass.
- Skinfold thickness: triceps skinfold thickness is a measure of subcutaneous fat stores.

Clinical syndromes of protein-energy malnutrition include:
- Marasmus: wasted (weight less than 60% of mean for age) wizened appearance, withdrawn, and apathetic.
- Kwashiorkor: occurs in children weaned late from the breast and fed on a relatively high-starch diet. It can be precipitated by an acute intercurrent infection. Features include wasting, edema, sparse hair and depigmented skin, angular stomatitis, and hepatomegaly.

Laboratory investigations
Useful laboratory tests include:
- Serum albumin: reduced in severe malnutrition.
- CBC: low hemoglobin and lymphocyte count.
- Blood glucose.
- Calcium, phosphate, and vitamin D levels.
- Serum potassium and magnesium levels.

Management
Nutrition can be supplied:
- Enterally, via the gastrointestinal tract: this route is preferred wherever possible.
- Parenterally, directly into the circulation.

In many cases, malnutrition is due to inadequate intake and can be managed by the provision of supplementary enteral feeds given via a nasogastric or gastrostomy tube.

Examples of chronic diseases requiring such supplemental feeding include:
- Cystic fibrosis.
- Congenital heart disease.
- Cerebral palsy.
- Chronic renal failure.
- Malignancy.
- Inflammatory bowel disease.
- Anorexia nervosa.

Vitamin deficiencies
Several important vitamin deficiency diseases still occur in childhood. These include in particular:
- Vitamin D deficiency: rickets.
- Vitamin A deficiency: blindness.
- Vitamin K deficiency: hemorrhagic disease of the newborn.

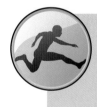

The most common dietary deficiencies in the USA are of iron and vitamin D. Scurvy due to vitamin C deficiency is now extremely rare in developed countries.

Vitamin D deficiency: rickets
The effects of vitamin D deficiency on growing bone cause rickets. The bone matrix (osteoid) of the growing bone is inadequately mineralized, giving rise to the clinical features described in

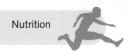

Clinical features of rickets
General Misery Hypotonia Developmental delay Growth failure
Skeletal Craniotabes (thin, soft skull bones) Enlarged metaphyses (especially wrists and knees) Rickety rosary (enlarged costochondral junction) Bowing of legs (caused by weight-bearing)

Fig. 27.7 Clinical features of rickets.

Fig. 27.7. The undermineralized bone is less rigid and bends and twists in an abnormal way.

The normal pathways of vitamin D absorption and metabolism are shown in Fig. 27.8.

The most common cause is nutritional deficiency. The minimum daily requirement of vitamin D is 400 international units (IU) and this may not be attained in infants who are breastfed for a protracted period. An additional important factor is decreased exposure to the sun, as vitamin D is synthesized from precursors in the skin under the effect of ultraviolet light. This can occur especially in:

- Infants with dark skin pigmentation.
- Urban living conditions.
- Winter.

Less common causes of rickets include:

- Inherited abnormalities of vitamin D metabolism or of the vitamin D receptor.
- Mineral deficiency (e.g., X-linked hypophosphatemia).
- Chronic renal disease.
- Decreased activity of 1α-hydroxylase in the kidneys leads to rickets as one component of renal osteodystrophy

Rickets of prematurity is a metabolic bone disease in the premature infant that occurs if the milk used contains inadequate calcium and phosphate (1α-dihydroxycholecalciferol levels are elevated because of the hypophosphatemic stimulus, but there is osteopenia and inadequate mineralization of growing bone).

Diagnosis

This is confirmed by x-ray imaging and blood biochemistry. X-ray of the wrist shows cupping and fraying of the metaphysis and a widened metaphyseal plate (Fig. 27.9).

The biochemical changes in classic nutritional rickets include:

- Serum calcium: low or normal (may be normalized by secondary hyperparathyroidism).
- Serum phosphate: low.
- Serum alkaline phosphatase: elevated.
- Serum parathyroid hormone (PTH): elevated.
- Serum 1,25-dihydroxycholecalciferol: low.

Treatment

Prevention is obviously preferred and is achieved by health education, exposure to sunlight, and supplementation of the diet with minerals and vitamin D when indicated.

Treatment of nutritional rickets is with vitamin D3 (1,25-dihydroxycholecalciferol) 5000–10,000 IU/day initially for several weeks, followed by provision of 400 IU/day in the diet.

Higher doses may be required in the inherited forms. Biochemistry and radiography monitor the effect of therapy.

Vitamin A (retinol) deficiency

Vitamin A is necessary for membrane stability and plays a role in vision, keratinization, cornification, and placental development. The body's need for vitamin A can be met by milk, butter, eggs, liver, and dark green or orange-colored (e.g., carrots) vegetables.

Worldwide, about 150 million children are at risk of vitamin A deficiency, and it has been calculated that up to a third of a million children go blind each year from vitamin A deficiency. In addition, vitamin A deficiency carries increased mortality from infection and poor growth.

The eye disease develops insidiously with impaired dark adaptation followed by drying of the conjunctiva and cornea (xerophthalmia).

Obesity

In 1998 the World Health Organization stated that obesity is a global epidemic. It results from numerous social and environmental factors that are difficult to alter. Obesity in children is increasing in prevalence, and treatment is often disappointing. Prevention of obesity remains the optimal solution.

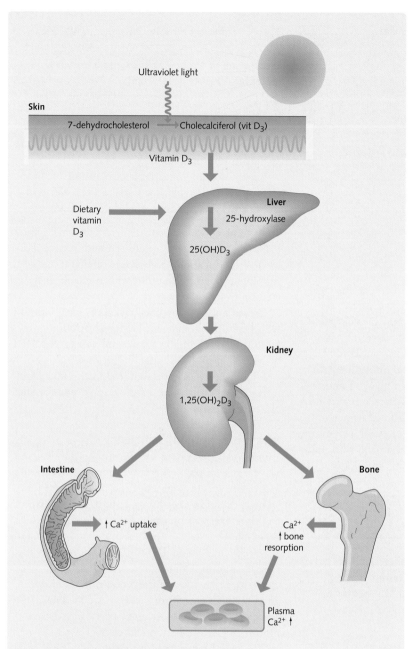

Fig. 27.8 Normal pathways of vitamin D metabolism and action.

- Most obese children are tall and above the 50th percentile for height.
- In Cushing syndrome or hypothyroidism, obesity is associated with low growth velocity and short stature.

The body mass index is a useful measurement of obesity and a BMI > 25 is considered obese. Etiologic factors include:
- Genetic factors.
- Excess carbohydrate intake.
- Reduced activity.

Rarely, an endocrine or chromosomal cause is present such as Cushing syndrome, hypothyroidism, or Prader–Willi syndrome.

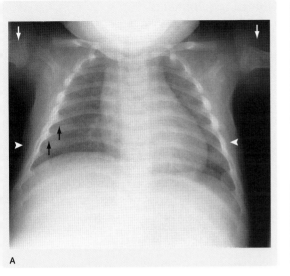

A

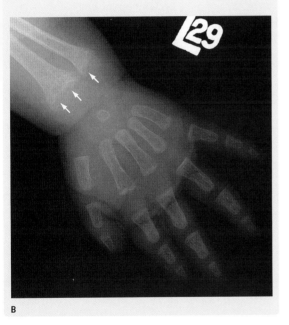

B

Fig. 27.9 X-ray appearance of rickets. (A) CXR of a young child with partially treated rickets. Note (i) changes at the metaphyses (white arrows), (ii) periosteal reaction on several ribs (white arrowheads), and (iii) bulging of anterior rib ends, the rickety rosary (black arrows). (B) Left wrist x-ray. Note the irregular "cupped" metaphyses with loss of bone density (white arrows).

Obesity has several deleterious consequences, including:
- Emotional disturbance: many psychological problems are associated with obesity.

Fluid and electrolyte balance in children
Children have a larger surface area to volume ratio than adults
Total body water is a higher percentage of bodyweight in children
The rate of turnover of fluids and electrolytes is higher in children.

Fig. 27.10 Fluid and electrolyte balance in children.

Clinical conditions associated with fluid and electrolyte disturbance
Gastroenteritis
Major burns
Diabetic ketoacidosis
Renal failure
Sepsis
Trauma

Fig. 27.11 Clinical conditions associated with fluid and electrolyte disturbance.

- Hypoventilation: obesity is the main cause of obstructive sleep apnea in the USA.
- Long-term complications: obese children are twice as likely to become obese adults.

Management
A large number of interventions have been tried and involvement of both parents and school is necessary. A reduced-calorie, balanced diet with increased exercise in combination with behavioral modification and psychological support offers the best way to manage obesity.

Fluids and electrolytes

Important physiologic factors render children more vulnerable than adults to disturbances of fluid and electrolyte balance (Fig. 27.10). Such disturbances are common in pediatric practice and occur in a number of important clinical contexts (Fig. 27.11).

Basic physiology
It is useful to know how fluid is distributed between the different compartments of the body and what the normal requirements for fluid and

electrolytes are. Important changes occur with age as the ratio of surface area to volume alters.

Fluid compartments

These are shown in Fig. 27.12. Infants are more "watery" and have a higher proportion of fluid in the extracellular space than adults. The percentages can be expressed as volumes: 70% is equivalent to 700 mL/kg bodyweight.

Blood volume is about 100 mL/kg at birth and falls to about 80 mL/kg at 1 year.

- As body density is close to that of water, and 1 liter of water weighs close to 1 kilogram, weights and volumes are freely interchangeable. For example, 1000 mL = 1000 g (1 liter = 1 kg).
- Changes in bodyweight are the best guide to short-term changes in fluid balance (e.g., a weight loss of 500 g indicates a fluid deficit of 500 mL).

Normal requirements

Fluid requirement is that needed to make up for normal fluid losses, which include urine output and "insensible" losses through sweat, respiration, and the gastrointestinal tract. In pathologic states there will be additional abnormal losses, such as those associated with diarrhea or vomiting.

A simple formula for calculating normal fluid requirements according to bodyweight is shown in Fig. 27.13.

There are obligatory electrolyte losses in the stools, urine, and sweat, and these require replacement. The electrolyte composition of various body fluids, which can be lost in excessive amounts, is shown in Fig. 27.14. The maintenance requirement for sodium is about 3 mmol/kg/day and for potassium is 2 mmol/kg/day.

Intravenous fluids

These can be divided into colloids, which include large molecules such as proteins, and crystalloids, which usually contain dextrose (glucose) and electrolytes. Although concerns about colloids have been raised, they are still in widespread use for volume expansion in sepsis.

The compositions of commonly available crystalloid fluids for intravenous use are shown in Fig. 27.15.

Important features of intravenous solutions

- They are isotonic or slightly hypertonic: their osmolality is close to that of plasma. A hypotonic (dilute solution) would lyse red cells and a very hypertonic solution would draw fluid

Body fluid compartments (as a percentage of bodyweight)			
Age	Total body water	Extracellular fluid	Intracellular fluid
Newborn	70	35	35
12 months	65	25	40
Adult	60	20	40

Fig. 27.12 Body fluid compartments (as a percentage of bodyweight).

Normal fluid requirements	
Bodyweight	Fluid requirement per 24 hours
First 10 kg	100 mL/kg
Second 10 kg	50 mL/kg
Further kg	20 mL/kg

Example: 24-hour requirement for child weighing 25 kg:
10 kg at 100 mL/kg = 1000 mL
10 kg at 50 mL/kg = 500 mL
5 kg at 20 mL/kg = 100 mL

Total = 1600 mL

Fig. 27.13 Normal fluid requirements.

Electrolyte content of body fluids			
Fluid	Na$^+$ (mmol/L)	K$^+$ (mmol/L)	Cl$^-$ (mmol/L)
Plasma	135–141	3.5–5.5	100–105
Gastric	20–80	5–20	100–150
Intestinal	100–140	5–15	90–130
Diarrhea	10–90	10–30	10–110

Fig. 27.14 Electrolyte content of body fluids.

Isotonic crystalloid fluids: composition				
Fluid	Sodium (mmol/L)	Potassium (mmol/L)	Chloride (mmol/L)	Energy (kcal/L)
0.9% saline	150	0	150	0
5% dextrose/0.45% saline	75	0	75	200

Fig. 27.15 Isotonic crystalloid fluids: composition.

into the circulation. Hypertonic saline has been used in raised intracranial pressure.

- Normal saline is useful for replacing deficits and for rapid volume expansion. However, it is not a maintenance fluid, as it contains too much sodium chloride.
- 5% dextrose and 0.45% sodium with potassium is the usual maintenance fluid. In neonates 10% dextrose solutions are used.
- Colloids are less frequently used except in septic shock. The best colloid in trauma is blood.

Specific fluid and electrolyte problems

These are mostly considered elsewhere:
- Dehydration (see Chapter 15).
- Diabetic ketoacidosis (see Chapter 26).
- Burns (see Chapter 26).

Important features concerning certain electrolyte disturbances are considered here.

Sodium

Serum sodium levels reflect extracellular water shifts:
- Hyponatremia is seen in the syndrome of inappropriate secretion of ADH (where excess extracellular water is present) and in gastroenteritis treated with water instead of salt solutions.

- Hypernatremia is less common but is seen in neonates who become dehydrated as a result of poor breastfeeding and in diabetic ketoacidosis.
- It is important to avoid rapid changes in sodium concentration because cerebral edema or myelinosis may result.

Potassium

Hypokalemia is usually a result of gastrointestinal loss (vomiting) or inadequate intake. It is treated by supplementing IV fluids or oral potassium.

Hyperkalemia is potentially dangerous, but children and neonates are less vulnerable to hyperkalemia than adults. The most common cause is renal failure, but it also occurs in:
- Severe acidosis.
- Hypoaldosteronism.
- Iatrogenic potassium overload.

Immediate management involves:
- Calcium gluconate to stabilize myocardium: this does not remove potassium
- Promotion of cellular potassium uptake by nebulized or IV albuterol. An alternative is insulin and dextrose.
- Ion-exchange resins (e.g., oral or rectal activated charcoal).
- Dialysis or hemofiltration if the above measures fail.

Bodyweight and body surface area by age

Age	Weight (kg)	BSA (m²)
Newborn	3.5	0.25
6 months	7.7	0.40
1 year	10	0.50
5 years	18	0.75
12 years	36	1.25
Adult	70	1.80

Fig. 27.16 Bodyweight and body surface area (BSA) by age.

Pediatric pharmacology and prescribing

Great variability exists between children and adults in the pharmacology of drugs; differences also exist between the preterm neonate, neonate, and older children (Fig. 27.16). It is therefore important that clinicians recognize that much of the information that applies to adults is not always applicable to children, and must be cautious in extrapolating adult data into pediatric use.

Water-soluble drugs (e.g., most antibiotics) require a larger initial dose in neonates because they have the greatest amount of total body water. The large volume also means delayed excretion so doses are less frequent

Many drugs currently used in pediatric practice remain unlicensed. Thus, pharmacokinetic and pharmacodynamic data are rarely available.

Absorption and administration

The oral route is most commonly used for administering medication because it is easy, safe, and cheap. Its limitations are that many children find certain drugs unpalatable and tablets need to be crushed. High doses are also not always possible and certain drugs (e.g., insulin) cannot be absorbed from this route.

The IV route is reliable and effective but requires venepuncture. The rectal route is useful in emergencies, and diazepam and divalproex (Depakote) can be given this way. Intramuscular injections are rarely used except for immunizations.

In neonates and infants, gastric absorption is altered as normal gastric acid secretion is reduced until 3 years of age; gastric motility is also delayed.

Distribution

The concentration of drug at the target organ depends on the solubility and protein binding of the drug and the characteristics of the tissues itself. At birth, there is a greater proportion of water in the extracellular fluid compartments and total body water is greater (85% compared with the adult 60%).

Protein binding of drugs differs as albumin concentrations reach adult levels at 1 year of age and binding capacity is different in children.

Metabolism and excretion

Hepatic metabolism differs from that in adults in that it is slow at birth but increases rapidly with age; the metabolic processes also differ. For example, acetaminophen is metabolized by sulfation, whereas adults use the glucuronidation pathway. Thus acetaminophen toxicity in children is less than in adults.

The renal handling of drugs also differs because the glomerular filtration rate in children does not approach adult levels until 9–12 months age.

- What are the benefits of breastfeeding?
- How is nutrition assessed in infants?
- What are the fluid requirements of a 3-year-old child weighing 15 kg?
- What intravenous fluids are available?
- How is the handling of drugs different in children compared to adults?
- What routes of administration are available for drug delivery?

HISTORY, EXAMINATION, AND COMMON INVESTIGATIONS

28. History and Examination

The art of taking a history from, and examining, a child shares some principles with the corresponding process in adult medicine. The young infant and neonate present special challenges, whereas the older child can often be interviewed in a similar manner to an adult. Most clinicians are concerned that children may not cooperate and communicate during the clinical assessment.

In many cases, the history will come predominantly from the parents but it is important not to overlook a communicating child, as he or she may offer a more accurate story than the parents! This is especially important in cases of child protection.

A problem-based approach

It is important to include a summary of clinical problems at the end of your evaluation in the notes. This shows that you are able to form a practical plan from your assessment and you have thought about the management of the patient. This is important, even when you are still a student—you may not always be right, but it is never too early to train yourself to think like a doctor. Failure to include a problem list and management plan is a common criticism of new house officers!

Pediatric history taking

The overall format is similar to that in adult medicine, but it is important to establish a rapport with parent(s) and child at an early stage. Ignoring the child when taking a history wastes a valuable opportunity to alleviate the anxiety that the child will have in this unfamiliar situation.

Ask the parents to help if the child is upset or shy.

The beginning
- Introduce yourself to the parents and the child. It is important to find out the name and sex of the child at this point.
- Make sure you know who is accompanying the child. Many parents are not married, or the child may have been taken to hospital by a relative.

Presenting complaint
Open-ended questions to start will put the parents at ease, and at this point they may volunteer both the presenting symptoms and the symptoms that caused them most anxiety. Often the symptoms that they are worried about are not the symptoms that most concern the doctor!

Once the main symptoms are established, details such as the nature of onset, duration and precipitating factors should be obtained by specific questioning. Associated symptoms and previous illnesses should be asked for at this stage.

Past history
Most children are healthy and have only minor illnesses in the past history but an increasing number with significant illnesses such as extreme prematurity, leukemia, and cardiac disease are surviving to older ages. Ask about:
- Immunizations.
- Hospital admissions.

Birth
A birth history includes:
- Gestational age at delivery.
- Mode of delivery (vaginal or c-section).
- Birth weight.
- Problems encountered at birth or during pregnancy.
- Mode of feeding (breast or bottle fed).

Developmental history
- Age at reaching milestones.
- Concerns about vision and hearing.

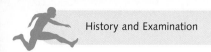

Family and social history

- Ask about any illnesses that run in the family and about recent infectious contacts.
- Make a family tree and ask about parental consanguinity (this increases the incidence of autosomal recessive conditions, which often present with neurologic or metabolic problems).
- Social circumstances: housing, parental occupations, and any difficulties at home. The family may be under the care of a social worker.
- Travel history: include foreign travel and contacts.

Review of systems

A systems review is not performed routinely because, with experience, the history of the presenting complaint should cover all relevant systems. However, a formal review of systems can be useful if the doctor feels that something may be missing in the history.

The history does not stop at one sitting—repeat questioning may produce information that was not volunteered the first time. There is no shame in reviewing the history and many parents do not give a complete picture at the beginning.

Neonatal history

When taking a neonatal history, more emphasis should be on the details of the birth. Many maternal conditions affect the newborn infant and the details of delivery and resuscitation are essential.

Pregnancy

- Maternal medical history (e.g., diabetes, HIV).
- Medication taken during pregnancy, including illicit drugs.
- Alcohol and smoking.
- Complications of pregnancy (e.g., pre-eclampsia).
- Results of any amniocentesis, chorionic villus biopsy, and ultrasound reports.

Maternal infections

Most mothers in the USA are tested in the antenatal period for HIV, hepatitis B, syphilis, and rubella. Ask if a high vaginal swab was taken for group B streptococci and maternal fever.

Birth

Important facts:

- Duration or rupture of membranes.
- Gestational age at delivery.
- Mode of delivery.
- Resuscitation of the baby (if needed).
- Birth weight.

Inquire about any problems after birth; for instance, feeding difficulties or admissions to the neonatal unit.

Examination

Older children are usually cooperative and an approach similar to that used in adults can be employed; young children and infants may be frightened and rather less cooperative. It is important to let the parents help you. They are the people the child is most comfortable with and it should be no surprise if a child is unwilling to let a total stranger approach if the parents are absent.

In children, most of the examination findings are obtained by observing the child interact with their environment. Watching a child play will give you almost all the information you need about his or her neurology!

Examination of children begins as they enter the room or when they play. Observing their spontaneous movements will provide more information than asking them to perform.

General examination

- Weight and height—plot on a growth chart with head circumference in infants.
- Temperature.
- Color.
- Posture, movements, and interaction with mother and observer.
- Rashes.

Respiratory rate at different ages	
Age	**Upper limits (breaths per minute)**
Newborn	>60
Infant	>40
Young child	>30
Older child	>20

Fig. 28.1 Respiratory rates at different ages.

Normal heart rates in children	
Age	**Beats per minute**
<1 year	120–160
2–5 years	90–140
5–12 years	80–120
>12 years	60–100

Fig. 28.2 Normal heart rates in children.

Respiratory system

Count the respiratory rate. Note the different normal values with age (Fig. 28.1). Note any cyanosis or finger clubbing.

Listen for

- Stridor (inspiratory) or wheeze (expiratory) sounds.
- Cough and its nature: barking cough is suggestive of croup.

Look for

- Nasal flaring and use of accessory muscles.
- Intercostal and subcostal retractions.
- Chest shape abnormalities.

Percuss

Percussion is more useful in the older child because it can be more sensitive than auscultation alone for detecting pulmonary abnormalities.

Auscultate

Auscultation can be done at any time that is suitable because the crying child will make auscultation impossible. Often, upper airway sounds will predominate and mask lung sounds. Listen for:

- Intensity of breath sounds on both sides.
- Presence of bronchial breath sounds.
- Wheeze and crackles.

Cardiovascular system

Similar to adults except that it is done as soon as the child is settled and not crying! (Fig. 28.2) Innocent murmurs are common in children and should be distinguished from pathological murmurs (Fig. 28.3). Palpation of the femoral pulse in

Features of innocent heart murmurs
Change with posture
Localized
Asymptomatic
Normal cardiac examination
Systolic only
No thrill

Fig. 28.3 Features of innocent heart murmurs.

neonates is mandatory to detect coarctation of the aorta. Hepatomagaly is one of the signs of cardiac failure.

Do not forget to measure blood pressure!

Abdomen

Observe for jaundice and abdominal distention. It is common for most infants to have a distended abdomen before they are walking. This alone is not pathologic.

Palpate

- The child must be as relaxed and as comfortable as possible. An unsettled anxious child will unconsciously tense their abdominal muscles.
- Abdominal masses: the liver is usually palpable until puberty.
- Peristalsis: this may represent obstruction or pyloric stenosis.
- Inguinal hernia.
- Umbilical hernias are common and not pathological.
- Watch the child's face for any sign of tenderness.

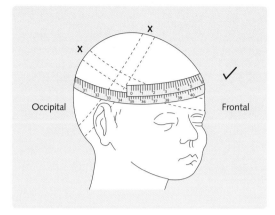

Fig. 28.4 Measuring head circumference.

Nervous system

Most children will give you a lot of information in their play and the examiner must observe how the child interacts with his or her surroundings. The assessment of the cranial nerves, tone, reflexes, strength, coordination, and sensation must be tailored to the individual child.

Observe

- The gait as the child walks in.
- Posture at rest.
- Level of alertness or consciousness.

Important points

- In infants, palpation of the fontanelle, sutures, and measurement of the head circumference is essential (Fig. 28.4).
- Presence of primitive reflexes in neonates and infants is normal.
- Meningism is usually not detectable until >2 years of age
- The plantar reflexes are predominantly extensor (down-going) in infants under 6 months, and the transition to flexor may be asymmetrical.

Ear, nose, and throat

This is often done at the end because it causes the most distress to the child (Fig. 28.5). It is vital that the examiner is helped by a parent who can hold the child still. The neck should be palpated for lymphadenopathy and then the ears should be examined. Looking at the throat should be done at the end because a wooden tongue depressor may be needed to visualize the throat. Wetting the tongue depressor will help ease the exam.

Never examine the throat if upper airway obstruction is suspected (e.g., epiglottitis or severe croup).

The neonatal examination

Neonatal history includes:
- Present complaint and its history.
- Maternal illness and drugs, including smoking and alcohol.
- Pregnancy: details of pregnancy, mode of delivery, and labor; include scans and any abnormal tests.
- Birth weight and the APGAR scores and/or need for resuscitation or admission to a neonatal unit.
- Feeding: breast or bottle.

All neonates should undergo a full examination within 24 hours. This allows any abnormalities to be detected early and also reassures parents of the numerous common normal variants that are found (Fig. 28.6).

Vital signs

Look at the baby's:
- Color.
- Heart rate.
- Respiratory rate.
- Weight and head circumference.

Skin

Observe:
- Many neonates show some jaundice, but this may be pathologic if seen in the first day or if severe.
- Erythema toxicum is a benign condition affecting approximately 50% of all infants. It presents as macular lesions with a central yellow papule.
- Cyanosis can be difficult to detect and should be observed on the tongue and lips. Peripheral cyanosis without central cyanosis is not pathologic (acrocyanosis).
- Pallor may represent anemia or illness; plethora may be due to polycythemia.
- Mongolian blue spots must be documented because they appear identical to bruising.

Fig. 28.5 Throat examination.

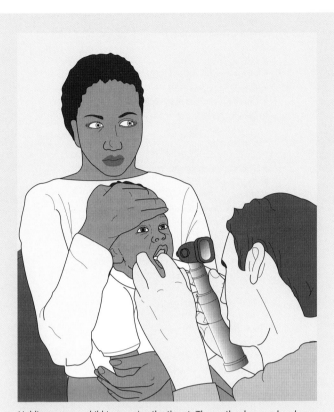

Holding a young child to examine the throat. The mother has one hand on the head and the other across the child's arms

- Mottling is often seen in healthy infants and alone is not suggestive of pathology.
- Vascular lesions such as strawberry hemangiomas and port wine stains.

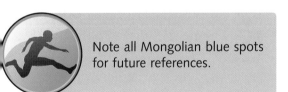

Note all Mongolian blue spots for future references.

Head

Note the shape and size of the head and fontanelle. The sutures should be palpable and head trauma from delivery may manifest as:

- Caput succedaneum: diffuse swelling that crosses the suture lines. It resolves in several days.
- Cephalohematoma: this never crosses the suture lines and is caused by subperiosteal hemorrhage; 5% are associated with fractures.

Neck

Sternocleidomastoid tumors or thyroglossal cysts may be palpable as neck lumps in the midline. The clavicles may be fractured but no treatment is necessary. Palpable lymph nodes are found in 33% of all neonates.

Face

Observe for symmetry when the infant cries or yawns. Facial nerve palsy is common after forceps delivery and is self-limiting:

- Eyes: look for the red reflex (if absent think of retinoblastoma) and evidence of conjunctivitis. A blue sclera is normal in infants <3 months.
- Ears: look at the position and for any skin tags.
- Mouth: loose natal teeth need removal. Palpate *and* look at the palate for cleft palate.

Chest

The following findings often cause concern among parents but have no clinical significance:

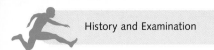

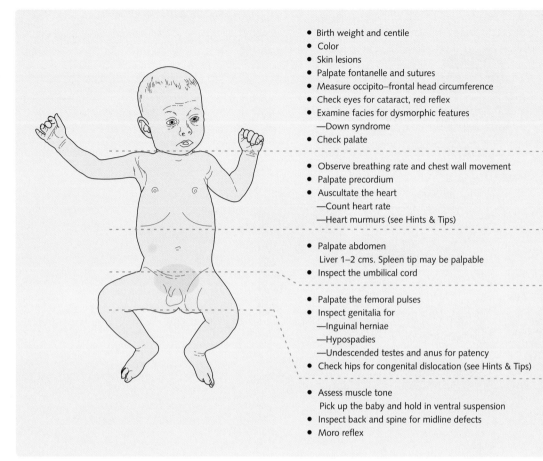

- Birth weight and centile
- Color
- Skin lesions
- Palpate fontanelle and sutures
- Measure occipito–frontal head circumference
- Check eyes for cataract, red reflex
- Examine facies for dysmorphic features
  —Down syndrome
- Check palate

- Observe breathing rate and chest wall movement
- Palpate precordium
- Auscultate the heart
  —Count heart rate
  —Heart murmurs (see Hints & Tips)

- Palpate abdomen
  Liver 1–2 cms. Spleen tip may be palpable
- Inspect the umbilical cord

- Palpate the femoral pulses
- Inspect genitalia for
  —Inguinal herniae
  —Hypospadies
  —Undescended testes and anus for patency
- Check hips for congenital dislocation (see Hints & Tips)

- Assess muscle tone
  Pick up the baby and hold in ventral suspension
- Inspect back and spine for midline defects
- Moro reflex

Fig. 28.6 Routine neonatal examination.

- Pectus excavatum.
- Breasts and milk production: caused by maternal estrogens.

Note that the normal respiratory rate in newborns is 40–60 breaths/minute and heart rate is 120–160 beats/minute. Commonly, periodic breathing can be seen, during which there are pauses lasting less than 10 seconds. This is normal and more common in preterm infants.

Auscultation for breath sounds and heart sounds should be done when the infant is quiet.

- Breath sounds: listen for presence and symmetry.
- Heart sounds: listen for the quality and intensity of the heart sounds.
- Murmurs may be heard but their presence does not always indicate heart disease.

 Murmurs are not always heard in the first 24–48 hours of life and cardiac problems do not usually present at this early stage.

The femoral pulses should be palpated and, if weak or absent, may indicate coarctation of the aorta.

Abdomen

Many infants have a small degree of abdominal distention and this is a normal finding. Observe for:

- Abdominal wall defects.
- Scaphoid abdomen suggests diaphragmatic hernia.

• Examine the umbilicus for three vessels. Single umbilical artery is associated with renal abnormalities. Also look for discharge and inflammation.

Genitalia

The clitoris and labia are normally enlarged, and vaginal bleeding may be observed. This is due to maternal estrogen withdrawal and requires no treatment.

In boys, the testes should be palpable, and phimosis is normal. The foreskin should never be retracted. A good urinary stream should be observed.

Anus

Check for patency of anus; meconium should be passed within 48 hours.

Urine should be passed within 24 hours and meconium within 48 hours.

Extremities

Examine all digits and for palmar creases. Supernumary digits (polydactyly) and abnormal fusion of the digits (syndactyly) are often familial.

Trunk and spine

Palpate the vertebrae, looking for scoliosis. Any abnormal pigmentation, dimples, or hairs over the lumbar region should raise the suspicion of spina bifida. A sacral dimple is common and usually normal if the base is seen.

The Barlow and Ortolani test should be performed to check for congenital hip dislocation. Observe for leg length discrepancy and range of abduction; only gentle force is needed.

Nervous system

The spontaneous movements of the infant should be observed and then examination of:

• Tone: look for both hypo- and hypertonia.
• Reflexes: both primitive and deep tendon reflexes.
• Cranial nerves.

A fine tremor and ankle clonus for 5–10 beats is normal.

Medical sample clerking

A sample of the medical history and exam is shown in Fig. 28.7. It illustrates some of the points discussed earlier in this chapter.

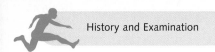

Hospital No. X349282
Baby, A 15/11/03
01/01/04 20:30 6wk old male

CC   Vomiting

> 1. Chief complaint should be brief, but it is helpful to mention relevant background information

HPI   Gradual onset over previous five days of intermittent vomiting.
          Usually occurs in period after feed.
          Vomit is milk only – no bile or blood staining
          Forceful vomiting – milk clears mother's lap
          Infant appears hungry and eager to feed. Breast fed
          Stool frequency reduced. No diarrhea

> 2. Past medical history should include details of birth and any neonatal problems

PMH   Born at St Elsewhere's Hospital
          Full term delivery (FTND)
          Birth weight 3650g
          Mild jaundice 3–5 days
          No significant perinatal problems

DH   Smiles in response
          Fixing and following
          Responds to sounds

Fam Hx   Siblings   1 brother aged 4 years—mild asthma
          1 sister aged 2 years—VSD. Under review
          Mother   Age 31 years. Well
          Operated on for 'bowel obstruction' at age 4 weeks
          Father   Age 33 years. Asthmatic

Social Hx Father electrician.
          Mother a nurse (not working)
          Living in own apartment

> 3. Always record the dose and frequency of any drugs – remember you'll be writing the drug chart later! Always document that you have asked about drug allergies

Drug Hx   Not on medication
          No known allergies

ROS   CVS —   No cyanotic episodes
          RS — Episodes of shallow breathing
          GIT —   Breast fed. No 'spitting up'. Stool frequency
                   previously X 5 per 24 hours
          GU —   Good urinary stream

          Medication — None

Fig. 28.7 Sample clerking.

PE   General: *Well infant*

Mild jaundice Dehydration 5%

Oral thrush

ENT: NAD

> 4. Record your initial observations – they are important. 'Alert and chatty' or 'Distressed and looks unwell' tell you a lot about the patient

        CVS   *Heart Rate 110/min. Peripheral pulses present.*

BP – 95/70 mmHg

Cardiac impulse–normal

Heart sounds 1 & 11. No murmurs

        Resp   *Respiratory rate 35/min*

No retraction

Breath sounds vesicular. No added sounds

> 5. You can use diagrams to clarify your examination findings

        Abdomen   *Not distended. No visible veins*

Visible peristalsis – intermittent

Soft. No masses

No hepatomegaly. No splenomegaly

Hernial ori ces – NAD

rectal – not done

        CNS   *Alert. Vigorous*

Anterior fontanelle – soft, slightly depressed

Tone; normal and symmetrical

Movements: symmetrical

Reflexes: not examined

Plan   *Diagnosis: Pyloric stenosis (PS)*

Plan   'test feed'

InvestigationsUrea and electrolytes

*   including serum HCO3*

*   Abdominal US (if 'test*

*   feed' equivocal)*

> 6. Always include a management plan – even when you are still a student. It might not be right but you need to start training yourself to think like a doctor

Inform pediatrics surgical team

Nursing plan: Nasogastric tube

*   Fluid balance chart*

*   Daily weight*

Site IV line. Intravenous rehydration

If PS diagnosis confrimrd, NPO ny mouth and schedule for

pylorotomy in 24–28 hours when rehydrated and metabolic alkalosis corrected

Pang 592

> 7. Sign your notes, including printed surname and beeper number

Fig. 28.7 Cont'd.

29. Developmental Assessment

Growing up involves the acquisition of new abilities and skills, as well as physical growth. The process by which an immobile, incontinent, and speechless baby develops into a mobile, communicating, socially interactive, and (hopefully!) well-behaved child involves a complex interaction between genes (nature) and environment (nurture).

Much study over many years has established the average rate and pattern of development and identified a very wide range of normal variation. A child may be far from average but still normal. A major challenge is to distinguish such normal variation from a significant problem requiring active intervention.

Developmental screening is offered routinely to all children in the USA. It is one component of child health surveillance, which also encompasses physical health and growth.

The aim is to identify developmental problems at an early stage to allow appropriate intervention. Any delay may be global or specific (see Chapter 8), but it is important to bear in mind the close interrelationships involved, e.g., hearing impairment can cause a delay in speech and language, with consequent disruption of social interaction and behavior.

Clinical assessment of a child's developmental status is based on a thorough history, physical examination, and observation of the child's performance and play.

History

Certain aspects of the history clearly assume special importance in assessing development. In particular, it is important to enquire about and document "risk factors" that contribute to vulnerability and poor outcome (Fig. 29.1). The history should therefore include inquiry into:
- Pregnancy and birth.
- Developmental milestones.
- Family and social history.
- Specific parental concerns.
- Child health record.

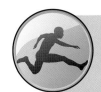

Milestones reflect the average age that a child acquires a particular ability:
- Motor problems often manifest in the first year.
- Talking and coordination problems often manifest in the second year.
- Behavioral and social problems often manifest in the third year.

Examination

Four aspects of development are routinely assessed:
- Gross motor.
- Fine motor and vision.
- Hearing and speech.
- Social behavior.

Routine surveillance is carried out during well-recognized stages of development:
- Newborn.
- Supine infant (6–8 weeks).
- Sitting infant (8–9 months).
- Mobile toddler (18–24 months).
- Communicating child (3–4 years).
- School-age child (5 years).

The milestones for each area in each of the above age groups are considered below.

Newborn
Gross motor
- Symmetrical movements in all four limbs.
- Normal muscle tone.

Fine motor and vision
- Fixes on mother's face and follows through 90° (to midline).

Hearing and speech
- Cries.
- Responds to bell.

271

Risk factors for developmental delay
Prematurity
Birth asphyxia
Dysmorphology
Psychosocial deprivation

Fig. 29.1 Risk factors for developmental delay.

Social
- Responds to being picked up.

Six weeks to 3 months
Gross motor
- Good head control at 3 months when pulled up to sitting (Fig. 29.2).
- When held in ventral suspension holds head transiently in horizontal plane (Fig. 29.3).
- Presence of the Moro response (Fig. 29.4).

> The Moro response consists of extension of the arms, then brisk adduction towards the chest when the infant is startled or the baby's head allowed to drop back slightly (see Fig. 29.4). It should be symmetrical and should have disappeared by 6 months. Persistence of this or any of the primitive reflexes beyond 6 months may indicate a cerebral disorder.

Fine motor and vision
- Stares at and follows mother's face past midline.

Hearing and speech
- Coos.
- Startles to loud noises.

Social
- Smiles in response.

At 4–6 months the ability to roll, sit, and use both hands is dependent on the disappearance of primitive reflexes and the appearance of head and trunk righting.

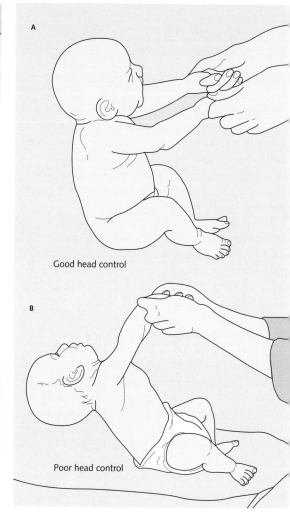

Good head control

Poor head control

Fig. 29.2 (A) Good head control at 3 months compared with (B) poor head control at 6 weeks.

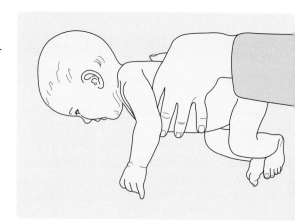

Fig. 29.3 Ventral suspension at 6 weeks.

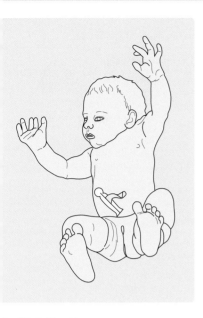

Fig. 29.4 The Moro response.

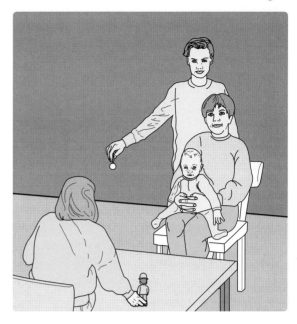

Fig. 29.5 Distraction test.

Eight months

Gross motor
- Sits unsupported.
- Weight bears on legs.
- Rolls. Starting to crawl.

Fine motor and vision
- Reaches out for toys and has a palmar grasp.
- Transfers objects hand to hand or hand to mouth.
- Follows fallen toys (and points).
- Fixes on small objects.

Hearing and speech
- Babbles (e.g., "dada").
- Distraction test (turns to sound) (Fig. 29.5).

Social
- Puts objects into mouth.
- Hand and foot regard.
- Plays peekaboo.
- Stranger awareness.
- Separation anxiety.

Eighteen months

Gross motor
- Walking.
- Climbs stairs two feet to a step.
- Climbs onto and sits on a chair.

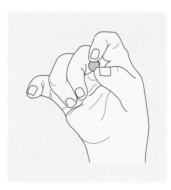

Fig. 29.6 Pincer grip.

Fine motor and vision
- Pincer grip (Fig. 29.6).
- Turns pages.
- Builds a three-brick tower.

Hearing and speech
- Uses three or more words.
- Points to parts of body or named objects.
- Understands simple instructions.

Social
- Uses a spoon.
- Domestic mimicry.

- Takes off socks and shoes.
- Developing toilet awareness.

Three years
Gross motor
- Runs, jumps.
- Throws and kicks a ball.
- Pedals a tricycle.
- Climbs stairs (like an adult).

Fine motor and vision
- Builds an eight-brick tower.
- Copies a line and a circle.

Speech and language
- Short sentences—using and understanding prepositions (e.g., "on").

Social
- Toilet trained: dry by day.
- Dresses with supervision.
- Plays with other children.
- Matches two colors.

Five years
Gross motor
- Skips.
- Catches a ball.
- Heel–toe walking.

Fine motor and vision
- Draws a man with all features.
- Copies alphabet letters.
- Snellen's chart test (by name or matching).

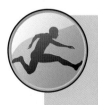

Hand preference develops at 18–24 months and is fixed at 5 years. Handedness in <1 year indicates a problem with the nondominant side.

Hearing and speech
- Comprehensive speech.

Social
- Plays games.
- Learning to read.
- Can tell the time.

Worrying signs at various ages	
Age	**Developmental sign**
6–8 weeks	Asymmetrical Moro Excessive head lag No visual fixation/following No startle or quietening to sound No responsive smile
8 months	Persisting primitive reflexes Not weight-bearing on legs Not reaching out for toys Not fixing on small objects Not vocalizing
10 months	Unable to sit unsupported
1 year	Showing a hand preference Not responding to own name
18 months	Not walking No pincer grip
3 years	Inaccurate use of a spoon Not speaking in sentences Unable to understand simple commands Unable to use the toilet alone Not interacting with other children

Fig. 29.7 Worrying signs at various ages.

Management options for concern over development:
- Reassure if within normal range.
- Review again.
- Refer for expert assessment.

Babies who were preterm need their development corrected for their gestational age, but this becomes less important after 2 years of age.

Signs of abnormal development: "limit ages"

Figure 29.7 lists the worrying signs at the ages given.

30. Investigations

Special investigations are often used to confirm, or refute, a diagnosis that is clinically uncertain and to monitor the progress of a disease or its treatment. They should be performed only when there are specific indications, not as a "routine." In all cases, the potential benefits must be weighed against any associated pain or discomfort.

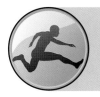

"Routine" investigation is rarely good practice.

In this chapter, the indications for and interpretation of common and important special investigations are considered.

Tests should be done for the benefit of the patient, not the doctor.

Imaging tests include the following:
- Ionizing radiation: chest x-rays (CXR), abdominal x-rays, skull x-rays, computed tomography (CT), and radionuclide scanning.
- Ultrasound: antenatal ultrasound, cranial ultrasound (newborn), and abdominal and renal ultrasound.
- Magnetic resonance imaging (MRI).

Blood tests may include:
- Hematologic tests: complete blood count (CBC), peripheral blood smear, sickle test, hemoglobin electrophoresis, coagulation studies.
- Biochemical tests: urea and electrolytes, creatinine, liver function tests, albumin, glucose, calcium and phosphate, magnesium, blood gases, and acid–base status.

- Immunology tests: tests for immunodeficiency, autoantibodies, diagnostic serology, and acute phase reactants.
- Microbiology tests: blood culture.

Urine tests include:
- Dipstick for protein, blood, glucose, and ketones.
- Microscopy and culture.

Tests for cerebrospinal fluid include:
- Microscopy and culture.
- Protein and glucose levels.
- Virology.

Imaging

All the major imaging methods are used in pediatric practice:
- Ionizing radiation: x-rays, simple or computed x-ray tomography, and nuclear medicine.
- Ultrasound.
- MRI.

The main circumstances in which each of these tests can be used are described in the following sections.

X-rays
Most commonly requested are:
- CXR.
- Abdominal x-ray.
- Skull x-ray.
- CT.

Chest x-ray
When inspecting a CXR, adopt a systematic approach for viewing and presentation:
- Check patient name, date, L/R orientation, posterior–anterior (PA), or anterior–posterior (AP).
- Note any striking abnormalities.
- Heart and mediastinum.
- Lung fields and pulmonary vessels.

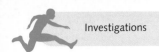

- Diaphragm and subdiaphragmatic areas.
- Bony thorax.
- Soft tissues.

The cardiac shadow is not always reliable in diagnosing heart disease. Look at the lung fields and hilar shadows.

Indications for doing a CXR

Acute:
- Pneumonia.
- Severe bronchiolitis.
- Asthma: severe or first presentation.
- Cardiac failure.
- Foreign body inhalation.
- Nonaccidental injury (old fractures).

Nonurgent investigation of:
- Cervical lymphadenopathy.
- TB.
- Cystic fibrosis.
- Cardiac disease.
- Malignant disease.

Abdominal x-ray

Supine AP is the standard plain film. A decubitus view is often requested. There is wide variation in the normal appearance of abdominal x-rays.

The checklist for an abdominal x-ray includes:
- Check patient name, date, erect, or supine.
- Note striking abnormalities.
- Hollow organs: stomach, bowel, and bladder.
- Solid organs: liver, spleen, and kidneys.
- Diaphragm.
- Bones.

Skull x-ray

The most common indication for skull radiography used to be head injury but CT scanning provides much more useful information (Fig. 30.1). These days, its primary use is in the diagnosis of non-accidental injury and craniosynostosis.

The presence of a skull fracture and/or neurologic signs increases the likelihood of intracranial damage.

Indications for head CT in trauma
GCS score less than 15
Any skull fracture
Focal neurologic signs or posttraumatic seizures
Clinical features of basal skull fracture
Persistent vomiting
Anterograde amnesia

Fig. 30.1 Indications for head CT in trauma.

Computed tomography

CT scanning uses multidirectional x-rays that, instead of falling onto film, are quantified by a detector and fed into a computer. Different readings are produced as the x-ray beam rotates round the body and the information is then presented as a two-dimensional image.

CT is a useful and widely available imaging modality for evaluating brain, chest, and abdominal disorders. These include:
- Brain: intracranial hemorrhage (e.g., head injury), tumors, intracranial calcification (e.g., tuberous sclerosis).
- Chest: mediastinal masses (e.g., lymphoma), lungs (e.g., bronchiectasis).
- Abdomen: masses (e.g., neuroblastoma or Wilms' tumor), injury (e.g., splenic rupture).

CT accurately assesses the nature of a mass (e.g., fluid, fat, necrosis, or calcification). Disadvantages include a disappointing lack of contrast between different organs. Intravenous contrast enhances the resolution between tissue planes.

Stabilization of any ill child must be done prior to a CT.

Ultrasound

Ultrasound (US) scanning uses ultra-high frequency sound waves to provide cross-sectional images of the body. In addition, Doppler ultrasound can be used for estimating the direction and velocity of blood flow.

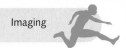

The advantages of US include:
- Noninvasive—no ionizing radiation involved.
- Portable equipment.

Body tissues reflect sound waves to different degrees and are therefore said to be of different echogenicity:
- Hyperechoic tissues appear white (e.g., fat).
- Hypoechoic tissues appear dark (e.g., fluid).

Ultrasound does not penetrate gas or bone and is therefore less useful for assessment of bony lesions. Intracranial contents are only accessible to ultrasound examination in young infants in whom the anterior fontanelle is still open.

The main applications include:
- Antenatal ultrasound.
- Cranial ultrasound in the neonate.
- Abdominal and renal ultrasound.
- Hip ultrasound.

Antenatal ultrasound

Initial ultrasound screening is carried out at 12 weeks with a detailed scan at 18–20 weeks' gestation. Antenatal US allows:
- Estimation of gestational age (less than 20 weeks).
- Identification of multiple pregnancies.
- Monitoring of fetal growth.
- Detection of structural malformations.
- Amniotic fluid volume estimation.

Neonatal cranial ultrasound

This is useful for the detection and evaluation of intracranial pathology (Fig. 30.2), including:
- Intracranial hemorrhage (e.g., intraventricular hemorrhage [IVH]).
- Periventricular leukomalacia.
- Hydrocephalus.
- Cerebral malformations.

 A cranial ultrasound is routine in all preterm babies under 32 weeks to look for hemorrhages.

Abdominal and renal ultrasound

Abdominal ultrasound is useful in the evaluation of:
- Abdominal pain: acute (e.g., identification of appendix abscess, intussception).

- Vomiting infant: ultrasound is the imaging of choice in pyloric stenosis.
- Liver disease: provides information on size and consistency of both the liver and spleen. The gallbladder and extrahepatic bile ducts can be visualized.

Renal ultrasound is very useful in the investigation of disorders of the genitourinary tract (Fig. 30.3). It provides information on:
- Kidney size.
- Structural abnormalities of the urinary tract (e.g., hydronephrosis, hydroureter, or increased bladder size).
- Gross renal scarring.
- Renal calculi.
- Tumors (e.g., Wilms' tumor).

 All infants and young children should have a renal US after a confirmed UTI. Its main role is to reveal structural abnormalities; it does not reliably detect vesicoureteral reflux or minor renal scars.

Hip ultrasound

Ultrasound is a useful modality for the investigation of hip disease. It is the imaging method of choice for assessing neonatal hip instability and is more reliable than plain radiography up to the age of 6 months. It allows evaluation of:
- Acetabular morphology.
- The degree to which the acetabulum covers the femoral head.

Ultrasound is also useful in the investigation of suspected hip pathology in young children. Even small effusions can be detected, and needle aspiration can be carried out under ultrasound guidance.

Magnetic resonance imaging

Magnetic resonance imaging (MRI) has several distinctive features that confer a number of useful advantages:
- No ionizing radiation.
- Images can be obtained in any plane.
- Excellent soft tissue contrast.

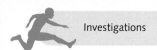

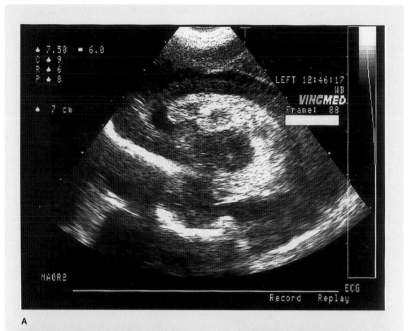

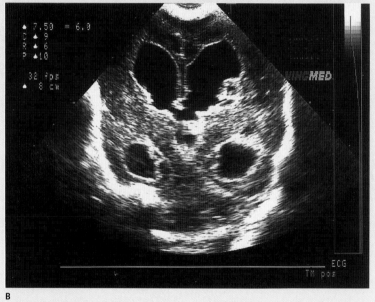

Fig. 30.2 (A) A parasagittal neonatal cranial ultrasound scan showing extensive intraventricular hemorrhage. (B) Coronal ultrasound scan of a neonatal brain with hydrocephalus.

It is the imaging modality of choice for many disorders of the brain and spine (in which sagittal views are particularly useful). MRI is also helpful in the evaluation of musculoskeletal disorders. It has not replaced other approaches, such as CT or ultrasound, in the imaging of many thoracic and abdominal disorders. Its main disadvantage in children is the need for sedation or general anesthesia because of the need to stay still for long periods.

Blood tests

Venous or capillary blood is usually satisfactory and can be obtained by venipuncture or capillary

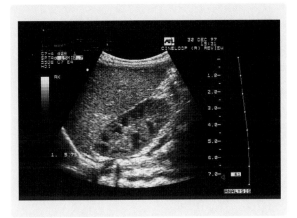

Fig. 30.3 Normal renal ultrasound. Normal prominent pyramids are demonstrated.

sampling. Arterial blood sampling is only occasionally necessary for blood gas analysis or estimation of acid–base status. (Pulse oximetry has rendered arterial sampling for determination of oxygenation rarely necessary.) With experience, skill, and local anesthetic cream, blood can be obtained quickly and with minimal discomfort from most infants and children.

Blood tests fall into the following general categories. See Fig. 30.4 for clinical chemistry reference values.

Hematology
Complete blood count (CBC)
This provides information about:
- Hemoglobin (Hb) (g/dL).
- Total white blood cell (WBC) count ($\times 10^9$/L).
- Platelet count ($\times 10^9$/L).

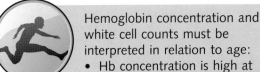

Hemoglobin concentration and white cell counts must be interpreted in relation to age:
- Hb concentration is high at birth (15–19 g/dL) and falls to a nadir at 3 months (9–13 g/dL).
- The total white cell count is high at birth and rapidly falls to normal adult levels. There is a relative lymphocytosis during the first 4 years of life after the neonatal period.

It can also provide:
- Red cell indices: MCV (fl), MCH (pg), MCHC (%).
- Reticulocytes (%).
- Differential WBC count: neutrophils, lymphocytes, eosinophils, monocytes (% or 10^9/L).

The examination of the film allows evaluation of:
- Red cell morphology (Fig. 30.5).
- Differential white cell count.
- Platelet numbers and morphology.
- Presence or absence of abnormal cells (e.g., blast cells).

See also Fig. 30.6, which shows important abnormalities that can be identified from a CBC.

Sickle test
This is a screening test for the sickle-cell trait or disease. Sickle cells are seen when the blood is deoxygenated with Na_2HPO_4.

Structure of hemoglobin:
- Fetal hemoglobin (HbF): $\alpha 2\ \gamma 2$
- Adult hemoglobin: HbA, $\alpha_2\ \beta_2$; HbA$_2$ $\alpha_2\ \delta_2$
- Sickle hemoglobin (HbS): $\alpha_2\ \beta_2^s$

Hemoglobin electrophoresis
The pattern of hemoglobin electrophoresis at different ages (birth and adult) and in different hemoglobinopathies is shown in Fig. 30.7.

Coagulation studies
Basic screening tests include:
- Prothrombin time (PT): usually expressed as international normalized ratio (INR).
- Activated partial thromboplastin time (PTT).
- Thrombin time (TT).

The evaluation of a bleeding disorder also requires an estimation of platelet numbers, morphology, and function.

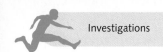

Clinical Chemistry		
Test		**Normal range (plasma or serum) SI units**
Sodium		133–145 mmol/L
Potassium	Infant Child	3.5–6.0 mmol/L 3.3–5.0 mmol/L
Urea	Newborn Infant Child	1.0–5.0 mmol/L 2.5–8.0 mmol/L 2.5–6.5 mmol/L
Creatinine	Infant Child	20–65 µmol/L 20–80 µmol/L
Osmolality		275–296 mosm/kg
Calcium (total)	24–48 h Child	1.8–3.0 mmol/L 2.5–2.60 mmol/L
Calcium (ionized)	24–48 h Child	1.00–1.17 mmol/L 1.18–1.32 mmol/L
Phosphate	Newborn Infant Child	1.4–2.6 mmol/L 1.3–2.1 mmol/L 1.0–1.8 mmol/L
Alkaline phosphatase	Newborn 2 years Adolescent female Adolescent male Adult	150–420 U/L 100–320 U/L 100–320 U/L 100–390 U/L 90–120 U/L
Albumin	Newborn Child	25–35 g/L 35–55 g/L
Creatine kinase	Infant/child	10–200 U/L
Glucose	Day 1 >1 day Child	2.2–3.3 mmol/L 2.6–5.5 mmol/L 3.0–6.0 mmol/L
Iron	Infant Child	5.0–17.9 µmol/L 10.0–21.5 µmol/L
Ferritin	Child	<150 µg/L
C-reactive protein	Varies by lab	
Blood gas (arterial, not preterm)	pH pO_2 pCO_2 Bicarbonate Base excess	7.35–7.45 11–14 kPa (82–105 mmHg) 4.5–6.0 kPa (32–45 mmHg) 18–25 mmol/L −4 to +4 mmol/L

Fig. 30.4 Normal ranges for blood tests (normal range for some tests varies between laboratories and must be checked with the local laboratory).

Common patterns of abnormality include:
- PT prolonged: liver disease.
- PTT prolonged: hemophilia (factor VIII), Christmas disease (factor IX).
- PT and PTT prolonged: vitamin K deficiency, liver disease.
- PT, PTT, and INR prolonged: disseminated intravascular coagulation (DIC).

von Willebrand's disease (VWD)

This is a heterogeneous group of inherited disorders with a defect in the von Willebrand factor (VWF)

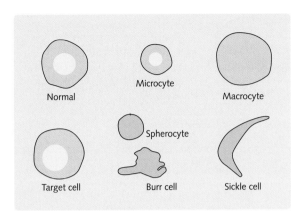

Fig. 30.5 Red cell morphology.

Important problems identifiable on a complete blood count
Anemia (e.g., iron deficiency)
Thrombocytopenia (e.g., idiopathic thrombocytopenic purpura)
Neutropenia (e.g., immunosuppression)
Pancytopenia (e.g., bone marrow failure)
Neutrophil leukocytosis (e.g., bacterial infection)
Lymphocytosis (e.g., *Bordetella pertussis*)

Fig. 30.6 Important problems identifiable on CBC.

which is important in platelet adhesion and as a carrier molecule for factor VIII. Bleeding time and PTT are prolonged. VWF levels can be measured directly.

Disseminated intravascular coagulation (DIC)

Uncontrolled activation of coagulation causes:
- Widespread intravascular fibrin deposition.
- Consumption of coagulation factors and platelets.
- Accelerated degradation of fibrin and fibrinogen.

In DIC the constellation of laboratory findings includes:
- Prolonged PT, PTT, and INR.
- Low fibrinogen.
- Elevated fibrinogen degradation products (FDPs) or D-dimers.
- Low platelets.
- Red cell fragmentation.

Further detailed investigations may be required—for example, when clinical evidence indicates a bleeding disorder but screening tests are normal. These tests may include:
- Assays of individual factors (e.g., factor XIII).
- Tests for the presence of endogenous anticoagulants.

Biochemical analysis

Most biochemical analyses are carried out on plasma rather than serum. The sample must be

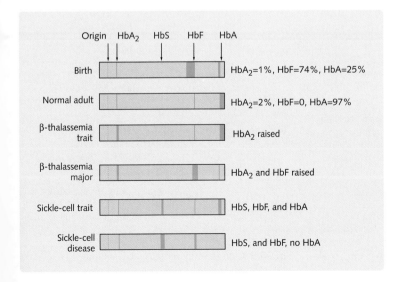

Fig. 30.7 Hemoglobin (Hb) electrophoresis.

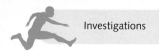

placed in a bottle containing anticoagulant (heparin in most cases—glucose estimations are a notable exception and should be placed in fluoride oxalate). It is important to know that reference values for children are often different to those in adults.

Chemistries

Urea and electrolytes (especially Na^+, K^+, Cl^-) are the most commonly requested biochemical analysis and can be useful in a host of circumstances including:

- Dehydration—diarrhea, vomiting.
- Ill patients on IV fluids—monitoring electrolyte status.
- Diabetic ketoacidosis.
- Renal disease.
- Diuretic therapy.

Urea

Urea is a major metabolite of protein catabolism. It is synthesized in the liver and excreted by the kidneys. The plasma concentration is influenced by:

- State of hydration.
- Protein intake.
- Catabolism.
- Glomerular filtration rate (GFR).

The creatinine concentration is a more reliable indicator of renal function. The most commonly encountered cause of a raised plasma urea is dehydration.

Sodium (Na⁺)

Changes in the plasma sodium concentration can reflect changes in either the sodium or water balance. Causes are shown in Figs. 30.8 and 30.9.

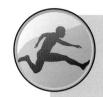

Concerning plasma sodium:
- Artifactually low plasma Na^+ concentration can occur with hyperlipidemia, as in diabetic ketoacidosis or parenteral feeding.
- A normal plasma Na^+ concentration may be found in salt depletion or overload if associated parallel changes in body water have occurred.
- Rapid falls in plasma Na^+ cause brain swelling.

Potassium (K⁺)

This is a predominantly intracellular cation. Plasma concentration is therefore influenced by exchange with the intracellular compartment as well as the whole-body potassium status. The causes of changes in plasma potassium are shown in Figs. 30.10 and 30.11.

Concerning plasma potassium:
- The intracellular K^+ concentration is very high: >100 mmol/L.
- Acidosis brings K^+ out of cells in exchange for H^+.
- Hemolysis releases K^+ from red cells and causes artefactual hyperkalemia.
- ECG changes reflect plasma K^+ concentration.

Causes of hyponatremia (Na⁺ < 130 mmol/L)	
Mechanism	**Cause**
Water excess	Iatrogenic: excessive hypotonic IV fluids Water retention due to inappropriate ADH secretion (e.g., postoperative, meningitis, head injury)
Sodium depletion	Diarrhea Diuretics Adrenal insufficiency (rare) Cystic fibrosis/sweating (rare)

Fig. 30.8 Causes of hyponatremia (sodium <130 mmol/L).

Causes of hypernatermia (Na⁺ > 150 mmol/L)	
Mechanism	**Cause**
Water deficit	Diarrhea Diabetes insipidus Excessive insensible water loss
Sodium excess	High solute intake Iatrogenic: excessive hypertonic IV fluids Child abuse: salt poisoning (rare)

Fig. 30.9 Causes of hypernatremia (sodium >150 mmol/L).

Causes of hypokalemia (K⁺ < 3.4 mmol/L)	
Mechanism	**Cause**
Potassium depletion	Diarrhea Diuretics
Inadequate intake	Daily need 2–3 mmol/kg
Redistribution	Metabolic alkalosis Glucose and insulin

Fig. 30.10 Causes of hypokalemia (potassium <3.4 mmol/L).

Causes of hyperkalemia (K⁺ > 5.5 mmol/L)	
Mechanism	**Cause**
Failure of renal excretion	Renal failure Adrenocortical insufficiency
Redistribution	Metabolic acidosis (e.g., diabetic ketoacidosis)
Excessive intake	Iatrogenic
Tissue injury	Hypoxia, catabolism
Artifact	Hemolyzed specimen

Fig. 30.11 Causes of hyperkalemia (potassium >5.5 mmol/L).

Plasma potassium in diabetic ketoacidosis:
- Whole-body K⁺ is always depleted.
- Plasma K⁺ concentration may be normal, high, or low, depending on the balance between acidosis and diuresis.
- Plasma K⁺ falls with treatment as redistribution into cells occurs.

Chloride (Cl⁻)
Hypochloremia is seen particularly in vomiting (e.g., associated with pyloric stenosis) and leads to a metabolic alkalosis.

Creatinine
Creatinine is a naturally occurring substance that is formed in muscles. The normal plasma concentration increases with age as muscle mass increases with growth. The plasma concentration of creatinine is a useful indirect measure of the glomerular filtration rate (GFR). In renal failure, the creatinine concentration increases steadily by more than 30 mmol/L/day.

Liver function tests
The basic biochemical tests of liver function include bilirubin, enzymes, and albumin and are outlined below.
Bilirubin:
- Conjugated and unconjugated.

Enzymes:
- Aspartate transaminase (AST).
- Alanine transaminase (ALT).
- Alkaline phosphatase (ALP).
- γ-glutamyltranspeptidase (γGT).

Additional investigations, which are useful for evaluating hepatic function and are abnormal in liver failure, include:
- Coagulation tests: PT, PTT.
- Ammonia.
- Glucose.

Bilirubin
Clinical evaluation of the severity of jaundice is unreliable, so it is important to document plasma levels of unconjugated and conjugated bilirubin. The normal proportion of conjugated bilirubin should not exceed 15% in infants. The causes of hyperbilirubinemia are considered elsewhere (see Chapter 9).

Excessive conjugated hyperbilirubinemia is a worrying sign in young infants as it may indicate biliary atresia.

Liver enzymes
Transaminases (aminotransferases). These intracellular enzymes occur in many tissues, including the liver, heart, and skeletal muscle. Normal plasma activity reflects release of enzymes during cell turnover and increases occur with tissue injury. Elevated serum aminotransferase activity is therefore primarily seen in hepatocyte damage, such as hepatitis (infection, drugs).

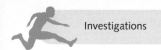

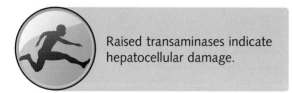

Raised transaminases indicate hepatocellular damage.

Causes of hypoalbuminemia (albumin < 30 g/L)	
Type	Cause
Decreased synthesis	Chronic liver disease Malnutrition (protein-energy malnutrition)
Increased losses	Nephrotic syndrome Burns Protein-losing enteropathy

Fig. 30.12 Causes of hypoalbuminemia (albumin <30 g/L).

However, elevation is not a specific marker of primary hepatocellular disease as it occurs in other forms of hepatobiliary disease (e.g., biliary atresia, cholecystitis) and also in nonhepatic conditions such as myocarditis and pancreatitis.

AST is the more sensitive indicator of liver injury but ALT is more specific.

Alkaline phosphatase. Isoenzymes of alkaline phosphatase are widely distributed in many organs including liver and bone. Normal activity levels change markedly throughout childhood and reference ranges are both age- and method-dependent. Activity is increased in:

- Biliary obstruction: intrahepatic or extrahepatic.
- Hepatocellular damage.
- Increased osteoblastic activity (e.g., rickets, normal growth, and pubertal growth spurt).

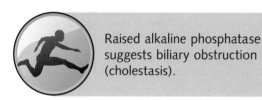

Raised alkaline phosphatase suggests biliary obstruction (cholestasis).

γ-glutamyltranspeptidase. Serum activity is commonly raised in liver disease especially when there is cholestasis. It may also be raised in the absence of liver disease in patients taking certain drugs, such as phenytoin, phenobarbitol, and rifampin (as a result of enzyme induction).

Albumin

Albumin is synthesized in the liver and is the main contributor to plasma oncotic pressure. It also has an important role as the protein to which many circulating substances are bound, such as:

- Bilirubin.
- Calcium.
- Drugs.
- Hormones.

Albumin has a long half-life of about 20 days.

Plasma albumin levels are a useful indicator of hepatic function. Low levels occur in several important clinical contexts (Fig. 30.12).

Prolonged hypoalbuminemia (e.g., in nephrotic syndrome) is associated with edema because fluid leaks into the extravascular space and hypovolemia triggers renal salt and water retention.

Glucose

Blood glucose concentrations are normally maintained within fairly narrow limits, which are lower in the newborn. Blood glucose can be estimated very rapidly at the bedside using test sticks but values should be verified by laboratory investigation.

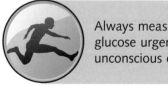

Always measure the blood glucose urgently in a seizing or unconscious child.

The only common causes of hyperglycemia in children are insulin-dependent type 1 diabetes mellitus and severe stress states. There are, however, many causes of hypoglycemia (Fig. 30.13).

Calcium and phosphate

Disorders of calcium and phosphate metabolism in childhood are uncommon and usually reflect abnormalities in the major controlling hormones, vitamin D, and parathyroid hormone. Laboratory estimations provide a measure of both total and

Causes of hyperglycemia and hypoglycemia	
Hyperglycemia	**Hypoglycemia**
Diabetes mellitus IDDM (most common) Secondary—pancreatic disease, Cushing syndrome **Stress-related** (e.g., postconvulsive) **Iatrogenic** Drugs (e.g., corticosteroids) Total parenteral nutrition	**Neonatal** Infant of diabetic mother Small for gestational age **Postneontatal** Ketotic hypoglycemia Hyperinsulinemia—known diabetic, pancreatic tumor (rare) ↓ GH, ACTH, cortisol—hyperpituitarism (rare), adrenal failure (rare)

Fig. 30.13 Causes of hyperglycemia and hypoglycemia.

Causes of hypocalcemia and hypercalcemia	
Hypocalcemia	**Hypercalcemia**

Rickets (low phosphate,
  high alkaline phosphatase)
Hypoparathyroidism (e.g.,
  DiGeorge syndrome)
Hypoalbuminemia
	Hyperparathyroidism
	Syndromic (Williams
	  syndrome)
	Vitamin D excess

Fig. 30.14 Causes of hypocalcemia and hypercalcemia.

ionized calcium. Changes in plasma albumin concentration affect total calcium levels independently of ionized calcium, leading to misinterpretation if serum albumin is outside the normal range. Therefore, the total calcium concentration needs to be corrected to give the expected value if albumin were in the normal range. Major causes of hypercalcemia and hypocalcemia are shown in Fig. 30.14.

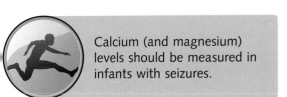

Calcium (and magnesium) levels should be measured in infants with seizures.

Blood gases and acid–base metabolism
Metabolism generates acid, which is eliminated via the lungs as carbon dioxide and via the kidneys as hydrogen ions. Acidosis, from whatever cause, is a much more common problem than alkalosis. Ideally, estimations of blood gas and acid–base

status are made on an arterial sample from an indwelling catheter, but capillary or venous blood can be useful for pH and pCO_2 measurements.

Where the main concern is oxygenation, non-invasive pulse oximetry is a valuable alternative to arterial blood gas analysis.

The pattern of changes seen in different forms of acidosis and alkalosis are shown in Fig. 30.15.

Common clinical contexts in which these disturbances occur include:
- Respiratory acidosis: hypoventilation (e.g., respiratory distress syndrome, severe asthma, neuromuscular diseases).
- Metabolic acidosis: diabetic ketoacidosis, hypoxia, circulatory failure.
- Respiratory alkalosis: hyperventilation (e.g., hysterical [rare in children], iatrogenic [ventilated patients]).
- Metabolic alkalosis: pyloric stenosis.

Immunology
Tests of the immune system carried out on the blood may be required in the following clinical contexts:
- Immunodeficiency.
- Autoimmune disease.
- Infection: diagnostic serology, acute-phase reactants.

Tests for immunodeficiency
Immunodeficiencies can be primary or secondary. The inherited primary deficiencies are rare; secondary causes are far more common (Fig. 30.16).

Immunodeficiency should be suspected in the following clinical circumstances:

285

Acid–base disturbances			
	pH	PaCO$_2$	HCO$_3^-$
Acidosis Respiratory Metabolic	Low Low	High Normal or low (compensation)	Normal or high (compensation) Low
Alkalosis Respiratory Metabolic	High High	Low Normal or high (compensation)	Normal or low (compensation) High

Fig. 30.15 Acid–base disturbances.

Causes of immunodeficiency
Primary Primary antibody deficiencies: • Common variable immune deficiency • X-linked antibody deficiency • IgG subclass deficiency • Specific antibody deficiency • Selective IgA deficiency Severe combined immunodeficiency Chronic granulomatous disease **Secondary** Malnutrition Infections (e.g., HIV, measles) Immunosuppressive therapy (e.g., steroids, cytotoxic drugs) Hyposplenism (e.g., sickle-cell disease, splenectomy)

Fig. 30.16 Causes of immunodeficiency.

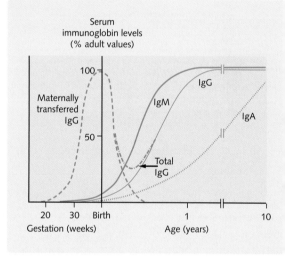

Fig. 30.17 Serum immunoglobulin (Ig) levels in fetus and infant.

• Recurrent severe infections.
• Infections with atypical organisms.
• Common infections with a severe or atypical clinical course.
• Failure to thrive.

Basic screening tests of immune function should include:
• Immunoglobulins.
• CBC, including differential WBC count and lymphocyte subsets.

Immunoglobulins

Serum immunoglobulin levels vary with age. Maternally transferred IgG is present at high levels at birth but has mostly disappeared by 6 months of age. This decline occurs before endogenous synthesis has fully developed, creating a physiological trough between 3 and 6 months of age. This is shown in Fig. 30.17.

IgG is the major immunoglobulin in normal human serum accounting for about 70% of the total pool. There are four distinct subclasses (IgG1 to IgG4), which have different functions. Specific IgM changes are very useful in the diagnosis of viral infections (e.g., rubella).

- IgG2 is the most common subclass deficiency and can be associated with IgA deficiency. The total IgG level may be normal. It causes recurrent respiratory infections (e.g., sinusitis, pneumonia).
- Selective IgA deficiency is common (1 : 700 population) and may cause no symptoms.

Differential WBC count

Immunodeficiency caused by marrow-suppressive cytotoxic or immunosuppressive therapy is related to the absolute neutrophil count. Patients with absolute neutrophil counts below 1.0×10^9/L are at increased risk of Gram-negative septicemia.

Lymphocyte subsets

Lymphocytes are further subdivided into T cells and B cells. T cells are categorized into:
- Cytotoxic T cells (TC), which are mostly CD8$^+$
- Helper T cells (TH), which are mostly CD4$^+$.

Cytotoxic T cells recognize infected target cells and lyse them. Helper T cells secrete regulatory molecules (lymphokines) that affect other T cells and cells of various lineages.

Monitoring absolute numbers of CD4$^+$ helper cells is useful in monitoring the progression of HIV-related diseases.

Autoantibodies

Autoimmune disease is uncommon in childhood but includes such entities as juvenile rheumatoid arthritis (JRA), systemic lupus erythematosus (SLE), and autoimmune thyroiditis causing juvenile hypothyroidism.

The following tests may be of value.

Antinuclear antibodies (ANA)

A broad group of antibodies present in 5% of normal children and induced by a wide spectrum of inflammatory conditions.
- High titers of ANA occur in 95% of SLE patients.
- The presence of ANA in subgroups of JRA is a risk factor for chronic anterior uveitis.

SLE is associated with antibodies against specific nuclear antigens such as double-stranded DNA.

Rheumatoid factors (RFs)

These are IgM autoantibodies against IgG. They should not be used to screen for JRA because they are neither sensitive nor specific. The majority of children with JRA are rheumatoid factor negative. Rheumatoid factors can be useful as a prognostic indicator in polyarticular JRA (their persistent presence is a poor prognostic factor).

Thyroid antibodies

Thyroid microsomal (peroxisomal) and thyroglobulin titers should be measured in suspected autoimmune thyroiditis.

Diagnostic serology

This is most widely used in the diagnosis of viral infections but is also of value in certain specific nonviral infections such as *Mycoplasma pneumoniae*, group A β-hemolytic streptococci, and *Salmonella* spp.

Viral antibody tests

Serological diagnosis depends on the detection of virus antibody. Diagnosis of recent infection requires the demonstration of a rising titer of specific IgM between the acute phase and convalescence. Methods used include:
- Immunofluorescence.
- Enzyme-linked immunoabsorbent assay (ELISA).
- Radioimmune assay (RIA).

Epstein–Barr virus (EBV)

Specific EBV serology is the most reliable diagnostic test. Antibodies to viral capsid antigen (VCA) are detected. IgG anti-VCA merely indicates a past infection. A positive IgM to VCA is diagnostic and is found early in the disease.

Tests for heterophile antibody, which agglutinates sheep red blood cells, are the basis of slide agglutination tests (monospot and Paul–Bunnell). However, this antibody does not appear until the second week or even later, and may not be produced at all in young children.

Mycoplasma pneumoniae

Diagnosis of infection with *Mycoplasma pneumoniae* is most quickly established by acute and convalescent serology: a four-fold rise in complement-fixing antibodies is diagnostic.

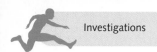

Antistreptolysin O titer (ASO)

Estimation of antibody to streptolysin O is a useful means of retrospectively diagnosing infection by group A β-hemolytic streptococci. The ASO is a valuable investigation in the evaluation of:

- Suspected acute nephritis.
- Rheumatic fever.
- Scarlet fever.

This test is being replaced by anti-DNAseB.

Acute-phase reactants

An inflammatory stimulus provokes the production of proteins in the liver known as the acute-phase response. This response is documented by the measurement of:

- C-reactive protein (CRP).
- Erythrocyte sedimentation rate (ESR).

The response is nonspecific and does not help in identifying etiology. However, if acute-phase reactants are elevated at the onset of disease, serial measurements are useful for monitoring progress.

The response times vary:
- CRP: elevated within 6 hours.
- ESR: peaks at 3–4 days.

Microbiology

Blood is normally sterile. Transient asymptomatic bacteremia can occur after dental treatment or invasive procedures such as catheterization. However, bacteremia leading to septicemia and shock can accompany a number of important childhood diseases such as pneumonia, meningitis, and typhoid fever.

Blood culture should be taken under the following circumstances:

- Fever of unknown origin.
- Clinical signs of septicemia.
- Febrile illness: in an immunodeficient child (e.g., sickle-cell disease, nephrotic syndrome, neutropenia) or in patients with a central catheter.
- Investigation of specific infections: meningitis, pneumonia, pyelonephritis, enteric fever.

The most common pathogens recovered from the blood are shown in Figs. 30.18 and 30.19. Most significant isolates will be obtained within 48 hours of inoculation, especially in septic neonates.

Common causes of septicemia in children after the newborn period
Streptococcus pneumoniae *Neisseria meningitidis* *Staphylococcus aureus* *Salmonella* spp. *Haemophilus influenzae* type B

Fig. 30.18 Common causes of septicemia in children after the newborn period.

Common causes of septicemia in the newborn
Group B streptococcus *Staphylococcus aureus* Coagulase-negative staphylococci Coliforms • Enterococcus • *E. coli* • *Klebsiella* spp.

Fig. 30.19 Common causes of septicemia in the newborn.

Upper respiratory culture

- Nasopharyngeal aspirates are best for diagnosing viral respiratory tract infections. They are sent for immunofluorescence and results are usually back on the same day. Rapid antigen tests for influenza are available and can offer a bedside diagnosis.
- Throat swabs are useful to diagnose pharyngeal infections.
- A pernasal swab is used to diagnose pertussis infection.

Urine tests

Urine samples are examined in the following ways:
- Dipsticks (sticks are available that test for: protein, glucose, ketones, blood pH, urobilinogen, leucocytes, and nitrites).
- Microscopy and culture (bacteria are easily identified on microscopy of an uncentrifuged sample; a centrifuged sample is necessary to examine the urinary sediment).

Dipstick testing

In certain clinical contexts, urine testing by dipstick is mandatory. These include:

- History of polyuria, polydipsia: diabetes mellitus?
- Generalized edema: nephrotic syndrome?

Microscopy and culture

Microscopy is required to look for casts and red cells in suspected glomerular disease, and is combined with culture in the investigation of suspected urinary tract infection (UTI).

Collection of an uncontaminated urine sample presents a problem in infants and young children. Alternative methods for collection in babies include:

- A clean-catch sample into a sterile pot.
- A pad system or an adhesive plastic bag applied to the perineum after careful washing ("bag" urine).
- Suprapubic aspiration (SPA): appropriate in a severely ill infant less than 6 months requiring urgent diagnosis.

The urine should be examined microscopically and cultured immediately, or refrigerated (to prevent overgrowth of contaminants) if there is unavoidable delay.

In UTI, pus cells and bacteria may be seen on microscopy. However, pyuria can occur with fever in the absence of UTI, and cell lysis may obscure pyuria if the sample is not examined immediately. The urine white cell count is not therefore a reliable feature in the diagnosis of UTI.

A mixed growth in the absence of pyuria usually represents contamination. Confident diagnosis of a UTI requires a bacterial culture of more than 10^8/L colony-forming units of a single species in a properly collected specimen.

Cerebrospinal fluid

Cerebrospinal fluid (CSF) is usually obtained by lumbar puncture. This is the critical investigation for the diagnosis of meningitis. The CSF can be evaluated in several ways including (Fig. 30.20):

- Appearance.
- Pressure.
- Microbiology: microscopy (white cell count/mm^3, organisms—Gram stain or acid-fast?), culture, and sensitivity.
- Biochemistry: protein (g/L), glucose (mmol/L).
- Rapid diagnostic techniques: countercurrent immunoelectrophoresis, latex agglutination, polymerase chain reaction.

Concerning meningitis:
- Infants may have nonspecific clinical signs; a high index of suspicion is therefore required, and a low threshold for performing a lumbar puncture.
- A missed diagnosis can be catastrophic.

Summary of the content and appearance of CSF in different types of meningitis				
Type	Appearance	WBC (m³)	Protein (g/L)	Glucose
Normal CSF (not neonatal)	Clear	0–5	0.15–0.4	>50% blood glucose
Bacterial meningitis	Turbid	500–10,000	0.4–3	Low
Viral meningitis	Clear	<1000	<10	Normal
TB meningitis	Clear/viscous	Up to 500 Usually <100	>10	Low

Fig. 30.20 A summary of the content and appearance of cerebrospinal fluid in different types of meningitis.

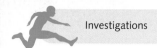

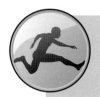

Lumbar puncture is contraindicated in the following circumstances:
- Signs of raised intracranial pressure.
- Focal neurologic signs.
- Rapidly deteriorating consciousness.
- Bradycardia.
- A coagulation defect.
- Skin infection at the lumbar puncture site.

Appearance

Normal CSF is clear. If the cell count increases to more than 500 cells/mm^3, it becomes turbid. Typically, this occurs in bacterial meningitis.

Microbiology
Microscopy

Normally, a few (<5 cells/mm^3) white cells can be found in CSF. The presence of polymorphs is always abnormal except in the neonatal period when up to 30 white cells/mm^3 can be physiologic. In the early stages of meningitis, white cells may not be detectable but classically very high counts are found.

Spun CSF is routinely Gram-stained:
- Gram-negative cocci: *Neisseria meningitidis*.
- Gram-positive cocci: *Streptococcus pneumoniae*.
- Gram-negative coccobacilli: *Haemophilus influenzae*.

Culture and sensitivity

This is always carried out even if the sample is clear and no white cells were detected on microscopy. Viral studies should be sent in encephalitis.

Biochemistry
Protein

Protein content of the CSF rises in bacterial meningitis. Note that in neonates the normal levels are high compared with older children and adults.

Glucose

Normal CSF glucose is approximately two-thirds of the blood glucose level. In bacterial meningitis, it drops to less than 40% of the blood glucose level.

Rapid diagnostic techniques

Bacterial antigens can now be detected by sensitive and rapid tests including:
- Countercurrent immunoelectrophoresis.
- Latex agglutination.

Sufficient antigen remains present even after treatment with antibiotics has been initiated and when direct culture is no longer possible. Unfortunately, neither test is reliable at detecting group B meningococcus, which is the most common type in the USA.

Polymerase chain reaction and DNA hybridization

New techniques that detect bacterial DNA, and viral DNA or RNA are becoming available. These tests are having an increasing role in early and more sensitive detection of infection.

Index

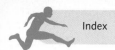

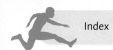

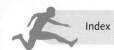

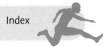

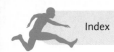

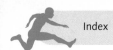

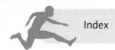

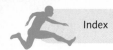

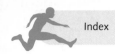

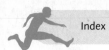